CANCER ETIOLOGY, DIAGNOSIS AND TREATMENTS

NEURO-ONCOLOGY AND CANCER TARGETED THERAPY

CANCER ETIOLOGY, DIAGNOSIS AND TREATMENTS

Additional books in this series can be found on Nova's website at:

https://www.novapublishers.com/catalog/index.php?cPath=23_29&seriesp=Cancer+Etiology%2C+Diagnosis+and+Treatments

Additional E-books in this series can be found on Nova's website at:

https://www.novapublishers.com/catalog/index.php?cPath=23_29&seriespe=Cancer+Etiology%2C+Diagnosis+and+Treatments

CANCER ETIOLOGY, DIAGNOSIS AND TREATMENTS

NEURO-ONCOLOGY AND CANCER TARGETED THERAPY

LUCÍA M. GUTIÉRREZ
EDITOR

NOVA BIOMEDICAL
Nova Biomedical Books
New York

Copyright © 2010 by Nova Science Publishers, Inc.

All rights reserved. No part of this book may be reproduced, stored in a retrieval system or transmitted in any form or by any means: electronic, electrostatic, magnetic, tape, mechanical photocopying, recording or otherwise without the written permission of the Publisher.

For permission to use material from this book please contact us:
Telephone 631-231-7269; Fax 631-231-8175
Web Site: http://www.novapublishers.com

NOTICE TO THE READER

The Publisher has taken reasonable care in the preparation of this book, but makes no expressed or implied warranty of any kind and assumes no responsibility for any errors or omissions. No liability is assumed for incidental or consequential damages in connection with or arising out of information contained in this book. The Publisher shall not be liable for any special, consequential, or exemplary damages resulting, in whole or in part, from the readers' use of, or reliance upon, this material. Any parts of this book based on government reports are so indicated and copyright is claimed for those parts to the extent applicable to compilations of such works.

Independent verification should be sought for any data, advice or recommendations contained in this book. In addition, no responsibility is assumed by the publisher for any injury and/or damage to persons or property arising from any methods, products, instructions, ideas or otherwise contained in this publication.

This publication is designed to provide accurate and authoritative information with regard to the subject matter covered herein. It is sold with the clear understanding that the Publisher is not engaged in rendering legal or any other professional services. If legal or any other expert assistance is required, the services of a competent person should be sought. FROM A DECLARATION OF PARTICIPANTS JOINTLY ADOPTED BY A COMMITTEE OF THE AMERICAN BAR ASSOCIATION AND A COMMITTEE OF PUBLISHERS.

LIBRARY OF CONGRESS CATALOGING-IN-PUBLICATION DATA
Available upon request

ISBN: 978-1-61668-708-3

Published by Nova Science Publishers, Inc. ✣ *New York*

CONTENTS

Preface		vii
Chapter 1	Trace Elements and Nanoparticles: Certain Approaches to Cancer Targeted Diagnostics and Therapy *Igor A. Khlusov, Professor, Galina B. Slepchenko, Georgy T. Dambaev, Professor, Leonid V. Zagrebin, Sergey S. Shestov, Sergey A. Antipov, Taisia A. Feduschak, Marina Yu. Khlusova, Oleg V. Kokorev, Anatoly Ye. Yermakov, Mikhail A. Uymin, and Anna M. Nekrasova*	1
Chapter 2	Brain Cancer Associated Tumor Marker Genes Expression Pattern in Humans *Harun M. Said, Carsten Hagemann, Adrian Staab, Buelent Polat, Mathias Guckenberger, Jelena Anacker, Michael Flentje, and Dirk Vordermark*	65
Chapter 3	Genetics of Rare Pediatric Brain Tumors of Childhood *Elvis Terci Valera, María Sol Brassesco and Luiz Gonzaga Tone*	99
Chapter 3	Mechanisms of Immune Evasion Exhibited by Different Rat Glioma Cell Lines *Martin R. Jadus, Lara Driggers, Neil Hoa, Jimmy T.H. Pham, Josephine Natividad, Christina Delgado, Edward W.B. Jeffes, Eric Giedzinski, Charles Limoli, and Lisheng Ge*	109
Chapter 5	Breaking the Barriers to Tumor-Targeting via Nanocarrier-Based Drug Delivery to the Tumor Microenvironment *Yusuke Doi, Tatsuhiro Ishida and Hiroshi Kiwada*	141
Chapter 6	Tumor Chemodosimetry: The Intersection of Imaging, Drug Delivery Vehicles and Targeted Therapies for the Improvement of Cancer Treatment *J. Hung, R. Daniel and B.L. Viglianti*	161

Chapter 7	Effects of Hypoxia on Angiogenesis and Survival of Glioblastoma Multiforme *Alok Bhushan, Sandeep Sheth, Aditi Jain and James C K Lai*	**183**
Chapter 8	Temozolomide in High-Grade Gliomas: Rationale, Schedules and Synergism with Radiation *Stefano Dall'Oglio, Anna D'Amico, Fabio Pioli and Sergio Maluta*	**199**
Chapter 9	Intra-Arterial Targeted Delivery of Lipophilic Photosensitizer for Photodynamic Therapy of Prostate Cancer *Ronald B. Moore; Zhengwen Xiao; Richard J. Owen; and John Tulip*	**213**
Chapter 10	Cervical Spine Deformity Associated with Laminoplasty for Resection of Spinal Cord Tumors in Children *Peter Kan and Meic H. Schmidt*	**227**
Chapter 11	Radionuclide Labeled Glucuronide Prodrugs for Imaging and Targeting Therapy of Cancer *Perihan Unak*	**239**
Index		**249**

PREFACE

Targeted therapy is a type of medication that blocks the growth of cancer cells by interfering with specific targeted molecules needed for carcinogenesis and tumor growth, rather than by simply interfering with rapidly dividing cells (eg. with traditional chemotherapy). Targeted cancer therapies may be more effective than current treatments and less harmful to normal cells. This book examines the various targeted therapies for cancer and also focuses on neuro-oncology, the study of cancer of the nervous system.

Chapter 1- Dissatisfaction with results of combined (surgery, chemotherapy, irradiation) cancer treatment determines relevance and availability of search new trends, such as development of immuno(bio)therapy methods. However, high theoretical and experimental antitumor potential of cancer immuno(bio)therapy haven't found its clinical confirmation yet.

One of basic reasons of unsatisfactory treatment results and poor forecast is considered as late disease diagnostics. Nanomedicine seems to be a way out of this situation. On the one hand, new scientific field is aimed at development of material and technical base of diagnostics and treatment of diseases. Analysis of nanomedicine publications showed that electrochemical methods were one of its leading analytical tools. On the other hand, address delivery (including ferreed delivery) of drugs and biological molecules into tumor tissue serves as its the most important therapeutic approach.

At the same time, proper value of trace elements and nanoparticles in organism vital activity, diagnostics and therapy of cancer has not yet been sufficiently studied.

In this connection, this chapter is devoted to: 1) our efforts to develop method of trace elements voltammeter control in biological substances for targeted cancer diagnostics; 2) finding out a role of trace elements imbalance in oncological patients and human tumor cell lines as a base of elaboration of approaches to cancer targeted diagnostics and therapy; 3) proper results of targeted magnetocontrollable delivery of cytostatic and nanoparticle composites into tumor cells and tissues.

Chapter 2- Hypoxia is an important phenomenon possessing a significant correlation with tumour progression, treatment result(s) and the overall disease prognosis.

Tumor oxygenation state leads to a series of genomic changes, enabling tumour cells survival or overcoming the oxygen deficient environment conditions. Tumour tissue growth requires a sufficient oxygen and nutrients supply. Tumor cell responses to hypoxic stress include adaptive proteomic changes allowing the cells to overcome nutritive deprivation or to escape their hostile environment by proliferation, invasion, or metastatic spread. Tumor cell proliferation requires rapid synthesis of macromolecules including lipids, proteins, and nucleotides.

Hypoxia-inducible factor 1 (HIF-1) is a multi-subunit protein that regulates transcription at hypoxia response elements (HREs) under hypoxic oxygenation conditions, while under normoxic oxygenation conditions, HIF-1α protein is subject to rapid degradation by a pVHL-mediated ubiquitin-proteasome pathway, while under it hypoxia blocks degradation leading to accumulation and translocation to the cellular nucleus and its binding together with HIF-1β on the so called Hypoxia responsive element within the hypoxia induced genes promoter region and thereby regulating the expression of the hypoxia responsive genes which proteins are expressed in human brain cancer especially in low grade astrocytoma and glioblatoma in a tumor stage and oxygenation specific manner. Genes which proteins are expressed in this manner are considered tumor marker genes as well as tumor therapeutic targets. Among the most important are Carbonic anhyrase 9 (CA9), N myc- Downregulated gene 1(NDRG1), Osteopontin (OPN), Vascular endothelial Growth Factor (VEGF) and Erythropoitin (EPO). HIF-1α is an important or the only regulator of these proteins under hypoxic conditions. CA9 is one of the most strongly hypoxia-inducible proteins but its expression pattern is not only related to its transcriptional induction by hypoxia in brain tumors, but also to effects of adverse microenvironmental stresses (such as diminished levels of glucose and bicarbonate. NDRG1 was shown at the same levels *in vivo* in normal human brain and human low-grade astrocytoma (WHO grade 2), while it showed a higher NDRG1 overexpression level in glioblastoma than in lowgrade astrocytoma. OPN was displayed a high level of cancer tissue expression specificity due to the favour expression in human GBM when compared to (LGA) based on the relative mRNA expression of hypoxia-related genes data. Regulation of OPN, mRNA and protein expression as a response to the hypoxic development in the tumor cell enviroment *in vitro* and *in vivo* represent an absolute phenomenon in human glioblastoma as a cell-specific post-transcriptionally regulated event. VEGF is a powerful hypoxia induced mitogen for endothelial cell growth and plays a critical role in the development of tumor vessels. OPN is a tumor-associated phosphoglycoprotein, has been described to be prognostic for tumor progression and survival in a number of solid neoplasms and linked to a "metastatic phenotype (Epo) is overexpressed at the mRNA level in human and mouse brain. Modulation of glycolysis reduces the hypoxic accumulation of HIF-1α protein in human tumor cells through a translational or post-translational process. Therefore, manipulation of tumor glucose levels represents a potential approach to therapeutically target HIF-1α.

In malignant glioma therapy, the main aim, as with all cancers, is to either eradicate the tumor or convert it into a controlled, quiescent chronic disease. Angiogenesis and hypoxia induced, HIF-1α regulated genes inhibition remains the main parts of therapeutic approaches in human oncology. It is well known that cancer cell metabolism can be perturbed specifically at the level of glycolysis leading to interesting therapeutic activities in cancer that can be displayed.

Chapter 3- Brain cancers are the most common solid tumors affecting children and adolescents. According to the last World Health Organization (WHO) classification of tumors of the central nervous system (CNS), more than one hundred different histological subtypes can primarily arise in the brain or spine. Cytogenetic and molecular information about these tumors is very heterogeneous and usually revised and pooled data about this topic are only available for the most prevalent subtypes. Although the molecular pathways involved in the initiation or progression of rare tumors may provide important evidence about the genetic mechanisms of tumorigenesis, the literature lacks systematic reviews of this topic. This chapter aims to gather and review recent information about conventional and molecular genetic findings for rare (1% or less) pediatric CNS tumors.

Chapter 4- Rat glioma cell lines could be considered the previous work horse of experimental glioma research. At least 9 established glioma cell lines exist and they have been used extensively to study many aspects of glioma biology and potential experimental therapeutics. These glioma cells have been defined as either being immunogenic or non-immunogenic, based upon empirical findings. The mechanisms of this immunogenicity/non-immunogenicity have not been fully elucidated. Traditionally, the major mechanisms by which murine tumors were viewed as being non-immunogenic was: by down-regulating the major histocompatibility complex (MHC) antigens, by lacking tumor specific antigens, or by making molecules that prevent the immune system from properly working. D74 glioma cells only showed low MHC class 1 (RT1-A) expression. Other non-immunogenic gliomas (F98, 36B10 and CNS-1) displayed equivalent levels of RT1-A, as their more immunogenic counterparts (RT2, BT4C, C6, 9L/T9). Human glioma cell lines possess numerous tumor-associated antigens. In contrast, rat tumor-associated antigens are relatively few. A plethora of immunosuppressive molecules are made by glioma cell lines. In this chapter we will examine why established rat glioma cell lines can grow in vivo, despite being considered "immunogenic". The intrinsic properties (lack of MHC molecules, self-defense molecules, production of immunosuppressive cytokines/enzymes, counterattack strategies, growth rates and resistance to cell-mediated killing) of these cells may allow various aspects of rat glioma immunology to be explained and may allow investigators to focus on their favorite mechanism of immune evasion.

Chapter 5- Nanocarrier-based cancer chemotherapeutics are thought to increase therapeutic efficiency and reduce the side effects of associated chemotherapeutic agents by altering the agents' pharmacokinetics and tissue distribution following intravenous administration. In spite of these favorable properties, nanocarrier-based cancer chemotherapeutics are not always effective because of their heterogeneous intratumoral localization. Accumulation of nanocarriers in solid tumors occurs passively via the highly permeable tumor angiogenic vasculature in a long-circulating property-dependent manner. Accumulation is therefore affected by the heterogeneity of the tumor vascularity and vascular permeability. Homogeneous intratumoral distribution of nanocarriers would improve the efficacy of nanocarrier-based cancer chemotherapeutics in some intractable solid tumors. In this review, we focus on the barriers in the tumor microenvironment that hinder extravasation through the tumor vasculature and penetration of nanocarriers in solid tumors. In addition, we describe and discuss some trials that attempt to manipulate these barriers. Alterations of the tumor microenvironment that relate directly to the intratumoral distribution of nanocarriers may be potential strategies to improve the delivery of nanocarrier-based cancer chemotherapeutics.

Chapter 6- Effective cancer treatment therapy requires drugs to be delivered to tumor cells at cytotoxic concentrations. The ideal goals for chemotherapy are to identify and modify drug distribution, deliver concentrated effective drug dosages to the tumor and/or predict the tumor effect, a concept termed as chemodosimetry [1]. This concept is analogous to radiation dosimetry, which is used when the radiation dose is administered in a prescribed manner based on calculated radiation intensity and known tissue dependent energy absorption. Radiation dosimetry has been successful in improving cancer therapy outcomes, but chemodosimetry has yet to achieve similar success [1-3]. Current non-targeted chemotherapy regimens require drug concentrations that cause dose limiting systemic side effects. With localized targeted drug delivery, mitigation of these systemic side effects is possible and, in the ideal case, chemodosimetry could be achieved.

Although advancements in current cancer therapy have allowed the development of localized treatment to the tumor via minimally invasive procedures, recent research in phase II/III clinical trials focused on molecular targeting and drug carriers for noninvasive target drug delivery. Most recently, data from preclinical trials have demonstrated the ability to monitor drug delivery in real time with nanoparticles, such as liposomes, drug-loaded polymers, polymersomes, and antibodies. Liposomes are small, self-assembling particles with diameters <400 nm, comprised of an outer phospholipid bilayer and an aqueous center capable of encapsulating and carrying water-soluble drugs (Figure 1)[4]. Since liposomes are the most mature form of nanoparticles in development, this review will primarily discuss liposomes to exhibit the combination of nanoparticle delivery, imaging, and selected drug deposition in conjunction with the use of local regional hyperthermia.

Chapter 7- Glioblastoma multiforme (GBM) is one of the most vascular, aggressive and malignant forms of primary brain tumors. The presence of pseudopalisading necrosis and glomeruloid microvascular hyperplasia distinguishes GBM from other lower-grade astrocytomas. In GBM, a critical correlation exists between the presence of hypoxic regions and its angiogenic phenotype. Pseudopalisading necrosis is the result of vascular pathologies and both can generate regions of hypoxia around them. Hypoxia can also be caused by high metabolic activity of the tumor. The presence of glomeruloid bodies in the regions adjacent to the necrotic foci indicates an aggressive angiogenic phenotype. Hypoxia seems to be an important physiological stimulus that gives rise to the incidence of necrosis, formation of pseudopalisading cells and glomeruloid bodies: these are the critical events in the progression of GBM. Hypoxia sets off various signals that initiate angiogenesis by upregulating the expression of hypoxia inducible factor-1 (HIF-1) and secreting pro-angiogenic growth factors like vascular endothelial growth factor (VEGF) and interleukin-8 (IL-8). This review will focus upon the emerging concept regarding mechanisms responsible for the accelerated growth in GBM, emphasizing a link between hypoxia and angiogenesis. Since no significant advances have occurred in the past twenty five years in the treatment of GBM, it is imperative to understand the underlying molecular mechanisms taking place in the development of GBM and then come up with a treatment strategy that can at least increase the survival rate of the patients if not eradicate the disease.

Chapter 8- High-grade gliomas (HGG)—glioblastoma multiforme (GBM) and anaplastic astrocytoma (AA)—are still characterized by a dismal prognosis despite recent advances in treatment options (new radiotherapy techniques including IMRT and radiosurgery, new alkylating agents such as Temozolomide [TMZ], molecular targeted drugs). Gold-standard therapy has involved maximum possible resection, followed by adjuvant irradiation plus TMZ followed by maintenance TMZ. TMZ has also proven its efficacy on tumors of oligodendroglial origin. The conventional "5 out of 28 days" schedule of TMZ achieved an overall survival rate at 2 years of 26.5%; in patients with methylation of methylguanine methyltrasnsferase (MGMT) promoter, better results can be achieved but MGMT methylation status determination is feasible only in a few centres. Dose- intensity TMZ schedules have the capability of depleting MGMT in tumor cells, thus promising a better outcome also in non-methylated patients. Alternative schedules, such as the "weekly alternating" or the "21 out of

28 days" ones, have been tried in relapsed patients and recently also in newly diagnosed ones. Sporadic cases of severe bone marrow aplasia with high doses of TMZ have been reported, which required bone marrow transplantation. This chapter tries to find a possible rationale for intensified regimens of TMZ administration and reviews its possible benefits and risks, focusing on results of clinical trials and reported toxicity cases.

Chapter 9- **Introduction**: Prostate cancer (PCa) is the most common malignancy in western men. The stage and grade of the disease at diagnosis directly determine survival. Recently widespread PCa screening has greatly improved the ability to detect small and early stage cancer. Consequently many men with low-risk cancers have undergone radical therapies, suffering side effects from treatments without significant survival benefits. Minimally invasive therapies are being developed that may offer options for men with low-risk disease who want to balance the benefits and risks of treatment. Interstitial photodynamic therapy (PDT) is one such option. PDT uses a photosensitizing drug (photosensitizer) that is activated in the prostate by laser light of a specific wavelength, delivered by optical fibers. In the presence of oxygen, tissue necrosis occurs at the site of interaction between the photosensitizer and light. Current limitations of interstitial PDT for treatment of prostate cancer include low drug selectivity after intravenous (i.v.) administration and incomplete ablation of glandular tissue. To overcome these limitations, we have been exploring intra-arterial (i.a.) delivery of photosensitizer into the prostate. We have tested this strategy in rat and canine models, as well as in humans. In this chapter we report our observations and propose future targeted therapies to the prostate.

Methods: Biodistribution studies of ^{99m}Technetium labeled Macro-Aggregated Albumin (^{99m}Tc MAA) were carried out using whole body scintigraphy and ex-vivo tissue imaging. Hypocrellin B derivative SL052 (a lipophilic photosensitizer), formulated in liposomes or dissolved in dimethyl sulphoxide (DMSO), was injected i.a. via the prostate arteries and compared to i.v. administration. Optical fibers were inserted into the prostate and 630nm laser light delivered through fibers in a cyclic fashion. Drug concentration (fluorescence) and light transmission in prostate tissue were monitored during the course of PDT. Side effect profile and completeness of prostate gland ablation were the major parameters compared between treatment groups.

Results and conclusion: Intra-arterial injection of ^{99m}Tc MAA or SL052 dissolved in DMSO selectively targeted the prostate and attained an extremely high therapeutic ratio (18:1). With PDT there was complete ablation of the prostate glandular tissue with a significant reduction of prostate volume when compared pre-PDT ($p < 0.0001$). PDT with i.a. injection of lipophilic SL052-DMSO has the potential to provide an effective treatment for both prostate cancer and benign prostate enlargement. Intra-arterial delivery of drugs has the potential to be extended to targeted gene and molecular therapies for diseased solid organs.

Chapter 10- Cervical deformity is a well-known complication of cervical laminectomy, especially for tumor resection in children. Despite the lack of evidence of its efficacy, cervical laminoplasty is often advocated in place of laminectomy in children to prevent such postoperative deformities. Our objective was to compare laminoplasty and laminectomy techniques in terms of postoperative spinal alignment and incidence of kyphotic deformity. The authors describe a case of a 28-year-old woman who developed a severe cervical kyphotic deformity after cervical laminoplasty for tumor resection performed 14 years earlier. The patient was treated with a posterior decompression and instrumentation, followed by multilevel anterior cervical discectomies and fusions. On the basis of our review of the literature, there appears to be no benefit to laminoplasty over laminectomy in terms of postoperative spinal alignment and incidence of kyphotic deformity.

Chapter 11- Glucuronide prodrugs may be useful tools to deposit the therapeutic and imaging agents in the target which enhanced enzyme β-glucuronidase. They can be synthesized through enzymatic, metabolic or chemical ways. The enzyme β-glucuronidase, which hydrolyses glucuronide conjugates, reversing one of the main detoxification and excretion pathways, was found to vary in concentration in different cysts and tumor tissues. Thus targeted delivery of cytotoxic agents and their retention in the tumor cells; decreased cytotoxicity and other side effects in normal tissues; decreased interference that caused by multi drug resistance; targeted delivery of therapeutic radionuclides; uptake and retention in the tumor cells with sitotoxic agents which they label; increased efficiency and synergic potentiation of therapeutic effects of sitotoxic agents and radionuclides can be possible.

The aim of this chapter is to provide a brief overview of current status of applications, advantages and up-to-date research and development of radiolabeled glucuronide prodrugs in cancer imaging and targeted therapy.

In: Neuro-Oncology and Cancer Targeted Therapy
Editor: Lucía M. Gutiérrez, pp. 1-63

ISBN 978-1-61668-708-3
© 2010 Nova Science Publishers, Inc.

Chapter 1

TRACE ELEMENTS AND NANOPARTICLES: CERTAIN APPROACHES TO CANCER TARGETED DIAGNOSTICS AND THERAPY

Igor A. Khlusov, Professor[1], Galina B. Slepchenko, D.Sc.[2], Georgy T. Dambaev, Professor[3], Leonid V. Zagrebin, Ph.D[4], Sergey S. Shestov[5], Sergey A. Antipov,[6] Taisia A. Feduschak,.[7] Marina Yu. Khlusova[8], Oleg V. Kokorev,[9] Anatoly Ye. Yermakov,[10] Mikhail A. Uymin,[11] and Anna M. Nekrasova[12]

[1] Deputy Director, FSE «Russian Ilizarov Scientific Centre «Restorative Traumatology and Orthopaedics», Tomsk Branch, Tomsk, Russia,
[2] Member of Council, Scientific Educational Center «Biocompatible Materials and Bioengineering», Tomsk Polytechnic University & Siberian State Medical University, Tomsk, Russia
[3] Chief, Hospital Surgery Department, Siberian State Medical University, Tomsk, Russia
[4] Deputy director, Limited Company "Center for Informational Cell Medicine", Moscow, Russia
[5] Director, Limited Company "Center for Informational Cell Medicine", Moscow, Russia
[6] Assistant, Hospital Surgery Department, Siberian State Medical University, Tomsk, Russia
[7] Researcher, Institute of Oil Chemistry SB RAS, Tomsk, Russia
[8] Docent, Department of Pathophysiology, Siberian State Medical University, Tomsk, Russia
[9] Researcher, Institute of Medical Shape Memory Materials, Siberian Physical-Technical Institute, Tomsk State University, Tomsk, Russia
[10] Institute of Metal Physics, Ural Department of RAS, Ekaterinburg, Russia
[11] Institute of Metal Physics, Ural Department of RAS, Ekaterinburg, Russia
[12] Limited company "SibMedCenter", Tomsk, Russia

---

1 Email: khl@ultranet.tomsk.ru   khlusov63@mail.ru

ABSTRACT

Dissatisfaction with results of combined (surgery, chemotherapy, irradiation) cancer treatment determines relevance and availability of search new trends, such as development of immuno(bio)therapy methods. However, high theoretical and experimental antitumor potential of cancer immuno(bio)therapy haven't found its clinical confirmation yet.

One of basic reasons of unsatisfactory treatment results and poor forecast is considered as late disease diagnostics. Nanomedicine seems to be a way out of this situation. On the one hand, new scientific field is aimed at development of material and technical base of diagnostics and treatment of diseases. Analysis of nanomedicine publications showed that electrochemical methods were one of its leading analytical tools. On the other hand, address delivery (including ferreed delivery) of drugs and biological molecules into tumor tissue serves as its the most important therapeutic approach.

At the same time, proper value of trace elements and nanoparticles in organism vital activity, diagnostics and therapy of cancer has not yet been sufficiently studied.

In this connection, this chapter is devoted to: 1) our efforts to develop method of trace elements voltammeter control in biological substances for targeted cancer diagnostics; 2) finding out a role of trace elements imbalance in oncological patients and human tumor cell lines as a base of elaboration of approaches to cancer targeted diagnostics and therapy; 3) proper results of targeted magnetocontrollable delivery of cytostatic and nanoparticle composites into tumor cells and tissues.

INTRODUCTION

Dissatisfaction with results of combined (surgery, chemotherapy, irradiation) cancer treatment [20,21] determines relevance and availability of search new trends, such as development of immuno(bio)therapy methods. However, high theoretical and experimental antitumor potential of cancer immuno(bio)therapy hasn't found its clinical confirmation yet [57].

Along with methods of adoptive cell therapy and vaccine therapy being actively developed in the last 20 – 25 years, achievements of molecular- and nanomedicine attract attention of researches at present increasingly.

On the one hand, new scientific field is aimed at development of material and technical base of diagnostics and treatment of diseases. At that, electrochemical methods are one of leading analytical tools of nanomedicine. On the other hand, address delivery of pharmaceuticals and biological molecules into tumor tissue is important therapeutic approach.

Analysis of 100 randomized Internet publications for clinical aspects of digestive tract cancer immunotherapy for years 2004 - 2007 carried out by us showed that along with vaccine therapy (31%), above all, with the use of lymphocytes and dendritic cells, hopes of biotherapy were connected with gene therapy and oncolytic viruses (29%), using cytokines (16%) and monoclonal antibodies (13%), search new targets and prognostic markers in immunotherapy (11%).

Nanoparticles well adsorbing biomolecules, such as hydroxyapatite nanoparticles, are actively developed for intracellular material delivery [43,99]. They can be used for increase of therapeutic specificity, for example, by means of suicidal genes [49]. At the same time, nanoparticles with size less then 50 nm penetrate natural barriers and can be accumulated in tissues including bone marrow and lymphoid tissue [46]. This implies their unpredictable side effect on antitumor organism resistance. In this connection, comparative research of antitumor activity and toxicity of nano-sized carriers of medicinal preparations and biological molecules allows to hope for creation of effective therapeutic protocols which will find their application in therapeutic practice.

Late cancer diagnostics is considered as one of the main reasons of unsatisfactory therapy results and poor forecast. In connection with enthusiastic search of specific antigenic cancer markers, many researches lose sight of the fact that 10-70% of disease cases are connected with nutrition habit [101] including its mineral constituent. Deficiency or excess of trace elements (copper, zinc, iron, selenium, chromium) initiates and provokes pathological processes such as structural-functional changes of digestive tract mucous membranes [91], tumor diseases [28].

In this connection, this chapter is devoted to: 1) our efforts to develop voltammetry method of trace elements control in biological substances for targeted cancer diagnostics; 2) finding out a role of trace elements imbalance in oncological patients and human tumor cell lines as base for elaboration of approaches to cancer targeted diagnostics and therapy; 3) proper results of targeted magnetocontrollable delivery of cytostatic and nanoparticle composites into tumor cells and tissues.

We suggest following content of this chapter: 1) possibilities of voltammetry methods for nano-sized objects control in biomedical diagnostics; 2) trace elements balance and patients' homeostasis indices as diagnostic and prognostic markers of progressive digestive tract cancer; 3) trace elements concentration in human tumor cell lines; 4) certain results of microelements application for correction of homeostasis in cancer patients; 5) experimental basis of biomedical use of ferreed nanoparticles; 6) antitumor and toxic effects of lipid composites of cisplatin and carbon-encapsulated iron nanoparticles in vitro and in vivo.

POSSIBILITIES OF VOLTAMMETRIC METHODS OF NANOSIZED OBJECTS CONTROL IN BIOMEDICAL DIAGNOSTICS

Electrochemical methods, first of all, voltammerty (VA), can be used for determination of traces both of organic and inorganic substances in medical objects on the level of maximum permissible concentrations, trace quantities in the range of concentrations of $10^{-5}....10^{-10}$ mole/dm^3 and lower. They compete with generally used physical methods (spectrophotometry, chromatography) in sensitivity of determination, expressivity and reliability of obtained data; they are inexpensive and simple to operate.

Detection limits of some trace elements in human biosubstrates obtained by means of different methods: flame atomic absorption spectrometry (AAS - flame), thermal-electric atomic absorption spectrometry (AAS - TE), atomic emissive spectrometry with inductively coupled plasma (AES - ICP), neutron-activation analysis (NAA) and voltammetry (VA) are shown in Table 1.

By comparison of detection limits in mentioned elements it is shown that voltammetry (with different polarography modes) successfully competes with universally recognized extremely sensitive AAS - TE method in sensitivity and significantly excels this method in simplicity and cheapness of used equipment.

Table 1. Detection limits (µg/l, µg/kg) of some chemical elements in human biological substrates (hair, urine, blood, cell suspension, biological tissues, etc.)

Element	AAS - flame	AAS - TE	AES - ICP	NAA	VA
Pb	10	0.5	20	300	0.001
Cd	2	0.002	1	2	0.004
Fe	5	0.05	1	5	0.02
Cu	1	0.02	2	0.1	0.01
Mn	2	0.005	0.2	0.003	0.3
Se	50	0.1	50	1	0.01
Zn	2	0.001	0.5	2.5	0.02

Among VA methods, such variants as adsorptive, inverse, cyclic, squarewave and differential pulse VA are used. First publications about inverse voltammetry (IVA) method as one of the variants of VA methods (synonym: amalgam polarography with accumulation) were issued by Yaroslav Geyrovskiy more than 80 years ago.

Substantial contribution into formation of IVA method, development of his theory and practical applications is made by schools of Russian scientists, such as A.G. Stromberg, S.I. Sinyakova, G.N. Vinogradova et al [13].

IVA is based upon effects of electrochemical reduction and oxidation of substances determined on electrode, where potential changing according to certain low is discharged. Obtained ratio of current and applied voltage – in form of peak or wave - depends on concentration of determined substance and its nature.

IVA method contains of two stages. The first stage is substance (ions) concentrating from large volume of solution into low volume of electrode or on its surface under constant potential. Anodic dissolution of substance concentrate under linear potential change is carried out in the second stage. As a result, analytic peak-like signal is obtained. Current-voltage peak height depends on ions concentration in solution, and peak potential is typical value for this element which is independent on its concentration.

In IVA method electrodes of different types are applied: mercury dripping, mercury membrane, pyrolytic graphite and glass carbon ones. Application of modified carbon paste electrodes sensitive to certain type of organic compounds is possible for analysis in some cases that allows avoiding stage of their release and separation.

In the opinion of analyst – ecologists (P. Bersier, Швейцария, J.Howell, C.Bruntlett, USA), VA method advantages over other analysis methods are following:

- wide range of concentrations being determined: from $10^{-5} \div 10^{-10}$ mole/l;
- opportunity of determination both of inorganic and metal-organic and synthetic substances;
- opportunity of determination of different forms (compounds) of one element;
- opportunity of simultaneous determination of 4-5 elements (by one VA-curve surveying);

- insensibility to presence of many inorganic salts;
- opportunity of analysis automation;
- simplicity and cheapness of equipment;
- wide range of indices being determined. Besides inorganic metal impurities (Zn, Cd, Pb, Cu, Hg, As et al.), it's possible to determine organic substances (antibiotics, phenols et al.). Along with toxic substances (metals, phenol, aniline), essential ones are determined (vitamins et al);
- using small shots (up to 0.1 g) of specimen that provides expressivity, minimum quantity of reagents being used, ecological cleanness of analysis.

More than 60 novel methods of quantitative chemical analysis of content not only metals (Zn, Cd, Pb, Cu, Sb, Sn, Tl, Bi, Mn, Hg, As, Se, Co, Ni, Fe, In, Pt, Ru, Rh, Ir, Os, Au, Ag et al) but also organic substances including aniline, phenol and its derivations, vitamin C and vitamins of B group (B_1, B_2, B_6, B_{12}), antibiotics (levomycetin, tetracycline, penicillin), uric acid, heart protectors (mildronate, obzidan et al.), iodantipirin and its derivates, flavonoids (quercetin, rutinum, hesperidin) were originated in Tomsk Polytechnic Unversity. Information about developed methods of analysis of samples of biological and medical character is shown in Table 2.

VA curves for concentration on the level of 10^{-7} -10^{-9} mole/l were obtained for the first time for many organic substances. Application of graphite electrodes modified with gold in "in situ" mode allowed improvement of metrological characteristics for selenium (obtaining reproducible results) and mercury (sensitivity increase).

Modified electrodes were applied at first in serial analyses due to the fact that conditions of their obtaining and regeneration were trained, and conditions of obtaining analytical signals of elements were optimized. Conditions of quantitative determination of water-soluble vitamin B1, B2, B6, C, PP, antibiotics - levomycetin, tetracycline hydrochloride, ftoruracil, adriablastin and other remedies, as well as flavonoids by means of VA method were established.

Quantitative determination of antibiotics and chemotherapeutical agents are relevant direction in toxic chemical, biopharmaceutical investigations, by estimation of malignant diseases treatment efficacy. Developed VA methods of antibiotics quantitative determination allowed carrying out remedies control by studying optimal doses, rhythm and ways of their administration in long-continued chemotherapy.

VA methods of multi-element analysis of hair specimens, healthy and tumor tissues for trace elements content (Cd, Co, Cu, Ni, Mn, As, Pb, Se, Zn, Cr) were developed on basis of available works [80]. The best 100 publications of the year 2007 given by Ion Channel Media Group Ltd., in journals with high impact-factor were studied. Analysis showed that electrochemical methods were the one of base instruments in nanomedicine infrastructure.

On the one hand, in connection with development of nanobiotechnologies, VA allows revealing nanoparticles and volume implants biodegradation products in different substrates. On the other hand, trace elements imbalance is important in development of human chronic and oncological pathology.

Table 2. Opportunities of application voltammetry methods for quantitative chemical analysis of pharmacological medications

Group of medications being determined (index)	Object of analysis	Detection limit
Antimicrobial, antiviral and antiparasitic agents	Remedies, foodstuffs, biological materials	From $2 \cdot 10^{-6}$ to $1.84 \cdot 10^{-10}$ mole/l
Agents regulating metabolic processes	Biological materials as well as in neoplasia, pharmacological medications	From $4 \cdot 10^{-5}$ до $5.9 \cdot 10^{-10}$ mole/l
Agents having impact on cardiovascular system	Blood, urine, remedies	From $4.0 \cdot 10^{-7}$ to $5 \cdot 10^{-10}$ mole/l
Remedies used for treatment of oncological diseases (fludarabin, colchicine)	Pharmacological medications, aqueous and biological mediums	0,4 ng/ml
Agents having impact on peripheral neurotransmitter processes (dopamine, piribedil, serotonin, famotidin, dimedrolum)	Pharmacological medications, urine, solutions and combined medications.	From $9 \cdot 10^{-8}$ to $1 \cdot 10^{-8}$ mole/l
Agents having impact on central nervous system	Pharmacological medications, blood serum, clean substances	From $1.7 \cdot 10^{-5}$ to $5.4 \cdot 10^{-11}$ mole/l
Agents having impact in field of sensitive nerve endings (ephedrine, novocain, galasolin)	Solutions, tablets, combined medications	From 3.9 to 5.1 pC
Medications of different groups Sugar (glucose, lactate, glutamate, fucosa), Hypolipidemic agent (betaine hydrochloride)	Rats' brain, medical products, biological liquids	From $3.18 \cdot 10^{-5}$ to $7.94 \cdot 10^{-6}$ M

TRACE ELEMENTS BALANCE AND HOMEOSTASIS INDICES IN PATIENTS AS DIAGNOSTIC MARKERS OF PROGRESSIVE GASTROINTESTINAL CANCER

In spite of particular progress of the last 15-20 years, population morbidity and survival rate in gastrointestinal tract (GIT) cancer are still on high level [21]. At the same time, morbidity rate in Tomsk is higher than in Russia on average [64,101]. Late stomach cancer detection leads to 54% one-year morbidity, low five-year survival rate of patients [101].

Detection of microelements in plasma and blood serum are used with the purpose of elaboration new directions in GIT cancer prophylaxis [53]. But their content varies significantly [35,53] that complicates results interpretation. Methods of body mineral homeostasis evaluation by means of detection of chemical elements level in hair actively develop in the last decade [78]. Nevertheless, such investigations are isolated instances in oncological cases [12,35].

The purpose of this work is determination of correlation between chemical composition of biological substrates (hair, tumor tissue), laboratory and clinical health indices for detection of pathogenetically proved predictors of stomach and large intestine oncological disease progressing.

Examination of 74 patients was carried out by authority of Ethics Committee (conclusion No. 583 from 19.03.2007) of Siberian State Medical University (SSMU) on the base of Surgical department of Tomsk Regional Oncological Dispensary and Research Institute of Gastroenterology of SSMU. Patient distribution according to tumor localization and growth stages is shown in Table 3.

Table 3. Distribution of patients according to localization and stage of gastro-intestinal tract tumor diseases

Disease stage	Stomach	Rectum	Sigmoid colon and segmented intestine
Benign changes (average patient age 57.26 ± 2.74 years)			
	17	3	-
Malignant neoplasia, 3^d clinical group (average patient age 62.32 ± 2.00 years)			
I	2	1	1
II	3	1	-
III	14	6	7
Malignant neoplasia, 4th clinical group (average patient age 61.39 ± 3.26 years)			
IV	11	5	3

Among benign changes are chronic erosion (10 %) and stomach ulcer (15 %), large intestine epithelium dysplasia (5%), glandular polyps of stomach (60%) and rectum (10%). Malignant neoplasia was represented as adenocarcinoma of different differentiation stage (85%), signet ring cell carcinoma (9%) and undifferentiated cancer (6%).

Group of healthy volunteers (average age was 36.77 ± 1.71 years) included 74 persons. Moreover, mineral composition of benign epidermis tumors histologically differentiated as papillomas was studied in 14 persons.

Content of chemical elements (zinc, copper, selenium, iron, iodine, mercury, cadmium, lead, arsenic) in hair and tissues was estimated by means of inversion voltammetry method [80]. The method was entered into the Public Register of measurement methods applied in spheres of State Metrological Control and Supervision. Hair has number of benefits in comparison with other biological objects (blood, urine, saliva etc.): material sampling simplicity, seable storage ability under room temperature during unlimited time, higher microelements concentration [78].

Determination of hexavalent chromium (Cr^{6+}) with 1.5-diphenylcarbazide was carried out by means of measurement of ion mass concentration after adsorptive concentrating of 1.5-diphenylcarbazonate Cr^{3+} on graphite electrode surface. It's formed in solution volume as a result of oxidation-reduction reaction of Cr^{6+} with diphenylcarbazide. Adsorbed chromium complex is exposed to cathode transformation. Maximum cathode current of chromium complex reduction depends on Cr^{6+} content in solution in direct proportion [54]. Preparation of samples was carried out with the use of "Temos-Express" complex; signals were measured by means of computerized voltammetry STA complex («ITM» Ltd, Russia) included in Public Register of measurement methods.

Hematologic (total amount of leucocytes and erythrocytes, hemogram, erythrocyte sedimentation rate, haemoglobin value) and biochemical blood indices (level of glucose, cholesterol, total protein, urea, creatinine, bilirubin; activity of amylase, alanine aminotransferase, aspartate aminotransferase and alkaline phosphatase) were determined by means of standard methods [98].

Membrane CD95 marker of leucocytes was determined by means of flow cytometry method (Coulter EPICS-XL-MCL complex) with the use of fluorescent monoclonal antibodies. Quantitative content of CA19-9 and CA242 oncomarkers, concentration of cortisol and somatotropic hormone (STH) in blood serum was estimated by means of immune-enzyme analysis methods with the use of specific monoclonal antibodies sets of the firms CanAg (Sweden) and DSL (USA). Cytochemical estimation of reduced sulfhydryl group (SH) content in erythrocytes was carried out according to [75].

Statistical results processing was made by means of variation statistics methods with the use of Student's t-criterion, Mann-Whitney U-criterion and Spearman's Rank Correlation.

Content of microelements in hair reflects microelemental body status as a whole, and hair tests are integral index of mineral metabolism [78]. According to views of A.V. Bgatov et al. [9], any disease is a consequence of internal body environment disturbance (its homeostasis); mineral balance is tolerance to diseases.

At the same time, official limits of "normal" content of the majority of chemical elements in hair is not determined up to now, in particular, in consequence of person's habitation region [65,79]. Scientific literature analysis has shown relativity of term "normal" microelement content in persons' hair. In this connection, average chemical elements levels in hair of inhabitants of different regions of Russia were used in work (Table 4).

Comparison of body microelements balance in men and women of Tomsk didn't reveal any statistical differences in level both of vitally necessary (zinc, copper, selenium, iron) and toxic metals (cadmium, lead, arsenic). In this connection, their results could be combined into one group and compared with other regions of Russia independently on sex (Table 4, 5). Results showed evident decrease of average content of essential elements such as zinc and selenium in Tomsk inhabitants in comparison with other regions. At that, zinc content, especially in men, decreases beneath all the values being recommended for normal vital activity (Table 4, 5).

At present time, multifactory of oncological morbidity problem is considered to be proved. Ones of the principal factors are nutrition and stress [101]. Relative urbanization of nutrition replacing natural products in some measure in rural areas and especially in Tomsk is to be related to peculiarity of multinational population of Tomsk region [64].

Table 4. Average levels of some chemical elements in hair of adult population of Tomsk and different regions of Russia (European part, Ural, Siberia), X ± m

Habitation region, sex	Average content, mg/kg							
	Zinc	Cadmium	Lead	Copper	Selenium	Iron	Arsenic
Recommended (normal) levels of microelements according to references [78,79]	140-280	less than 0.5-1.5	less than 5.0	6.5-15	0.8-5.0	15-60	less than 1-2
Recommended (normal) levels of microelements according to reference [65]	100-250	0.05-0.25	0.1-5.0	7.5-80	0.5-1.5	5.0-25.0	0.005-0.1
Women (n=28), Tomsk	125.83 ± 10.64 p<0.001	0.06 ± 0.03 p<0.01	2.13 ± 0.43	11.44 ± 2.35	1.01 ± 0.07 p<0.001	23.62 ± 1.70	< 0.002
Women (n=5211) in 30 towns of different regions of Russia	186.0 ± 3.52	0.21 ± 0.02	1.50 ± 0.11	10.81 ± 0.27	1.69 ± 0.05	24.01 ± 0.97	0.28 ± 0.06
Women (n=241) of Siberian region (Novosibirsk, Tumen' district, Krasnoyarsk, Irkutsk)	178.25 ± 4.60	0.17 ± 0.01	1.23 ± 0.32	10.39 ± 0.39	1.52 ± 0.13	22.55 ± 4.03	0.28 ± 0.09
Men (n=19), Tomsk	94.60 ± 9.64 p<0.001	0.08 ± 0.04 p<0.01	1.92 ± 0.32	10.26 ± 1.82	1.04 ± 0.07 p<0.001	24.08 ± 2.67	< 0.002
Men (n=1714) In 12 towns of different regions of Russia	174.58 ± 5.19	0.22 ± 0.02	1.97 ± 0.16	10.03 ± 0.29	1.94 ± 0.13	28.25 ± 1.99	0.27 ± 0.03
Men (n=136) of Siberian region (Novosibirsk, Irkutsk)	153 ± 5	0.27 ± 0.06	1.62 ± 0.12	9.25 ± 0.14	2.06 ± 0.25	21.12 ± 0.86	0.26 ± 0.07
Men and women (n=6925) in 42 towns of different regions of Russia	182.74 ± 3.00	0.21 ± 0.01	1.63 ± 0.10	10.59 ± 0.22	1.76 ± 0.05	25.22 ± 0.93	0.28 ± 0.05

Note: (p) – statistically significant differences of indices in Tomsk in comparison with correspondent groups in other regions; n – number of investigated. Data for other regions are calculated on the base of results [65,78,79].

Condition of homeostasis in patients with stomach and large intestine cancer (Table 3) with special stress on mineral substances balance was studied. The main microelements source in body is food; their intake occurs in stomach and large intestine [4], and is broken in diseases and gastro-intestinal tract disorders. At the same time, microelements (copper, zinc, iron, selenium, chromium) imbalance initiates and provokes development of different pathologies including structure-functional changes of GIT mucous membranes [91], which are able to provoke tumor diseases [28].

Statistical analysis of chemical elements concentrations showed following:

a) There were no significant group differences in corresponding values between men and women;
b) There were no significant indices differences in hair and tissue in patients with stomach and large intestine cancer.

It allowed combining groups being studied.

Data show that significant decrease (with respect to regional indices in healthy persons) of absolute concentrations both of vital important and toxic microelements: copper - 2 times less, iron, hexavalent chromium and lead – 2.5 times less; is noted in hair of patients with different stages of GIT cancer (Table 5). Progressive decrease of selenium content by 24-79% reached statistical differences in the stage IV not only with patients suffering from benign changes of GIT mucous membrane (as in case with copper), but also with patients with stages I-III, attracted special attention.

Microelements content in GIT tumor varies significantly in consequence of multifactorial interrelations of the whole body and tumor tissue [53]. In study having been carried out decrease of absolute content both of essential and toxic microelements which were monodirectional with hair in many respects took place in GIT malignant epithelium tumor (Table 6). At that, statistical differences in zinc and lead levels in comparison with analogue indices in benign pathology were noted. Obviously, it could be connected with deterioration of digestion and uptake processes as disease progresses.

Decrease of antioxidant activity and enhancement of lipid peroxidation processes against stress are of importance in disturbance of membrane structures [96]. Metal cations are specific regulators (catalysts) in the large family of metalloenzymes [24]. Superoxide dismutase (its activity is regulated with zinc and copper), catalase (contains iron), glutathione peroxidase (every of 4 subunits has one atom of selenium; is inhibited with chromium), cytochrome oxidase belong first of all to enzymatic component of antioxidant system (AOS) [32,101].

Practically equal average content of chemical elements being studied in benign neoplasia of skin epithelium and GIT mucous is of interest (Table 6). Perhaps, this fact reflects common mechanisms of mineral homeostasis imbalance and chemical carcinogenesis in different compartment of epithelium tissue. Leastways, mutant gene variants coding metal-dependent Mn-superoxide dismutase (SOD) and Zn-Cu-SOD, Se-glutathione peroxidase are considered as endogenous risk factors (markers) by mammary gland cancer development [35].

Table 5. Average levels of some chemical elements in hair of patients with benign and malignant changes of gastro-intestinal tract, $X \pm m$

Nr.	Investigated group	Elements content, mg/kg									
		Zinc	Copper	Selenium	Iron	Iodine	Chromium $^{6+}$	Mercury	Cadmium	Lead	Arsenic, x 10^{-3}
1	Healthy volunteers (51 women, 23 men)	122.66 ±6.73 n=70	12.13±1.37 n=73	0.90 ± 0.05 n=64	23.31±1.24 n=55	2.06 ± 0.38 n=19	1.36 ± 0.34 n=18	0.08 ± 0.03 n=10	0.07 ± 0.02 n=66	1.72 ± 0.24 n=65	2.90 ± 0.18 n=59
2	Benign changes of mucous membrane (10 women, 10 men)	143.77±18.43 n=14	11.18±2.03 n=15	0.44 ± 0.09 n=15 p1<0.006	19.50±5.50 n=10	2.32 ± 0.47 n=10	2.26 ± 1.22 n=11	-	0.17 ± 0.09 n=9	0.90 ± 0.31 n=9	less than 5 n=14
3	Cancer of stage I-III (18 women, 17 men)	118.63±8.71 n=33	6.20 ± 0.31 n=32 p1<0.001 p2<0.002	0.69 ± 0.08 n=27 p1<0.03	9.06±1.30 n=14 p1<0.001	2.74 ± 0.55 n=25	0.57 ± 0.09 n=31 p1<0.007	0.12 ± 0.05 n=6	0.05 ± 0.01 n=31	0.72 ± 0.10 n=30 p1<0.006	less than 5 n=24
4	Cancer of stage IV (12 women, 7 men)	126.31±14.45 n=14	6.01 ± 0.53 n=13 p1<0.04 p2<0.03	0.19 ± 0.05 n=10 p1<0.001 p2<0.05 p3<0.001	9.87±1.11 n=10 p1<0.001	3.46 ± 1.30 n=8	0.49 ± 0.12 n=12 p1<0.04	0.16 ± 0.09 n=5	0.05 ± 0.02 n=13	0.67 ± 0.19 n=12 p1<0.04	less than 5 n=9

Note: statistical differences according to Student's t-criteria p1 – with the 1st group; p2 – the the 2nd group; p3 – with the third group of observation are marked here and in Table 6

Table 6. Average content (mg/kg) of elements in epithelial skin and gastrointestinal tract (GIT) tumor, X ± m

Investigated group	Zinc	Copper	Chromium $^{6+}$	Cadmium	Lead
Benign skin tumor	16.11±5.69 n=8	1.84 ± 0.61 n=8	1.03 ± 0.18 n=13	0.020 ± 0.007 n=8	0.20 ± 0.06 n=8
Benign changes of GIT mucous	18.71±2.36 n=17	1.36 ± 0.16 n=15	1.84 ± 0.97 n=13	0.040 ± 0.012 n=13	0.20 ± 0.04 n=13
GIT cancer of stage I-III 3^d clinical group	12.04±0.74 n=26 p<0.003	1.22 ± 0.19 n=25	0.07 ± 0.03 n=11	0.020 ± 0.003 n=24	0.06 ± 0.02 n=24 p<0.001
GIT cancer of stage IV. 4th clinical group	10.48±0.87 n=7 p<0.04	0.95 ± 0.16 n=9	0.08 ± 0.03 n=7	0.018 ± 0.004 n=7	0.04 ± 0.01 n=7 p<0.015

Note: p – statistical differences with benign GIT changes

Sharp decrease of absolute concentration of essential microelements in tumor tissue in comparison with hair (Table 5, 6) stipulated comparison of their percentage with concentrations of toxic metals. Actually, 3-4-repeated summary accumulation (from 2-2.3% in hair up to 6.5-9.5% in tumor tissue) of toxic metals (chromium, cadmium, lead) in benign skin and GIT tumor in contrast to malignant one was noted. Related increase of hexavalent chromium level reached statistical differences (Table 7). At the same time, related content of cadmium (Table 7) increased in tumor cells probably due to its redistribution in the body as hair index (r = - 0.3; p<0.05, n=43) inversely correlated with disease stage.

Cadmium and chromium are carcinogenic elements for human being. At that, hexavalent chromium belongs to danger class I [14]. Pathogenesis of tumor transformation caused by microelements imbalance is incompletely known, but direct genotoxical action of hexavalent chromium and, presumably, cadmium and their ability to displace zinc from metal-dependent enzymes taking part in DNA reparation is determined [36]. According to [81,90], chemical elements imbalance underlies the initiation and promotion of tumor growth through modulation of nuclear and mitochondrial DNA metabolism and reparation and by means of regulation of different enzyme and peptide molecules (including lysosomal apparatus), immune cells and antioxidant system activity.

On the other side, chromium causes death of cells through activation of apoptosis. Carcinogenic/cytotoxic effects of chromium can be one of the mechanisms of tumor progression and selection of the most malignant strain of tumor cells burdening disease course and clinical prognosis. More than 1000-repeated variations of Cr^{6+} concentrations in benign GIT pathology leading to increase of average value mistake (Table 6) become clear from this point of view. Drop of chromium concentration (from 0.17 ± 0.05 mg/kg, $p < 0.001$ in comparison with content in benign skin tumor) practically up to the level marked in malignant neoplasia was noted in 8 cases; index growth up to 1-12 mg/kg – on the contrary - in 5 cases.

According to obtained results, parallel decrease of chromium concentration in hair and tumor tissue seems to be adverse sign associated with disease progressing. It is also interesting that proapoptotic signals disturbance is common mechanism of growth and progressing of different tumors [48,50].

Table 7. Relative content (%) of elements in hair and tissues in patients of different observation groups, X

Group being investigated	Biosubstrate	Zinc	Copper	Chromium $6+$	Cadmium	Lead
Healthy volunteers	hair	89	8.7	1	0.05	1.25
	benign skin tumor	84	9.5	**5.4***	0.1	1
Benign changes of GIT mucous	hair	91	7	1.4	0.1	0.5
	tumor tissue	84.5	6	8.5	0.2	0.8
GIT cancer of stage I-III, 3^d clinical group	hair	94	4.9	0.45	0.05	0.6
	tumor tissue	90	**8.9***	0.5	**0.15***	0.45
GIT cancer of stage IV, 4th clinical group	hair	94.5	4.5	0.45	0.05	0.5
	tumor tissue	90.5	8.3	0.7	**0.15***	0.35

Note: *) – statistically significant differences with correspondent indices in hair according to Mann-Whitney U-criterion

In that way, it is possible to define several pathophysiological processes in dynamics of tumor pathology:

1) Decrease of mineral substances entrance into body having negative consequences for blood cells including immunocompetent ones [17]. So, decrease of iron content in

hair of cancer patients was accompanied by sharp decrease of hemoglobin level in erythrocytes (Table 5, 8);

2) Redistribution of carcinogenic metals into tumor tissue, which was also revealed in other cancer forms, for example, mammary gland cancer [12];

3) Decrease of antioxidant elements (zinc, copper) absolute level in tumor cells. Nevertheless, relative copper quantity in tumor tissue increased practically by 2 times ($p<0.05$) in patients of the third clinical group in comparison with quantity of the last one in hair (Table 5) reflecting microelements level in the whole body. Processes of copper accumulation in tumor tissue have apparently general biological meaning inasmuch as they were earlier revealed in rapid growing transplantable adenocarcinoma in mice [85].

Obviously, redistribution of the element activating enzymes of antioxidant system reflexes tumor cells adaptation against deterioration of integral anticancer systems state caused by essential elements deficiency in body. Chromium and cadmium cause accumulation of oxygen and nitric oxide active forms in different ways. At that, cadmium accumulating in cancer cells (Table 7) blocks SH-groups of peptides [89], chromium suppresses glutathione reductase reducing oxidized glutathione [32].

This negative process may have a special significance in consequence of sharp decrease of selenium concentration in hair (body) in GIT tumors (Table 3). Such effect was noted in blood serum by other authors [26]. SH-groups and glutathione have conclusive meaning in cell energy keeping, enzyme inactivation prevention, oxidative peptide denaturation and membranes prevention from peroxide effect [61].

In this connection, comparison of microelement levels in hair with other laboratory indices as prognostic signs of unfavorable outcome was of apparent interest. Estimation of 52 homeostasis indices partially reflected in Table 8 showed that CD95 level on blood leucocytes increased by 72-76 % in patients with malignant epithelial stomach and intestine tumors.

CD95 (Fas, APO-1) is a receptor for Fas-ligand belonging to tumor necrosis factor (TNF) line; is homologous to TNF-α and TNF-β by 30% approximately. The level of soluble CD95 receptor correlates with stage of cancer [7] and deterioration of disease prognosis [55]. Direct correlation of CD95 expression on blood leucocytes with stage of tumor pathology ($r = 0.48$; $p<0.013$; $n=26$) was noted in our investigation.

At present time, search of specific oncologic markers for early diagnostics and prognostics of tumor pathology including digestive tract is still continued. Levels of carcinoma CA19-9 and CA242 markers were studied in our work. According to obtained data, excess of recommended oncomarkers levels reached 394 unit/ml maximum was noted only in 6 of 42 cancer patients (14%). Investigated indices had no prognostic meaning inasmuch as their values did not correlate with disease stage and clinical patient group.

Table 8. Some blood indices in patients of different observation groups, X ± m

Nr.	Investigated group	Investigated indices									
		SH-groups of erythrocytes, s.o.d.u.	Leucocytes, g/l	Haemoglobin, mmol/l	ESR, mm/h	CD95+ %	Cortisol, µg/dl	CTT, ng/ml	CA19-9, Units/ml	CA242, Units/ml	whole protein, g/l
1	Healthy volunteers (51 women, 23 men)	0.400 ± 0.014 n=25	-	-	-	-	14.51± 0.57 n=47	1.72 ± 0.14 n=47	-	-	-
2	Benign changes of GIT mucous membrane (10 women, 10 men)	-	6.29 ± 0.25 n=19	8.58 ± 0.26 n=20	10.05 ± 1.42 n=20	6.77± 0.74 n=18	32.95± 1.51 n=18 p1<0.001	4.46± 3.51 n=2	9.90 ± 6.41 n=2	10.61± 8.02 n=2	72.17± 2.22 n=18
3	GIT cancer of stage I-III, 3ᵈ clinical group (18 women, 17 men)	0.395 ± 0.030 n=28	7.17 ± 0.49 n=36 p2<0.007	7.10 ± 0.31 n=36 p2<0.003	25.25 ± 3.10 n=32 p2<0.001	11.64±1.50 n=22 p2<0.02	42.20± 2.18 n=29 p1<0.001 p2<0.03	1.79± 0.72 n=29	11.18 ± 3.15 n=29	13.14 ± 4.37 n=29	68.77± 1.26 N=36
4	GIT cancer of stage IV, 4ᵗʰ clinical group (12 women, 7 men)	0.399 ± 0.036 n=10	9.32 ± 1.02 n=19 p2<0.007	6.73 ± 0.36 n=19 p2<0.001	36.56 ± 3.79 n=18 p2<0.001	11.92±1.92 n=7 p2<0.03	39.12± 2.97 n=11 p1<0.001	1.15± 0.39 n=11	57.83 ± 35.90 n=11	35.77 ± 17.03 n=11	73.53± 1.79 n=19

Note: s.o.d.u. – standard optical density units

On the other side, statistically significant criteria of patients transfer from the 3^d (liable to anticancer therapy) into the 4th clinical group were following nonspecific indices: total amount of leucocytes in peripheral blood (correlation coefficient r = 0.28; p<0.039; n=54); erythrocytes sedimentation rate (r = 0.32; p<0.025; n=49); total protein amount in blood (r = 0.33; p<0.016; n=54); concentration of selenium in hair (r = - 0.48; p<0.002; n=38); correlation of Cr^{6+} level in hair with its content in tumor tissue (r = 0.54; p<0.011; n=21).

Thus, CD95 and microelements (Se, Cr^{6+}) have the biggest prognostic load in dynamics of progressing malignant GIT tumor in comparison with current laboratory indices. Whether decreased selenium content (and other elements) in blood serum is a factor facilitating carcinogenesis or a result of tumor development [4]? That is the question discussed in literature. In our appearance, "vicious circle" takes place starting with healthy people. Its prevention or tumor pathology inhibition is possible with the help of timely noninvasive diagnostics, application of preventive and curative doses of micronutrients. Leastways, selenium prescription in USA selenium-deficiency regions decreased cancer mortality by 50% and frequency of prostate, rectum, colon and lungs cancer by 63 %, 58 % and 46 % correspondingly [82].

TRACE ELEMENTS CONCENTRATION IN HUMAN TUMOR CELL LINES

Estimation of microelements content in different substrates is one of the most topical problems of modern medical-biological examination. According to views of A.V. Bgatov et al. (1999) [9], any disease is a consequence of body internal environment disturbances (its homeostasis), mineral balance determines resistance to diseases. As a rule, hypoelementoses are connected with deficiency of essential elements, such as iron, zinc, copper, selenium, and hyperelementoses – with accumulation of cadmium, lead, arsenic, titanium, vanadium, beryllium in organism. Deficiency or excess of trace elements (copper, zinc, iron, selenium, chromium) initiates and provokes pathological processes, such as structural-functional changes of gastrointestinal tract mucous membrane [91], tumor diseases [28].

In this connection, disturbance of chemical elements in different human tumor lines was of apparent interest.

Concentration of 7 microelements (Table 9) was estimated in vitro by means of inverse voltammetry (IVA) method. The method is entered in State Register of methods for carrying out measurements applied in scope of state metrological control and supervision. Results were expressed in grammes per every tumor cell (Table 9).

Investigation of microelemental composition of human tumor cell specimens showed essential fluctuations of their content both between inherently different tumor cells and within one kind of tumor. Individual concentration variations of one and the same substrate reached 10-100-fold, sometimes 1000-fold differences. It was reflected in essential mistakes of average values (Table 9).

Table 9. Concentration of microelements in cells of human tumor lines, X±m (average values of 3 measurements are presented)

Group	Histological type and quantity of investigated cell lines	Zinc 10^{-12} g/cell	Cadmium 10^{-15} g/cell	Lead 10^{-12} g/cell	Copper 10^{-12} g/cell	Iron 10^{-12} g/cell	Selenium 10^{-15} g/cell	Chromium 10^{-15} g/cell
1	Cancer of rectum and large intestine, n=5	2.46±1.41	0.34±0.07	0.082±0.023	0.176±0.066	1.38±0.20	4.25±1.89	20.91±2.23
2	Breast cancer, n=3	1.71±1.18	0.46±0.32	0.093±0.076	0.023±0.015	1.09±0.47	4.77±2.10	16.92±7.40
3	Stromal tumor cells n=4	1.66±0.18	0.20±0.03	0.074±0.024	0.097±0.046	0.63±0.12	7.78±5.65	14.88±2.44
4	Melanoma, n=5	14.18±9.77	26.67±12.38*	0.23±0.10	0.072±0.061	8.06±3.17*	23.95±10.39	110.32±50.80

Note: *) – statistically significant differences versus groups 1-3 according to Mann-Whitney U-criterion

Results of 4 groups of tumor cell lines were combined (Table 9):

1) cancer of large intestine and rectum;
2) breast cancer;
3) lines of stromal tumor cells (transformed fibroblasts, osteogenous sarcoma);
4) melanoma.

Statistical differences in average concentrations of investigated elements were not registered in epithelial and mesenchymal tumor cells. Levels of intracellular iron were the most stable in tumor cells. At the same time, content of all chemical elements in melanoma cells (tumor of neuroectodermal origin) was increased. At that, concentrations of cadmium and iron significantly exceeded such in epithelial and mesenchymal tumor cells (Table 9).

Thus, essential variations in cell concentration of chemical elements in different tumors prove necessity of diagnostics and treatment of tumor patients from the point of view of personalized and targeted medicine. Melanoma can be more sensitive to control of microelement balance in organism. Nano-sized iron particles and its oxides, taking into account their magnetosensitivity, can turn out optimal choice in development of ferreed composite systems for delivery of cytostatics and biological molecules for targeted therapy of tumors of different hystogenesis.

CERTAIN RESULTS OF USING MICROELEMENTS FOR HOMEOSTASIS CORRECTION IN CANCER PATIENTS

In connection with variety of neoplasia mechanisms, there are different approaches to antitumor therapy. One of the oldest methods of malignant tumors treatment is biotherapy - method of cancer treatment by means of activation of natural protective mechanisms or introduction of natural polymeric molecules (cytokines, growth factor) and antigens [10].

Vaccine therapy also remains promising clinical direction of gastrointestinal tract cancer biotherapy with enormous theoretical potential for 20-25 years [58]. However, vaccination regimes haven't reached sufficient clinical efficacy that demands a search of new molecular targets and development of new clinical protocols [57].

Thus, D. Nagorsen and E. Thiel (2006) [59] have carried out meta-analysis of 32 clinical results of I/II phases of active specific immunization tests (autologous tumor cells, peptide vaccine, dendritic cells, idiopathic antibodies, viral vaccines) in 527 patients with colon-rectal cancer according to WHO criteria. Immune response was fixed approximately in a half of patients: 59% - humoral reaction, 44% - cell reaction. Nevertheless, disease stabilization was noted only in 8.3% of patients, positive clinical response to vaccination didn't exceed 1% of cases.

In this connection, search of new approaches of cancer biotherapy is timely.

Peripheral blood erythrocyte suspension of adult volunteer in quantity of 25×10^6 cells in 6 ml RPMI-1640 was treated by means of mini-device (autonomous gastrointestinal tract electrostimulator, AES GIT) with sputtering of chromium ions (AES GIT-Cr) in vitro. The electrical stimulator generates pulse current with pulse duration of 5-7 msec., pulse amplitude of 9-15 mA, 16 pulse packets duration of 320-450 msec. Total energy density of electrical impulses varied in the range of W=0.1-3.6 Joule/cm^3.

Mini-device was removed, cell suspension was washed twice in balanced phosphate buffer under 500 G during 10-15 min. Supernatant was removed, water for injections 2 ml, was added to sediment. Osmotic erythrocyte hemolysis was carried out during 15 minutes under continuous suspension stirring. Suspension was centrifuged under 1500 vol./min. during 10 – 15 min, supernatant was collected in containers and kept under 4 °C temperature. Concentration of total chromium (4- or 6-valent) was determined in supernatants in 3 repeats by means of inversion voltammetry (IVA) method.

Subjective and objective evaluation (blood system, immune state, direction of base process) of condition of 10 patients with oncological pathology before and on different terms (1 week – 6 months) after implantation of hybrid implants was carried out in clinic. They were created by sowing of porous titanium carrier (PTC) with autologous blood cells, treated with AES GIT-Cr with W=1.8 Joule/cm^3 in vitro. Panel of hybrid implants is Know-How product permitted for clinical application by the order of Ministry of Public Health RF (protocol of Committee concerning new medical technique No. 11 from 23.12.1999). Implantation of PTC was carried out subcutaneously under local anesthesia.

Statistical results processing was carried out according to Student's t-criterion, Wilkokson's t-criterion (P$_T$) and Mann-Whitney U-criterion (Pu). Integral index (II) characterizing decrease (< 100 %) or increase (> 100 %) of sum of indices being investigated concerning their basic values was calculated as mentioned [25].

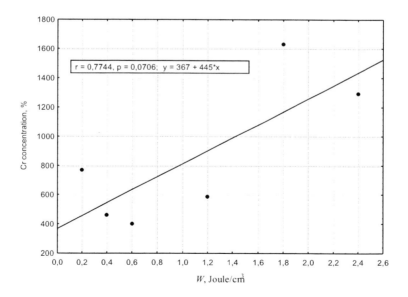

Figure 1. Level of chromium ions in erythrocytes after impact of autonomous gastrointestinal tract electrical stimulator with microelement sputtering in vitro.

Abscissa – total energy density of electrical impulses; ordinata – chromium ion concentration in cells, % of control (point 0). Data of 3 dimensions are represented.

Treatment of peripheral blood erythrocyte suspension of adult volunteer by means of AES GIT with sputtering of chromium ions in vivo has demonstrated practically rectilinear (in the range of W=0,2-2,4 Joule/cm^3) 4-16-fold increase of cation cell concentration (Figure 1). At that, similar treatment retards growth of pathogenic microbes, according to our previous data [45]. In this connection, this method could be used for controlled saturation of autologous cells with their consequent application as systems for chromium delivery into organism of tumor patients.

Cell and tissue transplantation is under view as prospective method of treatment of wide range of pathology [83], including oncological diseases [69].

Nevertheless, there are problems in cell therapy (strict selection of patients, host immune reactions, colonization of transplanted cells in organism, their fast utilization, and short-term treatment effect) which can be solved or minimized through application of scaffolds for cell material. They allow putting a question of prolongation opportunity for therapeutic effects of transplanted cells. Approach having been used can be considered as combined micro- (cells) and macro system (PTC) for delivery of chromium ions taking active part in metabolism of tumor cells and tumor-carrier organism (hereinabove).

On the other hand, one of difficult and unsolved immunotherapy questions explaining its low efficacy in cancer in some extent is creation of local therapeutic concentration of cytokines, activated immunocompetent cells, vectorial molecules in tumor tissue. Biotherapy principles take place in full in case with hybrid implants on PTC allowing concentration therapeutic efforts, having antitumor, immunomodelling and adaptogenous effects by experimental malignant growth [19]. At that, induction of autologous cells ex vivo is carried out by means of weak electromagnetic fields and microelements electrophoresis (chromium, zinc etc.) before implantation.

Opportunity of new technique for homeostasis correction in patients with inoperable tumors or tumors resistant to radio- and chemotherapy was determined in this investigation. Investigated group included 10 patients with solid tumors of different localization (pancreas, intestine, lung and bronchi, ovary, head-neck) of stage IV.

The method being developed by us is not to be considered as alternative for modern methods of cancer treatment. All of them are used as a whole supplementing each other. Thus, primary screening showed that hybrid delivery systems repaired blood system indices after implantation into oncological patients having massive courses of chemo- or X-ray therapy, which were important for antitumor therapy continuity.

On the other hand, hybrid delivery systems had active immunomodulatory properties: 3-month monitoring of 17 immune state indices showed that immune system response to implantation reminded stress reaction on extreme stimuli. Decrease of integral immunologic blood indices (shock phase) in peripheral blood (up to 71% of tumor control, $P<0.05$) in patients with solid tumors was noted during first two weeks. Indices increased (alert reaction) and stabilized on statistically reliable level of 140-160 % of tumor control (resistance phase) from the 3^d week during following 3 months.

Some cell immunity indices, in particular, spontaneous NBT-test, quantity of NK-cells, active (CD25+) and CD95-positive lymphocytes (Figure 2) increased most actively. Receptor-ligand CD95/FasL system underlies apoptosis of healthy and malignant cells [7]. CD95 (Fas/APO-1) antigen is receptor for Fas-ligand belonging to tumor necrosis factors family with cytotoxic, anti-inflammatory, antimicrobial and antitumor effect [7,55,92]. CD95 presents on membrane of activated (not quiescent) T- and B- lymphocytes; its stimulation leads to antigen-stimulated apoptosis of mature cells [70], on the one hand, and to "teaching" thymocytes in thymus (recruitment) – on the other hand [95].

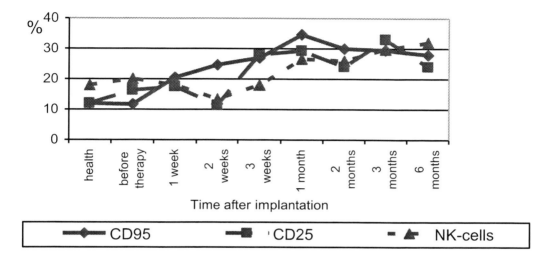

Figure 2. Some immunity indices on different terms after implantation of hybrid delivery systems in healthy and tumor patients.

Recruitment is considered as one of the mechanisms of antitumor action of organism's immunocompetent cells [87], probably, one of the ways to increase efficacy of (immuno)biotherapy method in advanced cancer forms. The last circumstance has important clinical value because, according to our data, number of patients in the 4th clinic group (who are subject to symptomatically supervision by reason of neglected tumor process) can draw up to 35 % of total number of suffering from malignant diseases of stomach and large intestine.

Level of humoral immunity (immunoglobulins, circulating immune complexes) increased from the 3[d] month of investigation of patients' immune state which can be critical point of repeated therapy in consequence of humoral factors' ability to promote tumor progression [8,72].

Clinical immunity activation was conducted with process stabilization or volume degradation and fragmentation of primary nodes of solid tumors, dehydration of malignant cells documented by means of X-ray, endoscopic methods and nuclear-magnetic resonance at least in 4 of 10 patients.

Thus, initial results show existence of proper niche and availability of hybrid implants on porous carrier combined with iontophoresis in complex treatment of metabolic and tumor diseases, correction of complications of classical methods of chemo- and X-ray therapy.

Several phenomena underlie mechanism of action of method being developed. On the one hand, mononuclear phagocyte system is activated in answer to scaffold's artificial material with formation of giant multinucleated cells of foreign bodies [45].

Regulatory action of electropulses, besides direct cell effect, is mediated through their secretory activity with production of stimulating or inhibiting cytokines depending on energy of effecting factor. Addition of ionic (chemical) component is able to inhibit vital activity of epithelial tumor cells effectively, in contrast to clear electrical (physical) factor [42]. In addition, essential trace elements, such as zinc, make systemic impact on organism [4], control activity of immunocompetent cells through gene expression for cytokines, enzymes of DNA reparation, signaling and transporting molecules [29].

EXPERIMENTAL JUSTIFICATION OF BIOMEDICAL APPLICATION OF FERREED NANOPARTICLES

Inclusion of nano-sized ferromagnetics in drug delivery systems allows obtaining their ferreed forms [39]. Nano-sized iron powders, its hydroxides and oxides usually serve as carriers of magnet properties [5,30]. It's well known that metal nanoparticles and metal nanopowders are characterized with high reactivity and catalytic activity [73]. At the same time, such ferromagnetics have their own toxicity relative to cells, tissues and components of biological liquids [62] conditioned with their participation in free radical processes, in accordance with conclusions of many authors [51].

In this connection, biological and toxicological properties of nano-sized, magneto-sensitive particles of iron and its composites which are prospective for targeted cancer therapy are doubtless of scientific-practical interest.

Isotonic sodium chloride solution (0.9 % NaCl) was used as a solvent for investigation of sanitary-chemical properties of nanoparticles by example of Fe_3O_4 magnetite according to ISO 10993-5 recommendations. For estimation of pH changes in Fe_3O_4 nanopowder extracts after 7 day - extracting its terminal dose of 0,3-3 mg/l that makes 1 – 10 maximum permissible concentrations (MPC) for iron was used [100].

For investigation of yield of iron ions by means of inversion voltammetry method [13] magnetite (100 mg/l) was solved under sterile conditions during 3, 8 and 20 days under the temperature of 37°C. In addition, solubility of magnetite nano-sized particles (average diameter of 40 nm) by 5-day impact of constant magnetic field strength of 0.13T was studied.

Cultural investigations were carried out with the use of marrow cell material of Balb/c line mice. Animals were devitalized with ether narcosis; marrow was extracted from femoral bone in concentration of 2.5×10^6 karyocytes/ml. Cell suspension was laminated on $MgFe_2O_4$ magnesium ferrite nanodispersion (average particle diameter was 5 nm, terminal particle concentration was 3 mg/l of cell culture, 10 maximum permissible concentrations for iron) and cultivated in 2 ml volume of cultural medium during 48 hours under 37 °C. Cultural medium of following composition was used: L-glutamin (Sigma) 280 mg/l, gentamicin sulphate 40 mg/l, 15 % of fetal bovine serum (ICN), 85 % of medium 199 (SPA "Vektor").

Appropriate volume of solvents: sodium chloride (0.9 %) (negative toxicity control, 0.33 ml) or 5% dimethyl sulfoxide (DMSO) (positive toxicity control) was added to control tubes. A half of investigated cultures were placed on magnetic mat with constant field strength 200 Oe (0.02 T).

Fraction of non-adhesive cells were extracted by means of mild pipetting, nanoparticles cytotoxicity was determined in staining test with trypan blue (0.4 %) according to ISO 10993-

5. Adhesive cells were air-dried, fixed with methanol during 3-5 min., stained with azure-II-eosin during 10 min (Figure 3). Optical density of cell cultures (D, s.u.o.d.) and area of adhered myelokaryocytes (S, mm^2) were evaluated in obtained preparations according to computer morphometry, as described [3,75].

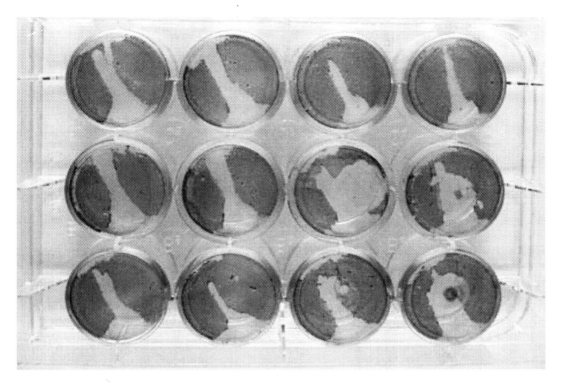

Figure 3. Preparation of myelokaryocytes adhering to plastic for evaluation of magnesium ferrite nano-sized particles effect. Staining with azure-II-eosin.

In preliminary investigations it was determined that 5 % DMSO solution may be considered as positive toxicity control relatively to marrow cells. On the one hand, it didn't inhibit mice marrow cells viability. Quantity of karyocytes stained with trypan blue was 90.78±3.36 % (n=5) versus 93.86±1.17 % in control (n=10). At the same time, DMSO disturbed marrow structural-functional organization decreasing quantity of unstained hemopoietic islets 2.5 times (with 72.22±1.39 × 10^3/femur in control up to 28.89±13.86 × 10^3/femur).

Quantitative composition of hemopoietic islets (HI) was investigated by means of modification of [75] method [18]. Balb/c line mice marrow from femoral bone canal was eluated into tubes with 1ml of RPMI-1640 medium. Nanodispersion of Fe$_3$O$_4$ magnetite or carbon encapsulated iron particles Fe(C) in terminal concentration of 3 mg/l obtained directly before blending with cells by means of ultrasonic treatment during 5 min was added to some tubes.

Suspension of megakaryocytes with 0.9 % NaCl added in 1/10 (100 μl) of complete volume of cultural medium served as negative control. Hydrogen peroxide with cytotoxic effect in terminal dilution of 1 mM was selected as positive control [56]. Components were mixed by means of pipetting of cell suspension through needle with diameter of 1 mm und cultivated in thermostat under 37°C during 1 hour.

Then, cell suspension was pipetted again, mixed with 0.1% solution of neutral red in 0.9% NaCl solution in proportion 1:1. Obtained mixture was put into Goryaev's camera, quantity of hemopoietic ilslets with stained and unstained central elements was counted along the full work surface before and after cultivation in thermostat. Supravital nuclear staining with neutral red increases with increase of their maturity [37]. Cell associations containing more than 3 myelokaryocytes connected with centrally placed monocytes/macrophage or stromal mechanocyte were taken as hemopoietic islets.

Absolute hemopoietic islets number in femoral marrow was determined according to formula:

$$X = (2N / 0.9) \cdot 10^3,$$

where N – number of HI calculated in Goryaev's camera; 0.9 (µl) – volume of Goryaev's camera; 2 – dilution coefficient.

Total karyocytes number (TKN) and number of dead cells stained with trypan blue (0.4 %) was estimated in Goryaev's camera before and after addition of nanodispersion according to [75].

Basic number of HI and TKN in femur is individual for every mouse. In this connection, obtained numerals were converted to percents from initial indices content (before 1-hour cultivation) for lightening the results analysis.

Statistical results processing was made by means of variation statistics methods with the use of Student's t-criterion, Mann-Whitney U-criterion and Spearman's Rank Correlation.

1. Magnetite Nanopowder Solubility Ex Vivo

Magnetite nanopowder degradation was studied in isotonic solution of sodium chloride (0.9 % NaCl) which is model biological liquid according to ISO 10993-5 recommendations. Obtained data showed that 7-day magnetite extracts insignificantly changed concentration of hydrogen protons in solvent (control) which pH was 6.94 units (n=4) at the average. Within magnetite nanoparticles dose interval of 1 – 10 MPC mean pH values modified in the range of 97.4-98.3 % of check value (n=6). At that, statistical dependence of pH change on nanoparticles dose wasn't ascertained. Influence of magnetite nanoparticles on model biological liquid doesn't exceed permissible limits for materials intended for medicine (±1.0 pH units).

Inversion voltammetry showed presence of Fe^{3+} ions in 3-200-day solutions of nano-sized Fe_3O_4 in the range of 42-56 µg/l by their concentration in pure solvent less than 1 µg/l. Such content doesn't exceed 1.4-1.9 % of theoretically possible pure iron output of solid phase into solution that was not of great biological importance by the use of Fe_3O_4 in the range of concentrations of 1 – 10 MPC. At that, in dissolution dynamics some decrease (with rate of 0.89 µg/day) of iron ions' level in solution was observed (Figure 4).

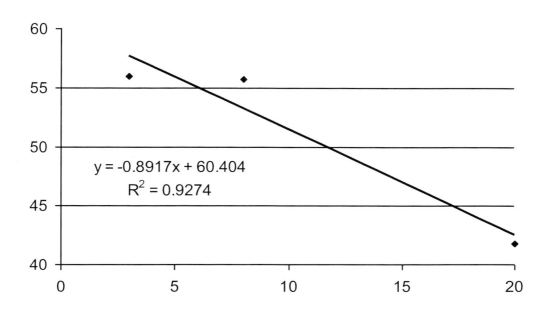

Figure 4. Dynamics of nano-sized magnetite particles dissolution.

Abscissa – dissolution time, days; ordinate – iron ions concentration in solution, µg/l. Every point is presented with data of four measurements.

Output of Fe^{3+} ions of nano-sized magnetite into solution also decreased in constant magnetite field. Accumulation of 5-day substance was 26 µg/l (n=4) by expected concentration of 54 µg/l according to regression equation on Figure 4.

Thus, sanitary - chemical investigations showed that synthesized ferromagnetic powders of ferric oxide were weak degenerative material, promising for development of magnet-sensitive delivery systems for medical and biological products. Direct effect seems to be the main influence component of surface of iron nanoparticles and its oxides on living systems within 1 month of their interrelation.

2. Influence of Magnesium Ferrite Nanopowder on Marrow Cells Adhesion to Plastic

Results showed that cultural medium dissolution with isotonic sodium chloride solution in proportion of 1/6 of terminal volume didn't influence significantly on indices of myelokaryocytes adhesion to plastic. At the same time, addition of magnesium ferrite nanodispersion in isotonic sodium chloride didn't have any visible effect on cell culture optic density as well as their liability (Table 10). At the same time, adhered cells area decreased by 20% in comparison with control (p_1=0.000008).

Direction of modulating nanopowder effect remains under constant magnetic field strength of 0.02 T. At that, myelokaryocytes adhesion area decreases less than by 10% in comparison with control, exceeds index in test cell culture out of magnetic field impact statistically significant (p_2=0.005).

Application of DMSO as a solvent for $MgFe_2O_4$ nanoparticles allowed determining its negative effect on functional activity of marrow nuclear cells. In comparison with cultural medium without addition of DMSO, adhesion area of myelokaryocytes decreased down to 87.5 % (p=0.0001) and came to 252.66±1.18 mm^2 (Table 11).

Table 10. Indices of Balb/c mice myelokaryocytes culture adhering to plastic after 48 hours of cultivation with magnesium ferrite nanoparticles (diameter 5 nm) in concentration of 3 mg/l, X± m, P

Observation group	Without magnetic field			Magnetic field strength 0.02 T		
	Viable cells, %	Culture optical density, D	Cells adhesion area, S, mm^2	Viable cells, %	Culture optical density, D	Cells adhesion area, S, mm^2
Check cell culture with 1/6 of NaCl (0.9 %) volume	58-61.5	41.44±1.20 n=6	293.64±3.23 n=4	55.5-78	46.67±2.64 n=6	316.62±2.04 n=4
Test cell culture with addition of $MgFe_2O_4$ nanoparticles in sodium chloride (0.9 %) solution	57-71	41.13±1.14 n=6	234.09±2.78* n=4 p_1=0.000008	55.5-57	48.91±1.62 n=6 p_2=0.003	286.75±11.78* n=4 p_1=0.05 p_2=0.005

Note: here and in Table 11 *) – statistically significant differences: p_1 – tests with control; p_2 – tests with results without magnetic field impact.

On the contrary, magnesium ferrite suspension in DMSO increased optical density and marrow cell culture area adhered to plastic by 16.5-21.5 %. Constant magnetic field leveled obtained effect (Table 11).

By interpretation of obtained data 3 circumstances are worthy of notice:

1) magnet-sensitive nanoparticles interact with cells because myelokaryocytes adhesion increases under conditions of additional magnetic field impact;
2) magnesium ferrite can't be used as magnetic-sensitive component in drug delivery systems because it has its own side effect on marrow cells functional activity;
3) negative magnesium ferrite effect on myelokaryocyte adhesion to plastic is, apparently, mediated through hydroxyl radical (HO$^\bullet$) generation, because DMSO is known as its effective catcher [54].

Table 11. Indices of Balb/c mice myelokaryocytes culture adhering to plastic after 48 of cultivation with magnesium ferrite nanoparticles (diameter 5 nm) in concentration of 3 mg/l, X± m, P

Check group	Without magnetic field			Magnetic field strength 0.02 T		
	Viable cells, %	Culture optical density, D	Cells adhesion area, S, mm^2	Viable cells, %	Culture optical density, D	Cells adhesion area, S, mm^2
Check cell culture with DMSO (5 %)	67-80	30.61±1.67 n=6	252.66±1.18 n=4	50-60	36.09±0.74 n=6	316.63±8.41 n=4
Test cell culture with addition of MgFe$_2$O$_4$ nanoparticles in DMSO solution (5 %)	60-83	37.17±1.19 n=9 p1=0.006	294.52±14.73 n=4 p1=0.049	80-100	38.91±1.14 n=6	321.67±16.20 n=4

Note: DMSO – dimethylsulfoxide.

3. Influence of Carbon Encapsulated Iron Nanopowder and Magnetite on Structural-Functional Marrow Organization in Vitro

Experiments showed (Table 12) that statistically significant differences weren't determined in morphological marrow culture indices in groups being investigated in vitro. Total number of karyocytes (TNK) and death of myelokaryocytes by dint of necrosis estimated by intracellular penetration of trypan blue varied in the range of values of negative and positive toxicity control after addition of nanoparticles.

At the same time, structural-functional marrow cells activity estimated by HI content practically decreased 1.5 – 2 times after addition of hydrogen peroxide into the culture (Table 13). Number of HI which central element was stained with neutral red decreased particularly sharply (by 45 % in comparison with negative control).

It ought to be remarked that magnetite nanoparticles had an effect on hemopoietic cells close to H_2O_2 effect on its own amplitude leading to decrease of HI summary content up to 70% (p=0.031) of negative toxicity control level.

Table 12. Number of stained nucleated cells (% of initial number) and total number of karyocytes (TNK) in Balb/c mice marrow culture in 1 hour after addition of nanopowders suspension in terminal concentration of 3 mg/l, X± m, P

Observation group	Stained cells	TNK
Negative toxicity control with addition of 0.9 % NaCl, n=5	138.73±24.92	81.25±7.73
Fe$_3$O$_4$ n=5	120.72±12.16	93.62±11.19
Fe(C) n=5	137.77±16.09	97.37±10.29
Positive toxicity control with addition of H$_2$O$_2$, n=6	157.82±11.59	81.96±9.97

Note: n – tests number.

Table 13. Content of hemopoietic islets (HI) (% of initial number) in Balb/c mice marrow in 1 hour after addition of nanopowders suspension in terminal concentration of 3 mg/l, X± m, P

Observation group	Content of hemopoietic islets		
	Stained HI	Unstained HI	Sum of HI
Negative toxicity control, n=5	126.15±15.27	224.38±28.27	161.06±14.42
Fe$_3$O$_4$ n=5	91.68±11.30	148.18±24.22	113.45±11.08* p$_1$=0.031
Fe(C) n=5	137.35±22.35# p$_2$=0.032	175.17±8.66	153.30±15.20# p$_2$=0.012
H$_2$O$_2$ – Positive toxicity control, n=6	69.03±16.21* p$_1$=0.032	142.18±30.51	92.78±10.74* p$_1$=0.006

Note: *) –statistically significant differences with negative toxicity control (p$_1$); # – statistically significant differences with positive toxicity control (p$_2$) according to Student's t-criterion; n – tests number.

On the other hand, direct contact of carbon coated iron nanoparticles with hemopoietic cells didn't lead to disturbance of intercellular associations playing important role in hemopoietic processes. HI content varied within the limits of negative toxicity control values and exceeded analogous indices (stained HI, sum of HI) in positive toxicity control (Table 13).

4. Influence of Carbon Encapsulated Iron Nanoparticles on Morphological-Functional Properties of Stromal Stem Cells in Vitro

Multipotent mesenchymal stromal cells (MMSC) are considered as cells with fibroblast-like morphology. In spite of numerous investigations, majority of sides of MMSC biology are still unclear [76]. Basic events connected with stem cells vital activity, tissue formation on the base of general-biological proliferation processes, commitment, differentiation and maturation take place on interface of artificial material (implant) and cell (tissue) [11,45].

None of antigen markers and cytokines being secreted can be reliable parameter for analysis of MMSC culture purity. On the one hand, even long-term cultures can show some heterogeniety (probably, because of marker expression connected with cell cycle) and, on the other hand, functionally different cell cultures can have similar immune-phenotypic profiles [60].

Purposeful design of scaffolds made of hydroxyapatite (HAP) and/or calcium phosphates allowed to reveal certain dependence of bone tissue growth on surface relief in vivo [44]. Certain MMSC tropia to artificial substrates is known. At that, only functional trials, such as alkaline phosphatase activity determination, allow characterizing MMSC maturation processes, first of all, in osteogenous direction [67]. Investigations of enzymatic cell activity by their direct contact with artificial surfaces [71] modeling local reactions on implanted articles are most wide spread.

In connection with absence of expressed effect of carbon encapsulated iron nanoparticles on structural-functional marrow organization, their influence on morphological-functional properties of stromal stem cell by their interaction with artificial materials is of interest for tissue bioengineering.

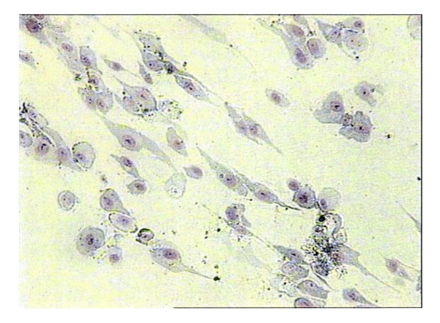

Figure 5. Culture of prenatal human lung cells. Staining with azure II-eosin. Magnification 400.

Characteristics of MMSC populations of different tissues are similar [77]. They are revealed in embryonic [1] and lung tissues [47]. In this connection, culture of prenatal fibroblastoid cells of human lung ("Stem cells bank" Co Ltd., Tomsk) used by us in experiments may serve as MMSC source. Preparations are population of cells of different shape and sizes (Figure 5), that is typical for MMSC pool [1], with limited life period, keeping stable karyotype by passages and carcinogenically safe. Cells are free from foreign viral (AIDS, hepatitis, herpes at al.) and bacterial agents (syphilis, mycoplasma, chlamydiae et al.). After unfreezing, cells viability determined according to ISO 10993-5 in test with 0.4 % trypan blue came to 91-93 %.

Discs made of pure titanium (diameter 12 mm, thickness 1 mm) carrying bilateral calcium phosphate (CP) coatings were used as artificial substrate for MMSC cultivation. Coatings were applied on titanium substrate by means of modification of anode-spark (microarc) oxidation method in 10% phosphoric acid solution containing suspension of nano-sized (20 – 40 nm) synthetic HAP particles.

Mechanical-chemical synthesis of nano-sized HAP was carried out as described above [15]. HAP of stoichiometric composition $Ca_{10}(PO_4)_6(OH)_2$ with particles diameter of 10 – 40 nm was synthesized. Phase composition and crystallinity of synthesized HAP nanopowder are confirmed with data of roentgen-phase analysis (RPA) and infrared microscopy (IRS).

Osteogenous medium includes differentiation inductors (as a rule, dexamethasone, beta-glycerophosphate and ascorbic acid), which concentrations differ by different authors [1, 23, 60]. For cell cultivation on calcium phosphate substrate we use following prescription: beta-glycerophosphate 10 mM, ascorbic acid 50 µg/ml, of dexamethasone 10^{-6} M, L- glutamine 280 mg/l, gentamicin phosphate 50 mg/l, HEPES buffer 10 mM, 20% fetal bovine serum, 80% DMEM/F12 (1:1) medium.

Discs were placed in wells (area 1.77 cm^2) of 24-well dishes (Costar); cell suspension in concentration of 3×10^4 viable karyocytes in complete cultural medium 1 ml was added. Suspension of carbon encapsulated iron nanoparticles Fe(C) (diameter was no less than 10 nm) in terminal concentration 3 mg/l (10 MPC for iron) was brought into some wells.

Implants with cells were removed in 3 days and air-dried. In the following, fixation of cells adhering to coating was carried out in formalin vapor during 30 sec. for cytochemical staining for alkaline phosphatase. Activity of alkaline phosphatase (ALP) in cells was determined according to [37] with the use of fast garnet staining agent.

Computer morphometry method was applied for detection of cell quantity parameters by means of measurement of their optical characteristic. Area and optical density of objects were calculated with the use of program Adobe PhotoShop 7.0 according to gray level statistics in modification [75] for non-transparent objects. Area was expressed in square nanometers, optical density – in standard units of optical density (s.u.o.d.).

Statistical results processing was made by means of variation statistics methods with the use of Student's t-criterion, Mann-Whitney U-criterion, Spearman's Rank Correlation and linear regression analysis.

It's known that stromal cells (fibroblasts, osteoblasts) produced by MMSC are positive stained for alkaline phosphatase [16,37]. At that, activity of ALP increases as cells mature [74]. Some authors consider significant staining for ALP as cytochemical characteristic of osteoblasts [67]. Erythroblasts, megakaryocytes, lymphocytes, monocytes and young granulocytes show negative reaction for AP [37].

According to data of computer morphometry, average density of distribution of cells positive stained for ALP was approximately 15 cells per 1mm^2 of disc surface with CP coating (Table 14, Figure 6). Addition of Fe(C) nanoparticles didn't practically influence morphological-functional indices (adhesion, maturing) of stromal cells culture adhered to discs surface. Increase of stained cells optical density could be connected with fixation of nanoparticles actively absorbing light in visible part of spectrum on them.

Table 14. Morphometric indices of prenatal human lung cells stained for alkaline phosphatase by different shot-term cultivation methods, X̄±m

Groups	Number of stained cells per 1 mm^2 of surface	Cell staining area (S), μm^2	Cell optical density (D), s.u.o.d.
Cells + disc, n=3	14.48±1.03 n_1=27	92.28±14.30 n_2=33	20.26±1.34 n_2=33
Cells + disc + Fe(C), n=3	18.51±2.30 n_1=18	71.75±9.49 n_2=29	24.66±1.12* n_2=29 $p<0.016$

Note: *) – statistically significant differences according to Student's t-criterion; n – discs number; n_1 – number of counted fields of vision; n_2 – counted cells number.

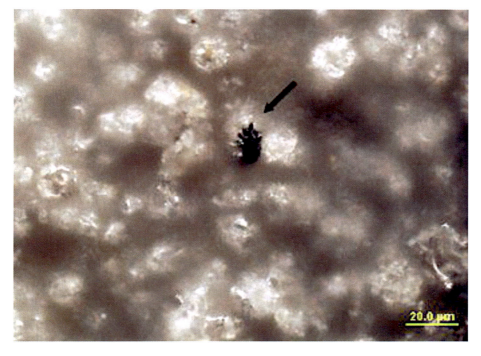

Figure 6. Optical microscopy of cell positive stained for alkaline phosphatase (marked with arrow) on surface of calcium phosphate coating. Magnification 1000.

Thus, Fe(C) nanoparticles in used concentration don't influence distinctly on adhesion and maturing of stromal stem cells by their in vitro interrelation with artificial CP surfaces modeling bone formation processes in vivo. In other words, application of Fe(C) nanoparticles in medical product delivery systems mustn't disturb osteogenesis processes in organism.

Thus, in vitro testing of toxicological properties of iron nanopowders and its oxides (magnetite, magnesium ferrite, carbon encapsulated iron) was carried out on stromal stem cells and hemopoietic elements of marrow being considered as target organ by particles dimension less than 50 nm [46]. It implies opportunity of nanoparticles' own side effect on organism antitumor resistance.

In this connection, carbon encapsulated iron nanopowders with bioinertness according to used toxicological tests are considered as optimal ones for creation of magnet-sensitive nano-sized carriers of antitumor drugs.

ANTITUMOR AND TOXIC EFFECTS OF CISPLATIN LIPID COMPOSITES AND IRON NANOPARTICLES WITH THIN CARBONIC COVER IN VITRO AND IN VIVO

Modern biotherapeutic approaches to systemic and regional treatment of oncological diseases imply realization of "address" delivery of pharmacological agents by means of attracting nano-sized carriers – polymer and metal nanoparticles, liposomes, niosomes, mycelium, quantum dots, dendrimers, microcapsules, cells, solid fats microparticles, lipoproteins and different nanoassemblies [88].

Liposome systems as delivery agents for drugs and biological molecules have been developed since the eighties of the 20th century [10]. Liposomes containing cytostatics are considered as prospective ones, from the point of view of system toxicity decrease and so-called "passive aiming" at tumor tissue [86]. Traditional raw material for liposome systems manufacturing is usually high-purity egg lecithin, phospholipids of phytogenous and animal origin [6]. Inclusion of nano-sized ferromagnetics in liposomes allows obtaining their ferreed forms [39].

Magnetic liquids on the base of micellar biopolymer solutions, remedies and nanoferromagnetics are no less interesting and simple in preparation. Their pharmacological activity is also a subject for rapt attention of researchers [94]. Effect of increased penetration and hold in tumor conditioning selective delivery by means of "passive aiming" mechanism realizes for micellar systems as well as for liposomes [52].

In spite of great success, it's early to draw final conclusions in the field of cancer nanotherapy. Although low toxicity and safety of biotherapy protocols were shown, efficacy of tests carried out for today leaves something to be desired [93]. In this connection, synthesis and biological properties of nano-sized, magnet-sensitive, lipid forms of antitumor preparations are of apparent scientific-practical interest.

It is not unreasonable to test nanoferromagnetics with surface being inert to chemical and biological substrates for medical aims. From this point of view, metal nanopowders coated with protective pyrocarbon coat preserving metal nucleus from impact of environment factors

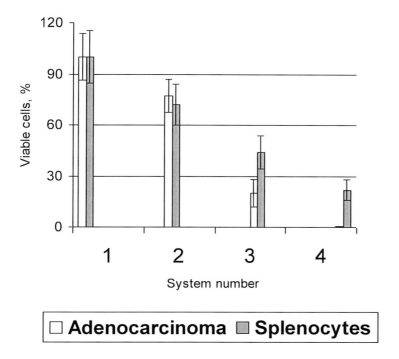

Figure 7. Viability of Ehrlich adenocarcinoma cells and mouse splenocytes in 24 hours of cultivation with lipid composites of cisplatin and carbon encapsulated iron nanoparticles. Abscissa –systems being investigated: 1 – phosphate buffer; 2 - phosphate buffer + cisplatin; 3 - phosphate buffer + phospholipid concentrate + cisplatin; 4 - phosphate buffer + phospholipid concentrate + cisplatin + Fe(C).

Sequential addition of phosphatidylcholine and Fe(C) nanoparticles to the system increased (more than by 20%) relative quantity of dead adenocarcinoma cells in comparison with splenocytes statistically significant. Building of trend lines (value of linear approximation R=0.96-0.99) by sequential addition of system's components showed that speed of increase of dead cells number was 36 % at 26% – for immunocompetent cells.

Thus, relative selectivity of toxic action of lipid composites of cisplatin and ferreed nanoparticles being investigated in relation to tumor cells was revealed. Terminal Fe(C) concentration used in vitro and in vivo (2 mg/kg) system is low.

Analysis of histological specimens showed (Figure 8) that by subcutaneous introduction Ehrlich adenocarcinoma cells tried to form gland-like structures. Tumor is built of sharply atypical glandular tubules of different size and shape. Some cavities have homogenous rose-pail mass looking like secretion. Glands are lined with cylindrical epithelium, partially multi-row. Cell deposition occurs in some atypical glandular structures. Signs of secretory process are determined in epitheliocytes.

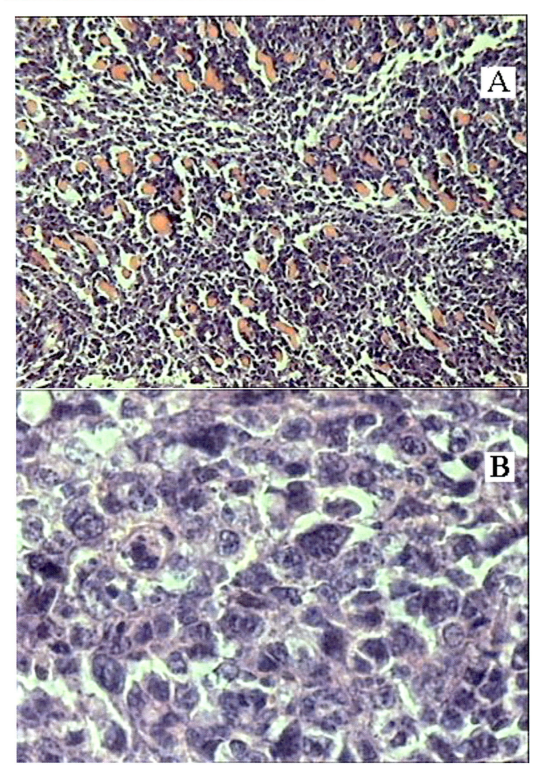

Figure 8. Morphological structure of tumor node after introduction of phosphate buffer. Staining with hematoxylin - eosin. Magnification 150 (A) and 700 (B).

Sharply marked cell atypism is determined in tumor tissue cells accompanied by formation of cells of different shape with aniso- and hyperchromic polymorphous nucleuses. Atypical giant cells with numerous nucleuses (4-6 nucleuses) are determined among tumor cells. Basal membrane outlines badly, partially misses. Focal polymorphocellular infiltrate is determined in tumor stroma.

Intratumor introduction of cisplatin in vivo caused statistically significant 2-3-fold decrease of size and mass of subcutaneous Ehrlich adenocarcinoma node (Table 16). Leukocytic infiltration increased by 80%, but glandular structure of tumor node persisted (Figure 9). It's built of sharply atypical glandular tubules of different size and shape. Glandules are lined with cylindrical epithelium which is partially multi-row. Some atypical glandular structures have cells deposition. Sharply frank cell atypism is determined in tumor tissue cells.

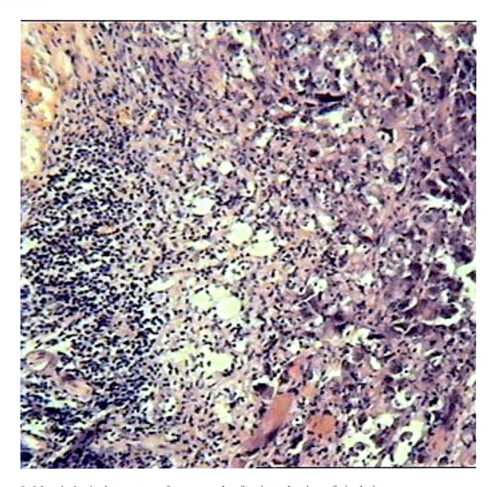

Figure 9. Morphological structure of tumor node after introduction of cisplatin.

Staining with hematoxylin - eosin. Magnification 150.

Table 16. Morphological and histological indices of Ehrlich adenocarcinoma subcutaneous growth after course introduction of medications, $X \pm m$

Group number, n=10	Tumor diameter, cm	Tumor relative mass (TRM), %	TGI, % by tumor weight	TRM × S of tumor on section, %	Tumor tissue area on section (S), %	Infiltrate area on section, %	Conjunctive tissue area on section, %	Foreign-bodies cell number pro 1 mm²
1	2.44±0.02	28.4	0	24±1.7	83±6	30±3	0	96.58±7.35
2	0.88±0.06 $p_1<0.01$	8.4 $p_1<0.01$	78 $p_1<0.01$	7.20±0.34 $p_1<0.01$	86±4	54±3 $p_1<0.01$	0	102.94±10.52
3	2.36±0.03 $p_2<0.01$	22.4 $p_2<0.01$	22 $p_2<0.01$	8.96±0.67 $p_2<0.01$	40±3 $p_2<0.01$	70±3 $p_2<0.01$	0	311.74±74.60 $p_2<0.01$
4	1.09±0.05 $p_3<0.01$	6.7 $p_3<0.01$	81 $p_3<0.01$	2.21±0.13 $p_3<0.01$	33±2	13±1 $p_3<0.01$	54±2 $p_3<0.01$	units

Note: n – number of animals and tumor nodes sections in each group; p_1 - p_3 – reliable differences with values in groups with correspondent number; group number to system number in Table 15; TGI – tumor growth inhibition.

Increase of tumor node size and mass can be connected not only with base process but also with organism reaction leading to edema, infiltration, necrosis and sclerosis of pathological focus. In particular, it's typical for micellar cytostatic form (Figure 10). In this way, the 3d system worsened cisplatin antitumor action according to morphological indices (size, tumor node mass, TGI) and enhanced the last one according to histological indices (tumor tissue area).

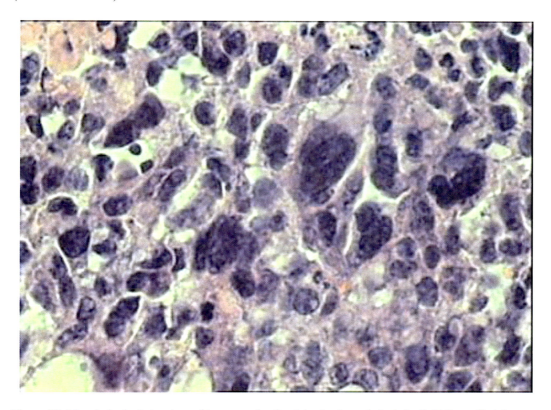

Figure 10. Morphological structure of tumor node after introduction of cisplatin lipid form. Staining with hematoxylin - eosin. Magnification 700.

Indices of tumor mass, size and TGI didn't correlate with tumor tissue area determined on sections which allowed multiplying their probabilities and introducing new efficacy index of investigated groups (RIM x tumor area on section). At that, number of giant cells increased in tumor tissue sections three times (Table 16).

The 4th composite system consisting of micellar form of cytostatic with pyrocarbonic iron nanoparticles had the most significant antitumor activity. In comparison with other supervision groups, fact of tumor node fibrosis more than 50% (Table 16, Figure 11) attracted great attention by small quantity of infiltrate and giant cells on histological sections.

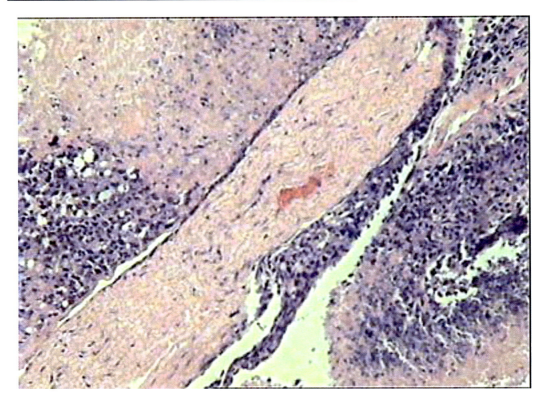

Figure 11. Morphological structure of tumor node after introduction of lipid composite of cisplatin and carbon encapsulated iron nanoparticles. Staining with hematoxylin - eosin. Magnification 150.

In experiments in mice it was shown (Table 17) that hepatocytes formed distinct hepatic lobule including general liver plates, triads, sinusoid capillaries and central veins in hepatic parenchyma of Balb/c tumor-carrier mice (Figure 12). Hepatic plates consist of 2 rows of hepatocytes and interconnect radially in central vein. Fine accumulations of lymphocyte-like cells (2-3 cells) are determined between hepatocytes.

These cell elements are of small size and have narrow cytoplasm limbus and small nucleus with pycnotic chromatin structure. Powder-like, fine, weakly basophilic granulosity can be distinguished in cytoplasm of some cells under big magnification. Functionally, these cells are related to natural killer cells.

Hepatic parenchyma triads keep normal structure and being presented with interlobular artery, vein and bile duct. Interlobular vein contains erythrocytes, polymorphonuclear leucocytes and lymphocytes. Sinusoid capillaries (spaces between hepatic plates) keep normal structure. Hepatocytes are cells of polygonal shape with distinct boundaries and centrally located nucleus. Staining of cytoplasm is homogenous with slight fine granulosity.

Chromatin structure in nucleus is reticular, uniform. Compact aggregations – nucleoluses (1-2 nucleoluses in nucleus of ordinary hepatocytes) are revealed in some hepatocytes. Single cells with dystrophic and necrotic changes (Figure 12) are revealed among hepatocytes of ordinary structure. Perls' reaction for iron is negative.

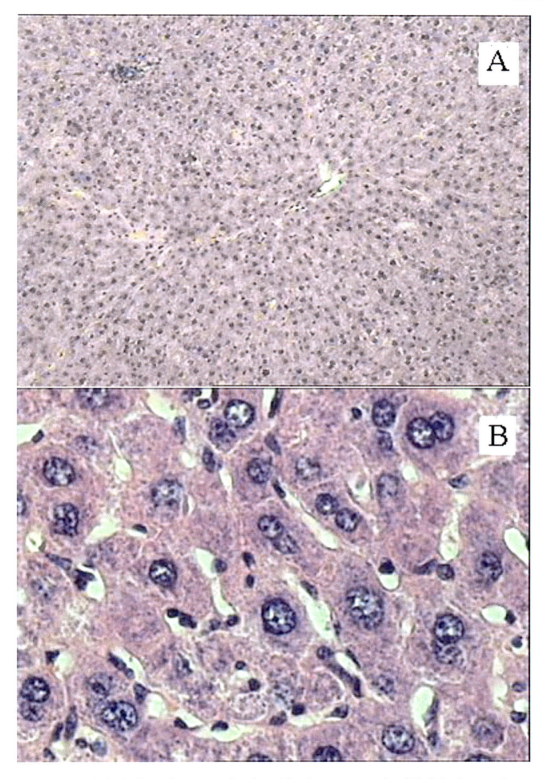

Figure 12. Morphological hepatic structure in mice with subcutaneous node of Ehrlich adenocarcinoma. Staining with hematoxylin - eosin. Magnification 150 (A) and 700 (B).

Intratumor cisplatin application (group 2) leaded to sharp increase of signs of compensatory-adaptive hepatic parenchyma rebuilt. Signs of central vein congestion were revealed in specimens (Figure 13). Sinusoid capillaries are dilated, endothelial cells are turgid. Polymorphocellular infiltrate is focal, localizes perivascularly.

Large number of hepatocytes with signs of granular degeneration, necrotized cells between which hepatocytes of normal structure were placed, as well as hypertrophied cells (large cells with uniform, homogenous cytoplasm staining, large nucleus with reticular chromatin structure in it) with multiple hypertrophied nucleoluses were determined. Binuclear hepatocytes with augmented nucleuses took place. Perls' reaction was negative.

Inflammatory process activity estimated on infiltrate density (practically, 2-fold), number of hepatocytes with morphological signs of dystrophy (785-fold) and death by dint of necrosis (1906-fold) significantly increased in comparison with tumor animals (group 1). As a result, signs of organ regeneration connected with binuclear hepatocytes number increase (749-fold) became stronger.

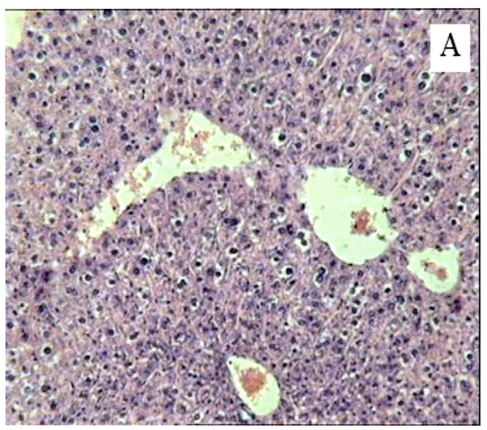

Figure Continued

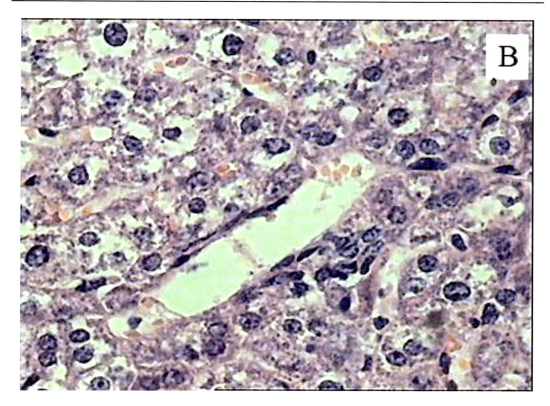

Figure 13. Morphological hepatic structure in mice after intratumor introduction of cisplatin. Staining with hematoxylin - eosin. Magnification 150 (A) and 700 (B).

Lipid cisplatin form (group 3) decreased systemic toxic effect of cytostatic by intratumor administration (Table 17). In comparison with group 2, statistically significant decrease (1.5 – 2 times) of necrotized and binuclear hepatocytes number, correspondingly, was observed.

Table 17. Morphological hepatic indices in Balb/c mice after course introduction of medications into subcutaneous node of Ehrlich adenocarcinoma, $X \pm m$

Group number, n=10	Infiltrate density in 1 mm^2	Hepatocytes with dystrophy signs, %	Necrotic forms of hepatocytes, %	Binuclear hepatocytes, %
1	126.23±12.2	6.14±0.68	0.89±0.31	2.22±0.22
2	234.55±38.9 $p_1 < 0.016$	48.23±7.47 $p_1 < 0.000026$	16.96±1.70 $p_1 < 10^{-6}$	16.63±0.71 $p_1 < 10^{-6}$
3	211.86±25.19	40.29±6.45	8.23±1.19 $p_2 < 0.0006$	10.27±1.75 $p_2 < 0.0036$
4	27.32±3.52 $p_1 < 10^{-6}$ $p_3 < 10^{-6}$	29.07±2.53 $p_1 < 10^{-6}$	2.19±0.44 $p_3 < 0.00015$	4.36±0.57 $p_1 < 0.0037$ $p_3 < 0.0037$

Note: n – number of animals and hepatic sections in every group; p_1 - p_3 – reliable differences with values in group with correspondent number; group number corresponds to system number in Table 15.

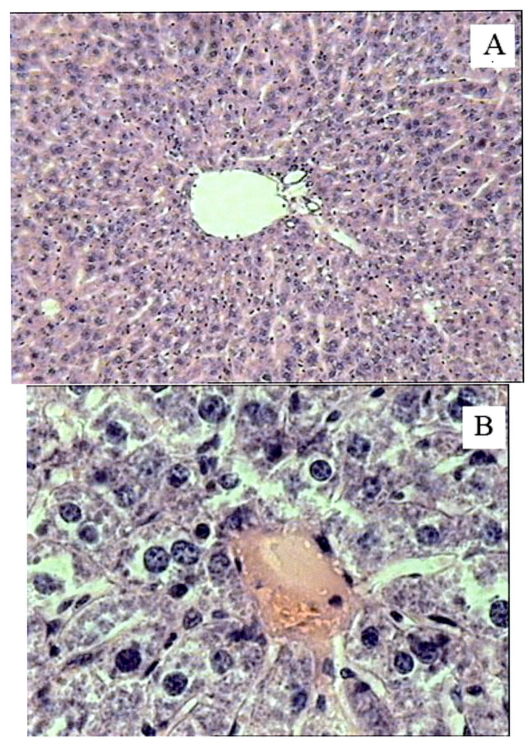

Figure 14. Morphological hepatic structure in mice after intratumor introduction of cisplatin lipid form. Staining with hematoxylin - eosin. Magnification 150 (A) and 700 (B).

Nevertheless, structure of hepatic parenchyma is disturbed, inflammatory and vascular changes dominate dystrophic processes in histological specimens (Figure 14). Hepatocytes don't form hepatic plates (girders) in hepatic lobules, but they are placed unordered and separately. Triads' structure (interlobular artery, vein and bile duct) is disturbed. There is congestion in interlobular veins. Marginal pool of leucocytes is noted. Focuses of fine (diapedetic) hemorrhages are noted between hepatocytes.

In connection with fact that hepatic plates' structure is disturbed, bile capillaries don't keep normal structure; bile accumulates in the form of focuses between hepatocytes, sinusoid capillaries and comes into blood.

Sinusoid capillaries are sharply dilated, overfull with blood; endothelial cells are turgid, lumens between them are dilated (Figure 14). The most part of cells among hepatocytes are destroyed, generally, as a result of disturbance of membrane continuity. The rest part of hepatocytes is pathologically changed. Sizes of these hepatocytes are enlarged due to small-drop and large-drop adipose degeneration. Focuses of lymphocytic - histiocytic infiltrate are noted. Cytoplasm of some cells is stained heterogeneously, with fine light vacuoles. Cells with cytoplasm occupied with one light vacuole can be met among these hepatocytes. Nucleuses in hepatocytes are placed eccentrically. Nuclear chromatin is compact, pycnotic. In some cells chromatin forms large lumps concentrating along nuclear membrane.

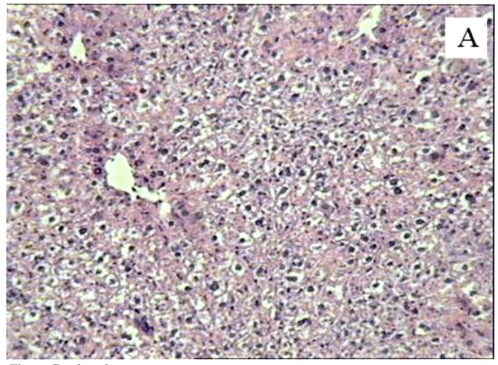

Figure Continued

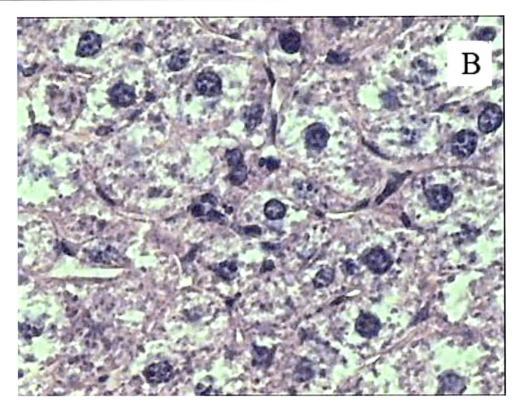

Figure 15. Morphological hepatic structure in mice after intratumor introduction of lipid composite of cisplatin and carbon encapsulated iron nanoparticles. Staining with hematoxylin - eosin. Magnification 150 (A) and 700 (B).

Systematic toxic action of cytostatic on mice liver decreased (Table 17) significantly by intratumor introduction of lipid composite of cisplatin and carbon encapsulated iron nanoparticles (group 4). The rest part of indices was significantly lower (2.5-7.5 times) than those in group 3, except hepatocyte dystrophy signs. At that, level of cells with signs of morphological necrosis in group 4 didn't differ from correspondent index in tumor-carrier animals receiving only solvent (phosphate buffer).

Qualitative changes of hepatic parenchyma on histological specimens turned out to be insignificant (Figure 15). Vascular changes are not evident. The most part of hepatocytes is in condition of albuminous and adipose degeneration. Evident fibrosis is revealed along periphery of hepatic lobules.

After local administration, nanoparticles of iron and its oxides can penetrate natural barriers, which presume opportunity of their systematic toxic effect on organs and tissues. Nevertheless, Perls' reaction on thin hepatic sections showed only single cells positively stained for iron (Figure 16) after local introduction of lipid composites of cisplatin and carbon encapsulated ferromagnetic nanoparticles into tumor node of Ehrlich adenocarcinoma.

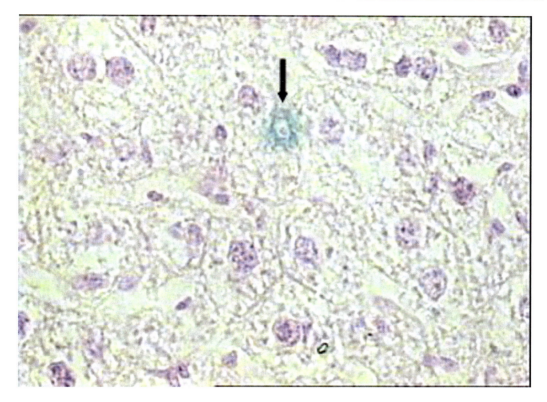

Figure 16. Histological hepatic picture after introduction of lipid composite of cisplatin and carbon encapsulated iron nanoparticles into tumor node. Localization of cell stained according to Perls' is marked with arrow. Magnification 700.

Histological sections analysis of lung of tumor-carrier mice receiving only solvent (phosphate buffer, group 1) showed fine diapedetic hemorrhages with small focal lymphocytic infiltrate in some areas of interalveolar spaces. Venous congestion is feebly marked. Bronchial tubes keep typical structure and consist of mucous, fibrocartilaginous and adventitious membrane (Figure 17).

Orientation of lung tissue structural changes in mice after administration of different forms of cytostatic is similar in many respects to disturbances fixed in liver. Evident lung congestion with sharply dilated venous vessels, diffusive polymorphocellular infiltrate localizing both in alveolar septum and in own plate of bronchus mucous tunic are determined by the use of groups 2 and 3. In some bronchi infiltration under basic membrane combines with exfoliation of bronchial epithelium into bronchus lumen. Accumulation of liquid with signs of edema is observed in separate alveoli (Figure 18).

Slight peribronchial fibrosis was determined in lung tissue by intratumor introduction of lipid composite of cisplatin and carbon encapsulated iron nanoparticles (group 4). Lumen of alveoli is emphysematous dilated in some regions; alveolar septums are degraded, where small number of leucocytes is revealed (Figure 19).

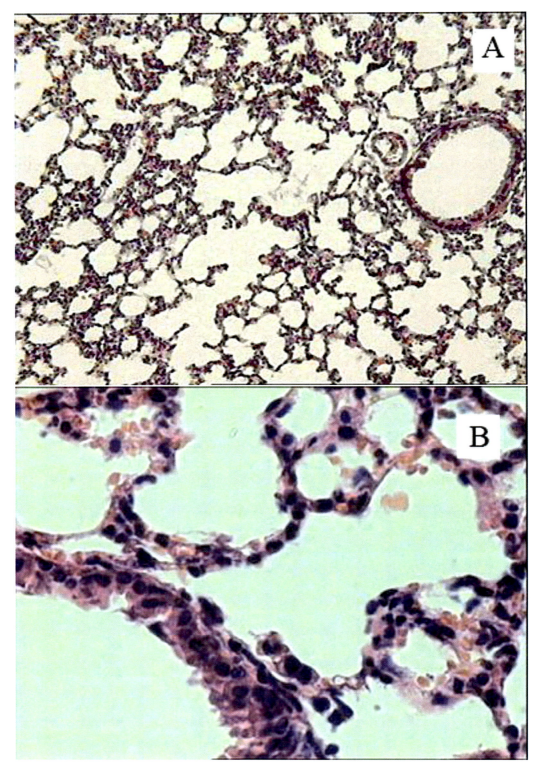

Figure 17. Morphological lung structure in mice with subcutaneous node of transplantable Ehrlich adenocarcinoma. Staining with hematoxylin - eosin. Magnification 150 (A) and 700 (B).

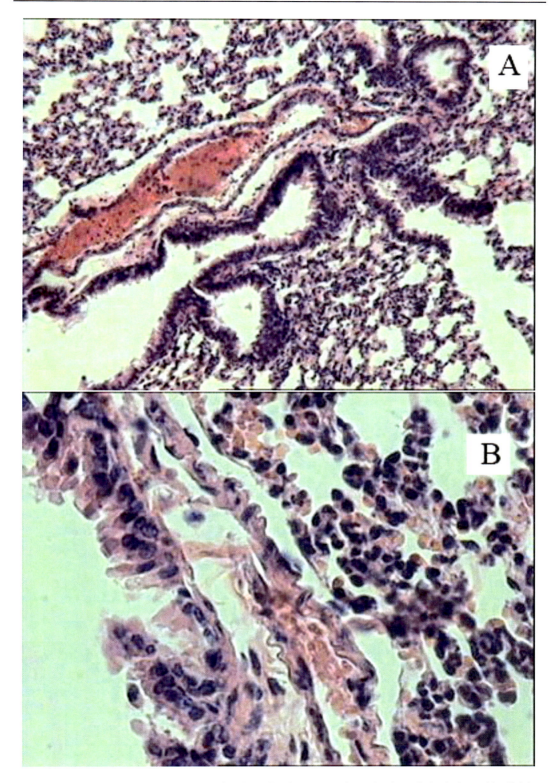

Figure 18. Morphological lung structure in mice after intratumor introduction of cisplatin and its lipid form. Staining with hematoxylin - eosin. Magnification 150 (A) and 700 (B).

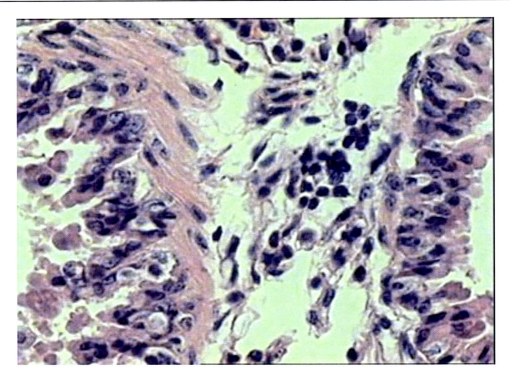

Figure 19. Morphological lung structure in mice after intratumor introduction of lipid composite of cisplatin and carbon encapsulated iron nanoparticles. Staining with hematoxylin - eosin. Magnification 700.

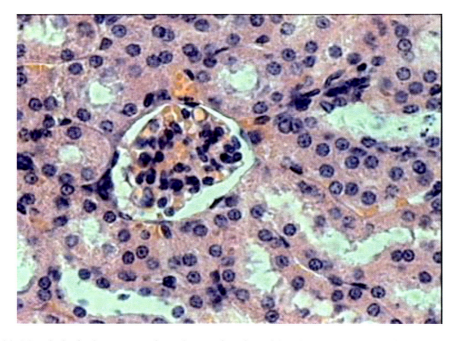

Figure 20. Morphological structure of renal tissue in mice with subcutaneous node of transplantable Ehrlich adenocarcinoma. Staining with hematoxylin - eosin. Magnification 700.

Cortical and medullary substances are determined in kidneys in mice with transplantable subcutaneous Ehrlich adenocarcinoma (investigation group 1). Cortical substance is presented with renal corpuscles, medullary substance - with renal tubules. Renal corpuscle is formed with glomerulus and Bowman's capsule lined with one layer of podocytes. Fine diapedetic hemorrhages are noted around the capsule. Renal tubules are lined with monolayer cylindrical epithelium. Lumen of some tubules is initially dilated, fine focal hemorrhages are determined between them (Figure 20).

Intratumor introduction of cisplatin (group 2) made systemic toxic effect on renal parenchyma (Figure 21). Evident congestion of renal cortical substance with focuses of hemorrhage into renal glomeruli took place in specimen. Lumen of tubules is dilated; accumulations of exfoliated cylindrical epithelium forming cylinders are determined in some of them. Focal infiltrate is determined between tubules.

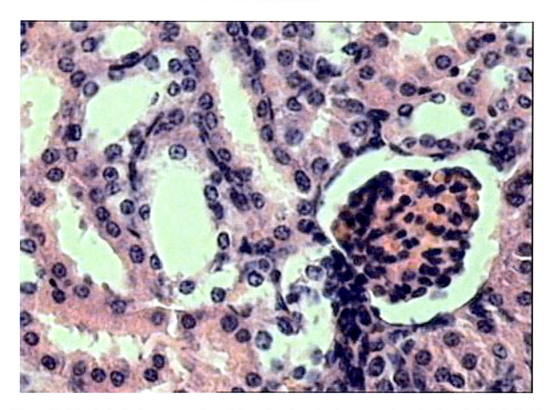

Figure 21. Morphological structure of renal tissue in mice after intratumor introduction of cisplatin lipid form. Staining with hematoxylin - eosin. Magnification 700.

Application of cisplatin lipid form (group 3) practically didn't change character of qualitative changes of renal parenchyma (Figure 22): renal cortical substance congestion with hemorrhages into glomeruli, polymorphocellular infiltrate, focuses of tubules' epithelium desquamation with formation of cylinders.

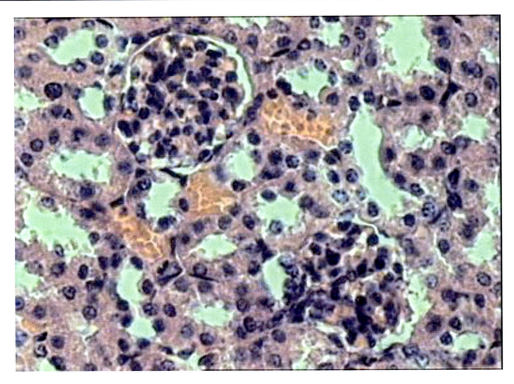

Figure 22. Morphological structure of renal tissue in mice after intratumor introduction of cisplatin lipid form. Staining with hematoxylin - eosin. Magnification 700.

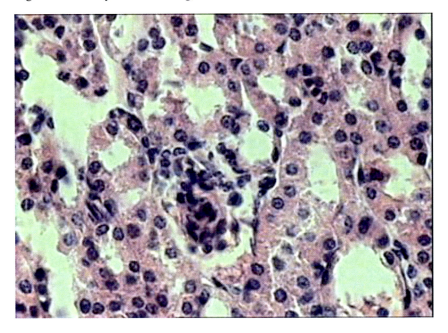

Figure 23. Morphological structure of hepatic tissue in mice after intratumor introduction of lipid composite of cisplatin and carbon encapsultaed iron nanoparticles. Staining with hematoxylin - eosin. Magnification 700.

At the same time, character of renal structure disturbances was sharply changed with underlying intratumor introduction of lipid composite of cisplatin and carbon encapsulated iron nanoparticles (group 4). Along with dilatation of tubules' lumen and degenerative changes of nephrocytes, vascular disturbances turned out to be feebly marked (Figure 23).

Questions concerning intercommunication of physical-chemical properties of metal nano-sized powders and their biological activity are not widely covered in modern literature. Set up of experiment in this work was planned as an effort to move forward in understanding of chemical condition of nanopowder surface and its biological properties.

Thermal effects registered for Fe(C) specimen in model reaction of isopropylbenzol oxidation can be corresponded to physical processes of wetting and adsorption on level of values, but they are not connected with flow of base reaction. In accordance with results of thermoprogrammed ammonia desorption, NH_3 molecules don't sorb onto surface of this specimen either.

IR spectrums of nanopowder don't show bands of functional groups. Consequently, Fe(C) nanopowder physical-chemical testing indicates absence of active centers which can determine display of reactivity in chemical reactions flowing by acid or free-radical mechanism. Investment of such mechanisms in realization of biological processes is of considerable value.

Electronic spectrum of cytostatical medication as a part of nanodispersion of cisplatin and nanopowder after keeping under temperature of 37°C during 24 hours doesn't undergo any changes. Apparently, cisplatin isomerization into pharmacologically inactive trans- isomer doesn't occur. This fact additionally demonstrates intactness of Fe(C) metal nucleus relative to environmental chemical factors under biological conditions.

It's known that phospholipids are substances with amphiphilic structure. Molecules' self-assembly in solution is conditioned with their dualism. This leads to formation of micelles where molecules' organic fragments are approached such a way that total contact area of hydrophobic groups of molecule dissolved in water is decreased. Lamellar (liquid-crystalline and gel phases) as well as volume hexagonal phases [33] are described for water-lipid systems as basic types of structural organization. Thus, combination of nano-sized ferromagnetic, phospholipid concentrate and cisplatin as a part of single composite will predispose to formation of micellar solution. Initial (lamellar type) and secondary (volume) structuring lipid composite of cisplatin with Fe(C) nanopowder with relatively uniform distribution of ferromagnetic in water-lipid phase is visible on Figure 24. Obtained micellar solutions of lipid composites kept their completeness without phase division under room temperature during several days.

As appears from Figure 7, only cisplatin in terminal dose of 1/10 LD 50 made approximately equal cytotoxic action on healthy and tumor cells fixed by increase of penetration their cytoplasmic membranes for staining agent in vitro. Consequent addition of phosphatidylcholine and Fe(C) nanoparticles in to system increased (more than by 20%) relative number of dead adenocarcinoma cells in comparison with splenocytes. Building of trend lines (value of linear approximation 0.96-0.99) under sequential addition of system's components showed speed of dead tumor cells number increase of 36%. At that, speed of dead immunocompetent cells number increase was 26%.

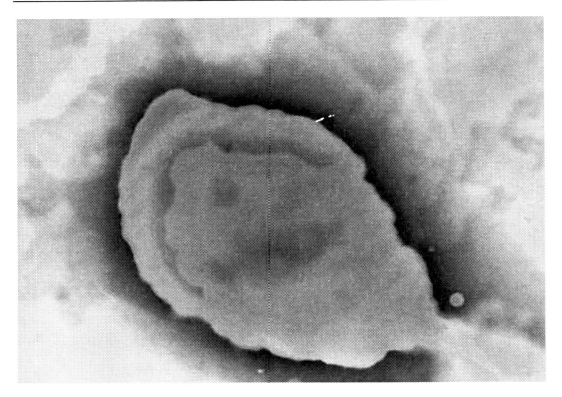

Figure 24. Electron microphotography of lipid composite of cisplatin and carbon encapsulated iron nanoparticles. Magnification 58000.

Thus, relative selectivity of toxic action of investigated composites relatively to tumor cells was revealed in vitro. Terminal Fe(C) concentration used in system in vitro and in vivo (2 mg/kg) is low. According to report [38], analogous doses (less than 10-50mg/l) of magnetite (Fe_3O_4) with particles of diameter 30-47 nm don't influence on cell morphology, mitochondrial function, formation of oxygen active forms and glutathione system in vitro. At the same time, Fe(C) nanoparticles of smaller diameter (no more than 10 nm) don't induce free radical processes either in reaction with cumene, as stated above, that excludes realization of their effect through oxidative process.

Majority of oncology treatment methods existing at present (irradiation, chemotherapy, massive operative intervention) induce immunosuppression [31] which impairs treatment efficacy and disease prognosis. In this connection, search of therapeutic solutions directed on preservation of immune system is urgent. One of directions is considered as regional application of cytostatic medications and biological molecules allowing creation of necessary local reactant concentrations without systemic toxic effect.

Intratumor administration of cisplatin caused statistically significant 2-3-fold decrease of size and mass of Ehrlich adenocarcinoma subcutaneous node (Table 16) in vivo. Leukocytes infiltration increased by 80%, but glandular structure of tumor node was kept (Figure 9). It's built of sharply atypical glandular tubules of different size and shape. Glands are lined with cylindrical epithelium which is partially multi-row. Cell deposition is observed in some atypical glandular cells. Marked cell atypism is determined in cells of tumor tissue.

Growth of size and mass of tumor node can be connected not only with basic process, but also with organism reaction leading to edema, infiltration, necrosis and sclerosis of pathological locus. In particular, it's typical for micellar cytostatic form (Figure 10). Thus, the 3d system impaired cisplatin antitumor action on grounds of morphological indices (size, mass of tumor node, TGI) and amplifies such on grounds of histological indices (area of tumor tissue).

Indices of tumor mass, sizes and TGI didn't correlate with tumor tissue area revealed on sections that allowed multiplying their probabilities and introducing new efficacy index for investigated groups (RIM x tumor area on section). At that, number of giant cells increased in sections of tumor tissue 3 times (Table 16).

In recent years, publications about macrophages and dendritic cells (DC), which are the most important antitumor effector elements along with natural killers (NK), natural killer T-cells (NKT) and cytotoxic lymphocytes CD8 (CTL) occur more often [56]. Their dysfunction in cancer doesn't raise any doubts [2].

Search of optimal intervals for introduction of DC [63] and their activation in situ [22] is being held. Cancer immunosuppression leading to hypo- and anergy of CTL and disturbance of DC migration into target organ in vivo leaded to idea of intratumor DC delivery [40]. However, clinical efficacy of therapy was proved only in 3 of 16 patients (19%) [84]. As a result, vaccination of DC is still far from therapeutic application, according to O. Proudfoot et al. [66].

Epithelioid and giant multinuclear cells of foreign bodies (GMCFB) are active participants of granulomatous inflammation tightly bound to DC, CD4-helpers and tumor necrosis factor (TNF) with outcome in fibrosis [11]. TNF is the most effective antitumor cytokine which facilitates migration of monocytes and formation of GMCFB which, in their turn, secrete TNF in pathological focus [97], facilitates functions of lymphocytes and fibroblasts [11]. TNF secretion and granulomatosis are facilitated by heavy metals [68].

Described mechanisms can underlie the most significant antitumor activity of the 4th composites system consisting of micellar cytostatic form with pyrocarbon encapsulated iron nanoparticles in vivo. In comparison with other supervision groups, fact of more than 50% tumor node fibrosis (Table 16, Figure 11) in small number of infiltrate and GMCFB on histological sections attracted attention.

Presented results allow implying acceleration of granuloma maturation by falling of carbon encapsulated iron nanoparticles into inflammation locus. In combination with data obtained in vitro, mechanism of antitumor effect of ultrafine-dispersed lipid composites of cisplatin and pyrocarbon encapsulated iron nanoparticles is conditioned with direct cytotoxic action on tumor cells and, on the other hand, with stimulation of cells of conjunctive tissue. Conceivably, target-cells are monocytes/macrophages which are able to catch liposomal forms of pharmaceutical substances actively [41]. In this connection, systemic fibrosis of internal organs (liver, lungs) revealed by administration of magneto-sensitive cisplatin lipid composite could be mediated, for example, through cytokine chain, particularly, through TNF family.

CONCLUSION

Technique of inversion voltammetry being developed by us allows estimation of trace elements content (zinc, copper, selenium, iron, iodine, mercury, cadmium, lead, arsenic, 6-valent chromium).

Results showed that following nonspecific values of 52 studied laboratory indices allowed to predict transfer of patients with malignant epithelial formations of stomach and intestines into incurable condition with 30-50% probability: total protein content in blood; concentration of selenium in hair; ratio of hexavalent chromium level in hair to its content in tumor tissue. According to correlation analysis, trace elements (selenium, hexavalent chromium) and CD95 have the most prognostic load in dynamics of progression of malignant gastrointestinal tumor in comparison with known laboratory indices. Blood markers CA19-9 and CA242 weren't of grate prognostic importance, because their values didn't correlate with disease stage and clinical group of patients.

Approach to creation and combined application of micro- (autologous cells) and porous macrosystem for delivery of ions taking active part in metabolism of tumor-carrier organism and human tumor cell lines was used thereupon. Initial results give evidence of existence of own niche and prospectivity of hybrid implants on porous carrier in combination with iontophoresis in complex treatment of human metabolic and tumor diseases, correction of complications of classic methods of chemo- and roentgenotherapy of cancer.

At that, significant variations in cell concentration of chemical elements in human tumor cell line revealed by us prove necessity of diagnostics and treatment of tumor-patients from the point of view of personalized and targeted medicine. Melanoma can be considered as more sensitive to mineral balance control in organism because it has high intracellular content of trace elements. At the same time, intracellular iron levels turned out to be stable in epithelial and mesenchymal tumor cells.

From this point of view, nano-sized particles of iron and its oxides can turn out to be optimal choice in development of ferreed composite delivery systems for cytostatics and biological molecules for targeted therapy of epithelial and mesenchymal tumors taking into account their magneto-sensitivity.

In vitro testing of toxicological properties of iron nanopowders and its oxides (magnetite, magnesium ferrite, and carbon encapsulated iron) was carried out on stromal stem cells and hemopoietic elements of marrow which is considered as one of target organs. It expects opportunity of evaluation of nanoparticles' own side effect on organism antitumor resistance. Results showed that carbon encapsulated iron nanopowders having bioinertness according to used toxicological tests were optimal ones for creation of magneto-sensitive nano-sized antitumor preparation carriers.

Ultrafine composites of phospholipids concentrate, cisplatin and nano-sized carbon encapsulated ferromagnetic were synthesized and testified on cells of Ehrlich adenocarcinoma in experiments *in vitro* and *in vivo* thereupon.

Local cisplatin introduction into subcutaneous node of Ehrlich adenocarcinoma leaded to inhibition of tumor growth. Nevertheless, evident toxic effect on mice parenchymatous organs (liver, kidneys, lungs) leading to their compensatory-adaptive reconstructions conditioned with infiltrative inflammation, dystrophy and cell death by dint of necrosis, reparative regeneration.

Lipid form of cysplatin and, especially, magneto-sensitive lipid composite of cytostatic sharply enhanced antitumor effect and decreased system toxic influence of cytostatic by intratumor administration. In other words, new cytostatic forms facilitated its relative localization in pathologic locus. Relative selectivity of toxic effect of ferreed lipid cisplatin composites studied in relation to tumor cells was confirmed in vitro.

On the other hand, nanoparticles of iron and its oxides are able to penetrate natural barriers that imply opportunity of their systemic toxic effect on organs and tissues. Nevertheless, after local introduction of lipid composites of cisplatin and carbon encapsulated nanoferromagnetics into Ehrlich adenocarcinoma, Perls' reaction on thin hepatic sections showed only separate cells staining positively for iron. Consequently, nanoparticles, as well as cisplatin, generally accumulated in place of their introduction.

Disproportion of antitumor/toxic reactions by existing classical and immuno(bio)therapeutic treatment schemes restrains development of modern oncology. Development and application of protocols directed on cardinal improvement of clinical results is required [55].

Offered biotechnological approaches using trace elements, low doses of cytostatics and nanoferromagnetic particles as components of micro- and nano-sized delivery systems can turn out be useful in plan of elaboration and development of clinical methods for targeted diagnostics and treatment of gastrointestinal tract cancer and its metastases.

ACKNOWLEDGMENTS

Work is carried out under support of Federal Target Program "Investigations and elaborations in priority directions of development of scientific-technological complex of Russia for the years 2007-2012" (State contract No. 02.512.11.2285 from 10.03.2009) of grant of the Russian Fund of Fundamental Investigations (project No. 09-04-00287-a).

REFERENCES

[1] Aerts, F., & Wagemaker, G. (2006). Mesenchymal stem cell engineering and transplantation. In: J.A. Nolta (Ed.), *Genetic Engineering of Mesenchymal Stem Cells* (pp. 1–44). Springer. Printed in the Netherlands.

[2] Aloysius, MM; Takhar, A; Robins, A; Eremin, O. Dendritic cell biology. Dysfunction and immunotherapy in gastrointestinal cancers. *Surgeon*, 2006, 4, 195-210.

[3] Avtandilov, GG. Fundamentals of quantitative pathological anatomy. Moscow: Medicine; 2002 (in Russian).

[4] Avtsyn, A.P., Zhavoronkov, A.A., & Sirochkova, A.S. (1991) *Microelementose of human: Aetiology, classification, organopathology*. Moscow: Medicine (in Russian).

[5] Babincova, M; Cicmanec, P; Altanerova, V et al. AC-magnetic field controlled drug release from magnetoliposomes: design of method for site-specific chemotherapy. *Bioelectrochemistry*, 2002, 55, 17-19.

[6] Babitskaya, SV; Zhukova, MV; Kisel', MA et al. Doxorubicin encapsulation in liposomes containing phosphatidylethanol. Antibiotic's influence on toxicity and its

accumulation in myocardium. *Chemical-pharmaceutical journal*, 2006, 3, 36–38 (in Russian).

[7] Baryshnikov, A.Yu. (2001). Programmed cell death (apoptosis): *Clinical oncogematology: Manual for doctors* (edited by M.A. Volkova). Moscow: Medicine.

[8] Berezhnaya, NM. Interleukins and immunological response formation by malignant growth. *Allergology and immunology,* 2000, 1, 45-61 (in Russian).

[9] Bgatov, A.V., Bgatov, V.I., & Novoselova, T.N. (1999). *Lithophagy phenomenon: Natural minerals working for human health*. Novosibirsk: Ekor (in Russian).

[10] *Biologic therapy of cancer: Second Edition*. Eds. V.T. DeVita, S.Hellmann, & S.A. Rosenberg. Philadelphia: Lippincott-Raven Publ.; 1995.

[11] *Biomaterials science: an introduction to materials in medicine. 2nd edition.* Ed. by B.D. Ratner, A.S. Hoffman, F.J. Schoen, & J.E. Lemons. San Diego: Elsevier Academic Press; 2004.

[12] Borella, P; Bargellini, A; Caselgrandi, E; Piccinini, L. Observations of the use of plasma, hair and tissue for trace elements status evaluation in cancer. *J. Trace. Elem. Med. Biol.*, 1997, 11, 162-165.

[13] Braynina, HZ. Inversion voltammetry of solid phases. Moscow: Chemistry; 1972 (in Russian).

[14] Bystrykh, VV; Tin'kov, AN; Makshantsev, SS et al. Metals and carcinogenic risk for population of agroindustrial region. *Bulletin of OSU*, 2004, 4, 21-22 (in Russian).

[15] Chaykina, MV; Khlusov, IA; Karlov, AV et al. Mechanical-chemical synthesis of nonstoichiometric and replaced apatites with nano-sized particles for using as biocompatible materials. *Chemistry in the interests of sustainable development*, 2004, 12, 389-399 (in Russian).

[16] Chertkov, I.L. & Friedenstein, A.J. (1977). *Cellular foundations of haemopoiesis.* Moscow: Medicine (in Russian).

[17] Choi, JW; Kim, SK. Relationships of lead, copper, zinc, and cadmium levels versus hematopoiesis and iron parameters in healthy adolescents. *Ann.Clin.Lab. Sci.*, 2005, 35, 428-34.

[18] Crocker, PR; Gordon, MY. Isolation and characterization of resident stromal macrophages and hematopoietic cell clusters from mouse bone marrow. *J. Exp. Med.* 1985, 162, 993-1014.

[19] Dambaev, GT; Gyunter, VE; Zagrebin, LV et al. Influence of transplantation of fetal liver cells on porous scaffold made of titanium nickelide on hematoimmunological indices in malignant growth. *Shape memory implants,* 2000, 1-36 (in Russian).

[20] Das, P; Ajani, JA. Gastric and gastro-esophageal cancer therapy. *Expert Opin. Pharmacother.*, 2005, 6, 2805-2812.

[21] Davydov, MI. Encyclopedia of clinical oncology. Moscow: Medicine; 2004.

[22] Den Brok, MH; Nierkens, S; Figdor, CG et al. Dendritic cells: tools and targets for antitumor vaccination. *Expert Rev. Vaccines*, 2005, 4, 699-710.

[23] Di-Silvio, L., & Gurav, N. (2002). Osteoblasts. In: M.R Koller, & B.O. Pallson (Eds.), *Human Cell Culture* (JRW. Masters, pp. 221–241). Kluwer Academic Publishers.

[24] Dixon, M., & Webb, I.E. (1958). *Enzymes.* N.Y.: Academic Press.

[25] Dygay, AM; Khlusov, IA; Aksinenko, SG et al. Adrenergic control of humoral hemopoiesis regulators production in cytostatic myelodepression. *Bul. of experimental biology and medicine*, 1995, 135-140 (in Russian).

[26] Federico, A; Iodice, P; Federico, P et al. Effects of selenium and zinc supplementation on nutritional status in patients with cancer of digestive tract. *Eur. J. Clin. Nutr.*, 2001, 55, 293-297.

[27] Fedushchak, TA; Ermakov, AE, Uymin, MA et al. Physical-chemical properties of copper nanopowders obtained by means of methods of conductor electric explosion and gas-phase synthesis. *Journal of Physical Chemistry*, 2008, 4, 708-712 (in Russian).

[28] Fox, JG; Wang, TC. Inflammation, atrophy, and stomach cancer. *J. Clin. Invest.*, 2007, 117, 60-69.

[29] Fraker, PJ; King, LE. Reprogramming of the immune system during zinc deficiency. *Annu. Rev. Nutr,* 2004, 24, 277-298.

[30] Galanov, AI; Yurmazova, TA; Savel'ev, GG et al. Deveolpment of ferreed system for delivery of chemical medications based on nano-sized iron particles. *Siberian oncology journal*, 2008, 3, 50-57.

[31] Garin, A.M., & Bazin, I.S. (2003). *Malignant gastrointestinal tumors.* Moscow: Infomedia Publishers (In Russian).

[32] Gavrilov, O.K., Kozinets, G.I., & Chernyak, N.B. (1985). *Marrow and peripheral blood cells.* Moscow: Medicine (in Russian).

[33] Genis, R. (1997) *Biomembranes: Molecular structure and functions.* Moscow: Mir (in Russian).

[34] Grass, RN; Athanassiou, EK; Stark, WJ. Covalently functionalized cobalt canoparticles as a platform for magnetic separations in organic synthesis. *Angew. Chem,* 2007, 46, 4909–4912.

[35] Gròmova, OA. Threpsology importance in prevention and treatment of mastopathy. *Aesthetic medicine*, 2006, 2, 216-225 (in Russian).

[36] Hartwig, A. Carcinogenicity of metal compounds: possible role of DNA repair inhibition. *Toxicol Lett*, 1998, 102-103, 235-239.

[37] Hayhoe, F.G.J,& Quaglino, D. (1980). Hematological cytochemistry. Edinburgh, London & N.Y.: Churchill Livingstone.

[38] Hussain, SM; Hess, KL; Gearhart, JM et al. In vitro toxicity of nanoparticles in BRL 3A rat liver cells. *Toxicol In Vitro,* 2005, 19, 975-83.

[39] Ismailova, GK; Efremenko, VI; Kuregyan, AG. Biotechnology for obtaining ferreed liposomes. *Chemical-pharmaceutical journal*, 2005; 39, 47-49 (in Russian).

[40] Kanazawa, M; Yoshihara, K; Abel, H et al. Two case reports on intra-tumor injection therapy of dendritic cells. *Gan.To Kagaki Ryoho,* 2005, 32, 1571-1573.

[41] Kaplun, AP; Le Bang Shon; Krasnopolskiy, YuM; Shvets, VI. Liposomes and other nanoparticles as agents for pharmaceutical substances delivery. *Problems of medical chemistry*, 1999, 1, 3-12 (in Russian).

[42] Khlusov, IA. Opportunities of physical-chemical regulation of stem cell pool. *Bulletin of Siberian medicine,* 2007, 6, 7-12 (in Russian).

[43] Khlusov, IA; Karlov, AV; Chaykina, MV et al. Influence of alpha-fetoprotein and nano-sized hydroxyapatite particles on colony-forming marrow activity. *Bulletin ESSC SB RAMS,* 2007, 4, 135-139 (in Russian).

[44] Khlusov, IA; Karlov, AV; Sharkeev, YuP et al. Osteogenic potential of mesenchymal stem cells from bone marrow in situ: role of physicochemical properties of artificial surfaces. *Bulletin of Experimental Biology and Medicine*. 2005, 140, 144-152 (in Russian).

[45] Khlusov, IA; Zagrebin, LV; Shestov, SS; Naumov, SA. Physical-chemical manipulations with microbial and mammalian cells: from experiments to clinic. In: Burnsides WB, Ellsley RH editors. *Stem cell applications in disease and health*. N.Y.: Nova Science Publishers Inc.; 2008; 37-80.

[46] LaConte, L; Nitin, N; Gang Bao. Magnetic probe nanoparticle. *Nanotoday*, 2005, 3, 32-39.

[47] Lama, VN; Smith, L; Badri, L et al. Evidence for tissue-resident mesenchymal stem cells in human adult lung from studies of transplanted allografts. *The Journal of Clinical Investigation*, 2007, 117, 989-996.

[48] Lin, WW; Karin, M. A cytokine-mediated link between innate immunity, inflammation, and cancer. *J. Clin. Invest*, 2007, 117, 1175-1183.

[49] Liu, T; Zhang, G; Chen, YH et. al. Tissue specific expression of suicide genes delivered by nanoparticles inhibits stomach cancer growth. *Cancer Biol.Ther*, 2006, 5, 1683-1690.

[50] Lushnikov, E.F., & Abrosimov, A.Yu. (2001). *Cell death (apoptosis)*. Moscow: Medicine (in Russian).

[51] Lystsov, V.N., & Mursin, N.V. (2007). *Problems of nanotechnology safety*. Moscow: MIFI (in Russian).

[52] Maeda, H; Wu, J; Sawa, T et al. Tumor vascular permeability and the EPR effect in macromolecular therapeutics: a review. *J Control Release,* 2000, 65, 271 – 284.

[53] Magalova, T; Bella, V; Brtkova, A et al. Copper, zinc and superoxide dismutase in precancerous, benign diseases and gastric, colorectal and breast cancer. *Neoplasma*, 1999, 46, 100-104.

[54] Malakhova, NA; Chernysheva AV; Braynina KhZ. Inversion voltammetry of chromium with diphenylcarbazide. *Journal of analytical chemistry,* 1987, 42, 1636 – 1640 (in Russian).

[55] Marshall, JL. Novel vaccines for the treatment of gastrointestinal. *Oncology,* 2005, 19, 1557-1565.

[56] Men'shhcikova, E.B., Lankin, V.Z., Zenkov, N.K. et al. Oxidative stress. Prooxidants and antioxidants. Moscow: Firm "Slovo"; 2006 (in Russian).

[57] Mocellin, S. Novel strategies to improve the efficacy of colorectal cancer vaccines: from bench to bedside. *Curr. Opin. Investig. Drugs,* 2006, 7, 1052 - 1061.

[58] Mocellin, S; Campana, LG. Trends in colorectal cancer vaccination. *Recenti Prog. Med,* 2005, 96, 338-343.

[59] Nagorsen, D, Thiel, E. Clinical and immunological responses to active specific cancer vaccines in human colorectal cancer. *Clin. Cancer Res,* 2006, 12, 3064-3069.

[60] Nardi, N.B., & da Silva Meirelles, L. (2006). Mesenchymal stem cells: isolation, in vitro expansion and characterization. *HEP, 174,* 249–282.

[61] Novitskiy, V.V., Stepovaya, E.A., Goldberg, V.E. et al. *Erythrocytes and malignant neoplasms*. Tomsk: STT; 2000 (in Russian).

[62] Oberdorster, G; Oberdorster, E; Oberdorster, J. Nanotoxicology: an emerging discipline evolving from studies of ultrafine particles. *Environ Health Perspect*, 2005, 113, 823-839.

[63] Okovityy, SV. Clinical pharmacology of antioxidants. In: *Collection series for practical doctors, Issue 5: Therapy*. Moscow: "PharmIndex-Practic"; 2003; 85-111.

[64] Okulov, VB; Zubova, SG. Adaptive cell reactions as a basis of tumor progression. *Problems of oncology*, 2000, 46, 505-512 (in Russian).

[65] Oosterling, SJ; van der Bij, G.J; Mels, A.K; Beelen, R.H; Meijer, S; van Egmond, M; van Leeuwen, PA; Perioperative IFN-alpha to avoid surgically induced immune suppression in colorectal cancer patients. *Histol.Histopathol*, 2006, 21, 753-760.

[66] Park, MY; Kim, CH; Sohn, HJ et al. The optimal interval for dendritic cell vaccination following adoptive T cell transfer is important for boosting potent anti-tumor immunity. *Vaccine*, 2007, 25, 7322-7330.

[67] Pisareva, LF; Choynsonov, EL; Boyarkina, AP et al. Characteristic of oncological morbidity among the population of Tomsk region (1990-2001). *Bulletin of Siberian medicine*, 2003, 4, 86-96 (in Russian).

[68] Preobrazhenskiy, V.N., Ushakov, I.B., & Laydov, K.V. (2000). *Activation therapy in system of medical rehabilitation of persons in hazardous occupation*. Moscow: Paritet (in Russian).

[69] Proudfoot, O; Pouniots, D; Sheng, KC et al. Dendritic cell vaccination. *Expert Rev. Vaccine*, 2007, 6, 617-633.

[70] Riggs, B.L., & Melton III, L.J. (2000). *Osteoporosis: translation from English*. SPb.: ZAO "Publishing House BINOM". "Nevskiy dialekt" (in Russian).

[71] Rolfe, MW; Paine, R; Davenport, RB; Strieter, RM. Hard metal pneumoconiosis and the association of tumor necrosis factor-alpha. *Am. Rev. Respir. Dis.*, 1992, 146(6), 1600-1602.

[72] Rummel, SA; van Zant, G. Future paradigm for autologous bone marrow transplantation: tumor purging and ex vivo production of normal stem and progenitor cells. *J. of Hematotherapy*, 1994, 3, 213-218.

[73] Russell, JH; Rush, B; Weaver, C et al. Mature T-cells of autoimmune lpr/lpr mice have a defect in antigen-stimulated suicide. *Proc. Natl. Acad. Sci. USA*, 1993, 90, 4409 - 4413.

[74] Santis, D; Guerriero, C; Nocini, PF et al. Adult human bone cells from jaw bones cultured on plasma-sprayed or polished surfaces of titanium or hydroxyapatite discs. *J. mater. Sci. Mater. Med*, 1996, 7, 21-28.

[75] Sepiashvili, RI; Shubich, MG; Kolesnikova, NV et al. Apoptosis in immunological processes. *Allergology and immunology*, 2000, 1, 15-23 (in Russian).

[76] Sergeev, GB. Nanochemistry. Moscow: MSU Publishing House; 2003 (in Russian).

[77] Serov, V.V., & Shechter, A.B. (1981). Conjunctive tissue (functional morphology and general pathology). Moscow: Medicine (in Russian).

[78] Shakhov, V.P., Khlusov, I.A., Dambaev, G.Ts. et al. Introduction into methods of cell culture, bioengineering of organs and tissues. Tomsk: STT; 2004 (in Russian).

[79] Shumakov, VI; Onishchenko, NA; Krasheninnikov, ME. Bone marrow as a source of obtaining mesenchymal cells for reparative therapy of damaged organs. *Bulletin of transplantology and artificial organs*, 2002, 4, 7 – 11(in Russian).

[80] Silva Meirelles, L; Chagastelles, PC; Nardi, NB. Mesenchymal stem cells reside in virtually all post-natal organs and tissues. *Journal of Cell Science*, 2006, 119, 2204-2213.

[81] Skal'niy, A.V., & Bykov, A.T. (2003). *Ecological-physiological aspects of macro- and microelements application in restorative medicine*. Orenburg: DPC SEI OSU (in Russian).

[82] Skal'niy, A.V., Bykov, A.T., Serebryanskiy, E.P., & Skal'naya, M.G. (2003). *Medical-ecological estimation of hypermicroelementose risk in population of megapolis*. Orenburg: DPC SEI OSU (in Russian).

[83] Slepchenko, GB; Zakharova EA; Cherempey, EG. Opportunities and application of inversion voltammetry method as estimation indicator of content of microelements in hair. *College news: Chemistry and chemical technology*, 2002, 45, 89–94 (in Russian).

[84] Snow, ET. Metal carcinogenesis: mechanistic implications. *Pharmacol Ther.*, 1992, 53, 31-65.

[85] Stein, J. Consequences of increase of recommended daily dose of micronutrients: folic acid and selenium. *Problems of feeding*, 2000, 3, 50-53.

[86] Sukhikh, TT. Fetal cells transplantation in medicine: present and future. *Bul. of experimental biology and medicine*, 1998, Annex 1, 3-13 (in Russian).

[87] Takeda, T; Makita, K; Okita, K et al. Intratumoral injection of immature dendritic cells (DC) for cancer patients. *Gan.To Kagaki Ryoho*, 2005, 32, 1574-1575.

[88] Timakin, NP; Shemetova, II; Ivanova, EV. Effect of combined impact of 5- fluorouracil with different kinds of ionizing radiation on content and distribution of microelements between adenocarcinoma HK and the whole organism. *Problems of radiobiology and biological effect of cytostatics*, 1974, 6, 44-54 (in Russian).

[89] Tolcheva, EE; Oborotova, NA. Liposomes as transport agents for bioactive molecules delivery. *Russian biotherapeutical journal*, 2006, 5, 54 – 61 (in Russian).

[90] Topalian, SL. Adoptive cell therapy: preclinical investigations. In: DeVita VT, Hellmann S, Rosenberg SA editors. *Biological methods of cancer treatment: Translation from English*. Moscow: Medicine; 2002; 484-503.

[91] Torchilin, V P. Targeted Pharmaceutical Nanocarriers for Cancer Therapy and Imaging. *The AAPS Journal*, 2007, 9 (2), 15.

[92] Valko, M; Morris, H; Cronin, MT. Metals, toxicity and oxidative stress. *Curr. Med. Chem.*, 2005, 12, 1161-1208.

[93] Valko, M; Rhodes, CJ; Moncol, J et al. Free radicals, metals and antioxidants in oxidative stress-induced cancer. *Chem. Biol. Interact*, 2006, 160, 1-40.

[94] Vasilevskaya, LS; Orlova, SV; Do Thi Kim Lien et al. Importance of zinc in metabolism. *Trace elements in medicine*, 2004, 5, 25-26 (in Russian).

[95] Vladimirskaya, EB. Mechanisms of cell apoptotic death. *Gematology and transfusiology*, 2002, 35-40 (in Russian).

[96] Vogiatzi, P; Cassone, M; Claudio, PP. Personalizing gene therapy in gastric cancer. *Drug News Perspect*, 2006, 19, 533-540.

[97] Wang, J; Mongayt, D; Torchilin, VP. Polymeric micelles for delivery of poorly soluble drugs: preparation and anticancer activity in vitro of paclitaxel incorporated into mixed micelles based on poly(ethylene glycol)-lipid conjugate and positively charged lipids. *J Drug Target*, 2005, 13, 73 – 80.

[98] Watanabe-Fukunaga, R; Brannan, CI; Copeland, NG et al. Lymphoproliferative disorder in mice explained by defects in Fas antigen that mediated apoptosis. *Nature*, 1992, 356, 314-317.

[99] Weinstein, SG; Zvershkhanovskiy FA. Condition of lipid peroxidation in patients with ulcer and cancer of stomach. Problems of oncology, 1984, 30, 39-41 (in Russian).

[100] Yanagishita, T; Watanabe, D; Akita, Y et al. Construction of novel epithelioid cell granuloma model from mouse macrophage cell line in vitro. *Arch Dermatol Res.*, 2007, 299, 399-403.

[101] Yeliseev, YuYu. Analyses: The complete reference-book. Moscow: EKSMO; 2006 (in Russian).

[102] Zhu, S; Zhou, K; Huang, B et al. Hydroxyapatite nanoparticles: a novel material of gene carrier. *Sheng Wu Yi Xue Gong Cheng Xue Za Zhi*, 2005, 22, 980-984.

[103] Zlobinskiy, B.M., Ioffe, V.G., & Zlobinskiy, VB. (1972). Inflammability and toxicity of metals and alloys. Moscow: "Metallurgy" Publishing House (in Russian).

[104] Zyryanov, B.N., Kolomiez, L.A., & Tuzikov, S.A. (1998). Stomach cancer: prophylaxis, early diagnostics, combined treatment, rehabilitation. Tomsk: Tomsk University Publishing House (in Russian).

In: Neuro-Oncology and Cancer Targeted Therapy
Editor: Lucía M. Gutiérrez pp.65-98

ISBN 978-1-61668-708-3
© 2010 Nova Science Publishers, Inc.

Chapter 2

BRAIN CANCER ASSOCIATED TUMOR MARKER GENES EXPRESSION PATTERN IN HUMANS

Harun M. Said[1]*, Carsten Hagemann[2], Adrian Staab[1,6,7], Buelent Polat[1], Mathias Guckenberger[1], Jelena Anacker[2,3], Michael Flentje[1], and Dirk Vordermark[1,4#]

[1]. Dept. of Radiation Oncology, University of Würzburg,
[2]. Dept. of Neurosurgery, University of Würzburg
[3]. Dept. of Gynecology and Obstetrics, University of Würzburg
[4]. Dept. of Gynaecology and Obstetrics, University of Würzburg, Germany
[5]. Dept. of Radiation Oncology, Martin-Luther-University-Halle-Wittenberg, Germany
[6]. Dept. of Radiation Oncology, University of Zürich, Switzerland
[7]. Paul Scherer Institut - Proton Radiation Human Therapy Center - 5232 Villingen –Switzerland

ABSTRACT

Hypoxia is an important phenomenon possessing a significant correlation with tumour progression, treatment result(s) and the overall disease prognosis.

Tumor oxygenation state leads to a series of genomic changes, enabling tumour cells survival or overcoming the oxygen deficient environment conditions. Tumour tissue growth requires a sufficient oxygen and nutrients supply. Tumor cell responses to hypoxic stress include adaptive proteomic changes allowing the cells to overcome nutritive deprivation or to escape their hostile environment by proliferation, invasion, or

---

* Correspondence to: Harun M. Said, Ph.D.
Dept. of Radiation Oncology
University of Würzburg
Josef – Schneider - Str. 11
97080 Würzburg
Tel: ++ 49-0931-201-28402
Fax: ++ 49-0931-201-28396
E-mail: said_h@klinik.uni-wuerzburg.de
# Equal contributor

metastatic spread. Tumor cell proliferation requires rapid synthesis of macromolecules including lipids, proteins, and nucleotides.

Hypoxia-inducible factor 1 (HIF-1) is a multi-subunit protein that regulates transcription at hypoxia response elements (HREs) under hypoxic oxygenation conditions, while under normoxic oxygenation conditions, HIF-1α protein is subject to rapid degradation by a pVHL-mediated ubiquitin-proteasome pathway, while under it hypoxia blocks degradation leading to accumulation and translocation to the cellular nucleus and its binding together with HIF-1β on the so called Hypoxia responsive element within the hypoxia induced genes promoter region and thereby regulating the expression of the hypoxia responsive genes which proteins are expressed in human brain cancer especially in low grade astrocytoma and glioblatoma in a tumor stage and oxygenation specific manner. Genes which proteins are expressed in this manner are considered tumor marker genes as well as tumor therapeutic targets. Among the most important are Carbonic anhyrase 9 (CA9), N myc- Downregulated gene 1(NDRG1), Osteopontin (OPN), Vascular endothelial Growth Factor (VEGF) and Erythropoitin (EPO). HIF-1α is an important or the only regulator of these proteins under hypoxic conditions. CA9 is one of the most strongly hypoxia-inducible proteins but its expression pattern is not only related to its transcriptional induction by hypoxia in brain tumors, but also to effects of adverse microenvironmental stresses (such as diminished levels of glucose and bicarbonate. NDRG1 was shown at the same levels *in vivo* in normal human brain and human low-grade astrocytoma (WHO grade 2), while it showed a higher NDRG1 overexpression level in glioblastoma than in lowgrade astrocytoma. OPN was displayed a high level of cancer tissue expression specificity due to the favour expression in human GBM when compared to (LGA) based on the relative mRNA expression of hypoxia-related genes data. Regulation of OPN, mRNA and protein expression as a response to the hypoxic development in the tumor cell enviroment *in vitro* and *in vivo* represent an absolute phenomenon in human glioblastoma as a cell-specific post-transcriptionally regulated event. VEGF is a powerful hypoxia induced mitogen for endothelial cell growth and plays a critical role in the development of tumor vessels. OPN is a tumor-associated phosphoglycoprotein, has been described to be prognostic for tumor progression and survival in a number of solid neoplasms and linked to a "metastatic phenotype (Epo) is overexpressed at the mRNA level in human and mouse brain. Modulation of glycolysis reduces the hypoxic accumulation of HIF-1α protein in human tumor cells through a translational or post-translational process. Therefore, manipulation of tumor glucose levels represents a potential approach to therapeutically target HIF-1α.

In malignant glioma therapy, the main aim, as with all cancers, is to either eradicate the tumor or convert it into a controlled, quiescent chronic disease. Angiogenesis and hypoxia induced, HIF-1α regulated genes inhibition remains the main parts of therapeutic approaches in human oncology. It is well known that cancer cell metabolism can be perturbed specifically at the level of glycolysis leading to interesting therapeutic activities in cancer that can be displayed.

INTRODUCTION AND BACKGROUND

Hypoxia is an important phenomenon possessing a significant correlation with tumour progression, treatment result(s) and the overall disease prognosis [Wang GL 1995 Kallio PJ 1997], representing an important tumour microenvironment factor that significantly influences tumour cells behaviour via activation of genes encoding proteins involved in hypoxic stress adaptation. Tumor hypoxia is an important cancer prognosis indicator associated with aggressive growth, metastasis, and poor treatment response [Höckel M 1996, Brizel D M 1996], with further association with malignant progression and human cancers poor outcome. Tumor oxygenation state is leading to a series of genomic changes, enabling tumour cells survival or overcoming the oxygen deficient environment conditions. Hypoxia tumour tissue growth requires a sufficient oxygen and nutrients supply. Tumor cell responses to hypoxic stress include adaptive proteomic changes allowing the cells to overcome nutritive deprivation or to escape from their hostile environment by proliferation, invasion, or metastatic spread [Fandrey J, 1995]. However, proliferating tumour cells quickly overgrow the oxygen diffusion distance from the nearest blood vessel (100 - 150 μm), leading to a highly irregular tumour vasculature, with arteriovenous shunts, blind ends, and incomplete endothelial linings. Blood flow, as a consequence becomes less efficient than in normal tissues [Richard DE 1999]. Hypoxia-inducible factor 1 (HIF-1) is a multi-subunit protein that regulates transcription at hypoxia response elements (HREs) and is composed of 2 basic helix-loop-helix proteins: the α subunit, HIF-1α, and the constitutively expressed HIF-1β (also known as aryl hydrocarbon receptor nuclear translocator [ARNT]), during normoxia HIF-1α is hydroxylated on several proline and asparaginyl residues, which enables high-affinity binding of HIF-1α to von Hippel – Lindau tumor suppressor protein (vHL), a component of a ubiquitin ligase complex that ubiquitinates and thereby targets HIF-1α for proteosomal degradation. Under normoxic oxygenation conditions, HIF-1α protein is subject to rapid degradation process by pVHL-mediated ubiquitin-proteasome pathway, Under hypoxic conditions the O_2-dependent hydroxylation of HIF-1α is decreased, which prevents its degradation. whereas hypoxia blocks degradation leading to accumulation and translocation to the cellular nucleus and its binding together with HIF-1β on the so called Hypoxia responsive element within the hypoxia induced genes promoter region [Huang LE 1996, Kallio PJ 1997].

The association of HIF-1α with pVHL is triggered by the post-translational hydroxylation of proline residue that is mediated by prolyl hydroxylase (PHD) or HIF prolyl hydroxylase (HPH). The hypoxia-inducible factor (HIF-1) is an oxygen-dependent transcriptional activator, which plays crucial roles in the angiogenesis of tumours and mammalian development. HIF-1 consists of a constitutively expressed HIF-1β subunit and one of three subunits (HIF-1α,

HIF-2 α or HIF-3α). The stability and activity of HIF-1α are regulated by various post-translational modifications, hydroxylation, acetylation, and phosphorylation. Therefore, HIF-1α interacts with several protein factors including PHD, pVHL, ARD -1, and p300/CBP. Under normoxia, the HIF-1α subunit is rapidly degraded via the von Hippel - Lindau tumor suppressor gene product (pVHL)- mediated ubiquitin-proteasome pathway. The association of pVHL and HIF-1α under normoxic conditions is triggered by the hydroxylation of prolines and the acetylation of lysine within a polypeptide segment known as the oxygen-dependent degradation (ODD) domain. On the contrary, under hypoxic conditions, HIF-1α subunit becomes stable and interacts with its co-activators such as p300/CBP to modulate its transcriptional activity. Eventually, HIF-1 acts as a master regulator of numerous hypoxia-inducible genes under hypoxic conditions. The target genes of HIF-1 are especially related to angiogenesis, cell proliferation/survival, and glucose/iron metabolism. Moreover, it was reported that the activation of HIF-1α is closely associated with a variety of tumors and oncogenic pathways. Blocking of HIF-1α itself or HIF-1α interacting proteins inhibit tumor growth. Based on these findings, HIF-1 can be a prime target for anticancer therapies. It has been shown that carbonic anhydrase IX (CA IX) represents an important intrinsic marker of hypoxia. Carbonic anhydrase IX (CA IX) is one of the most strongly hypoxia-inducible proteins. Due to its different characteristics it is considered as an intrinsic marker of hypoxia. Carbonic anhydrase IX (CA - IX) belongs to an -carbonic anhydrase family of metalloenzymes that catalyse the reversible hydration of carbon dioxide to carbonic acid and play important roles in various biological processes related to acid-base balance [Chomczynski P 1987].

Several genes are regulated via the hypoxia induced HIF- 1α activation. Among these important genes, which is CA IX which is a transmembrane N - glycosylated isoenzyme localised at the cell surface in a trimer form composed of monomeric subunits of 58/54 kDa [Pastorek J 1994]. The large CA IX extracellular molecular part contains an N - terminally located proteoglycan-like region that is missing from other CAs and possessing adhesion capacity [Závada J 2001, Wingo T 2000]. The central carbonic anhydrase domain exhibits high enzymatic activity and has a structural predisposition to serve as a receptor site [Ivanov S 2001]. The intracellular CA IX C-terminus is linked to the extracellular part by a single hydrophobic transmembrane anchor [Pastorek J 1994, Opavsky R 1996]. CA IX is frequently present in different types of tumor cells and absent from their normal counterparts [Závada J 1993]. Natural CA-IX expression occurs only in few normal tissues like the; stomach epithelia, small intestine and gallbladder [Pastoreková S 1997]. CA IX is a recognised target of HIF-1 transcriptional complex that is highly responsive to changes of the oxygen levels in tumor cells *in vitro* and shows a typical hypoxic pattern of distribution in a wide variety of tumor tissues [Wykoff C 2000, Ivanov S 2001].

CA IX expression pattern is not only related to its transcriptional induction by hypoxia, but also to effects of adverse microenvironmental stresses (such as diminished levels of glucose and bicarbonate) and to high protein stability in reoxygenated cells. This suggests that CA IX potentially detects also the tumor regions that have experienced hypoxia either alone or in combination with low glucose or low bicarbonate before the tissue removal. Therefore,

CA – IX is serving as a marker of actual intra-tumoral microenvironment. Also, CA - IX serves as a 'record' of the expired hypoxia and stresses related to hypoxia. CA-IX expression occurs in different tumour tissues where CA - IX expression is normally absent like; bladder, kidney, breast, lung, head and neck, and cervix uteri, i.e. [Pastorekova S 2004] CA IX expression also occurs in mouse brain [Hilvo M 2004]. For human brain, CA IX expression was only shown in normal human brain tissue only as a slight or no expression in epithelial cells of the choroid plexus [Ivanov S 2001], and increasingly shown in high grade astrocytomas (Grade III and Grade IV) [Said HM 2007].

A further level of O_2-dependent regulation exists: the hydroxylation of an asparagine residue by factor inhibiting HIF-1α (FIH) blocks the interaction of HIF-1α with p300/CBP transcriptional coactivator proteins, thereby decreasing transcription of HIF-1α-regulated genes at normoxia. When HIF-1α levels increase in response to hypoxia in tissues, functional HIF-1 regulates transcription at HREs of target gene regulatory sequences, which results in the transcription of genes such as Carbonic anhydrase 9 [Bunn HF 1996, Fandrey J 1995].

Cellular pH level and carbon content influence expression of HIF-1α [Svastová E 2004], and CA-IX in tumour cells to overcome the stress situation by providing an energy source needed for their various activities [Svastová E 2004] and therefore contributing to the resistance of these cells towards radiation therapy and being therefore resistant to radiation therapy since, tumor hypoxia is well recognized as a major factor contributing to radioresistance [Overgaard J 1989, Knisely J 2002, Koukourakis MI 2006], the interference into this process through glycolysis inhibition [Nodin C 2005, Alabovskii VV 2004] represent an important issue.

Vascular endothelial growth factor (VEGF) is a powerful hypoxia induced mitogen for endothelial cell growth and plays a critical role in the development of tumor vessels]. Osteopontin (OPN), a tumor-associated phosphoglycoprotein, has been described to be prognostic for tumor progression and survival in a number of solid neoplasms and linked to a "metastatic phenotype Erythropoietin (Epo) has been reported to be overexpressed at the mRNA level in human and mouse brain (Said HM 2007).

Hypoxia induced regulation of another hypoxia induced gene, NDRG1 was shown at the same levels *in vivo* in normal human brain and human low-grade astrocytoma (WHO grade 2), while it showed a higher NDRG1 overexpression level in glioblastoma than in lowgrade astrocytoma (Said HM 2009)

Glycolysis inhibiton is effective against cancer cells under hypoxic conditions, which is frequently associated with cellular resistance to conventional anticancer drugs and radiation therapeutic approaches. Otto Warburg demonstrated that ascites tumor cells had high rates of glucose consumption and lactate production despite sufficient oxygen availability necessary for complete glucose oxidization [Hedeskov CJ 1968]. The so called "Warburg effect" represent a metabolic hallmark of aggressive tumors; however, the phenotype is also observed in non transformed cells during rapid proliferation [Hedeskov CJ 1968, Wang T, 1976]. Glycolytic enzyme inhibitors functional actions are based primarily on ATP depletion including:

A) Hypoxia-linked cancer-cell resistance reduction,
B) Anabolic and Energetic processes inhibition;
C) Improvement of drug selectivity by exploiting particular glycolysis dependency of cancer cell
D) ATP-dependent multi-drug resistance reduction,
E) Cytotoxic synergism with conventional cancer treatments [Scatena R 2008].

Hypoxia is an adverse prognostic factor in many tumor entities and tumor hypoxia has been associated in particular with poor response to radiotherapy [Evans SM 2003, Grumann T 2006, Höckel M 1993, Höckel 1996, Höckel M 2001 Mayer R 2005, Molls M 1998, Nordsmark M 2005, Rohrer Bley C 2006, Vaupel P 2006]. In order to improve the therapeutic efficacy of radiotherapy and to overcome the radioresistance of hypoxic tumors, a modification of tumor oxygenation and targeting of hypoxia-related molecules have been investigated [Hagen T 1975, Molls M 1998, Sakata K 2006]. The transcription factor hypoxia-inducible factor-1 (HIF-1) is one potential target molecule to improve the radio sensitivity of hypoxic tumors and consists of the two subunits HIF-1α and HIF-1β. It activates over 60 known genes regulating multiple functions relevant to cellular survival and proliferation in an oxygen-dependently manner [Lee JW 2004]. HIF-1α degradation is O_2-dependent by the prolyl hydroxylases activity. HIF-1 is associated with poor outcome for multiple cancer types and high HIF-1 expression is a predictor of poor prognosis after radiotherapy [Aebersold DM 2001, Birner P 2001, Bos R 2003, Giatromanolaki A 2001]. Cancer cell energy metabolism deviates from that of normal tissues by maintaining high glycolytic rates which has also been associated with disease progression in several tumor entities [Brizel DM 2001, Galarraga J, 1986 Isidoro A 2005]. Hypoxic accumulation of HIF-

1α occurs in a cell-type-specific manner [Vordermark D 2004], and is strongly dependent on glucose availability [Sobhanifar S 2005, Vordermark D 2004].

As it could be seen in the direct inhibition of a hypoxia induced gene like NDRG1 Said HM 2009) via siRNA or indirect inhibition through interfering with the cancer cell glycolytic activities via application of IAA (Said HM 2007, Staab A 2007) might be a potential therapeutic tool for regulating the expression of this gene in glioblastoma. Detailed understanding of how hypoxia regulates transcription of the NDRG1 gene increase knowledge of the cellular responses of normal and cancer cells towards low oxygen tension.

BIOCHEMISTRY OF HUMAN BRAIN TUMOR CELLS

Metabolism in Human Brain Tumor Cells

Tumor cell proliferation requires rapid synthesis of macromolecules including lipids, proteins, and nucleotides. Many tumor cells exhibit rapid glucose consumption, with most of the glucose-derived carbon being secreted as lactate despite abundant oxygen availability (the Warburg effect). (DeBerardinis RJ, 2007). Ordered pattern of metabolic and morphologic changes occurs during neoplastic cell transformation. Apparently, an increase in the flux of certain metabolic pathways such as the hexose - monophosphate shunt and glycolysis develops during transformation of many cell types. This metabolic aberration is conventionally explained as a consequence of a higher metabolic requirement (Banash P 1986). Gliomas represent 50% of primary brain tumors, and their prognosis remains poor despite the advances in diagnosis and therapeutic strategies (Lamari F, 2008). Positron emission tomography is used to study abnormalities in the glucose oxidative metabolism in human cerebral gliomas. It was possible to see that tumor regional cerebral glucose consumption was not depressed and regional glucose extraction ratios were similar for tumor and brain tissue, (Rhodes CG, 1983). Acidic pH1 decreased Lactate / pyruvate ratio and ATP level while both markedly increased by basic pH1 (Miccoli L, 1996). In some other experimental analysis, it was observed in human xenografted gliomas that Lactate / pyruvate ratios increased 3 - 4 fold and HK activity was of 2 - 4 fold lower than that of normal rat brain tissue, used as the control. The mitochondria-bound HK (mHK) fraction varied considerably and represented 9 to 69% of the total HK of that normal rat brain (Oudard S, 1997). Further in another series of experiments, Lactate to pyruvate ratio was >1, suggesting that the energy metabolism in LGG is glycolytic in nature, particularly in the tumors centre. Peripheral samples of tumors showed increased glucose consumption and cytochrome c - oxidase activity (Lamari F, 2008).

Hexokinase bind to a mitochondrial porin involving peripheral benzodiazepine receptors.

HK and peripheral benzodiazepine receptors inhibition by lonidamine and diazepam led to synergistic anti tumoral activity in xenografted gliomas. Co-inhibition of these two receptors will lead to a decrease in glycolysis, often elevated in these tumors, without modifying energetic metabolism of normal cells (Oudard S, Miccoli L, 1998).

Potential Role of Glycolytic Inhibitors in Human Brain Cancer Treatment

Glycolysis, the transformation of glucose to pyruvate, is a key step for the acquisition of ATP in all mammalian cells, including cancer tissues. Glucose transporters are commonly overexpressed in human malignancies enhancing glucose influx in the proliferating cancer cells (Macheda ML 2005). Glycolytic inhibitors are particularly effective against cancer cells with mitochondrial defects or under hypoxic conditions, which are frequently associated with cellular resistance to conventional anticancer drugs and radiation therapy (Pelicano H, 2006). Energy metabolism is considered for brain cancer treatment through metabolic targeting in the normal orthotopic tissue. The glucose transporter, GLUT-1, is enriched in the brain capillary endothelial cells and mediates facilitated glucose diffusion through the blood brain barrier. Glucose is metabolized mostly, to pyruvate, which enters neurons and glia mitochondria and is converted to acetyl-CoA before entering the TCA cycle. In well-oxygenated normal cells, pyruvate enters the mitochondria where, by the enzymic activity of pyruvate dehydrogenase, it is transformed to acetyl - Co A, the substrate for ATP production through the Krebs cycle (Harris RA 2002). Under normal conditions, 13% of glycolytic pyruvate is converted to lactate (Clarke DD 1999). Because intracellular acidosis triggers apoptosis blocking increased glycolytic activity by down regulating HIF-1α may reduce apoptosis of the hypoxic cells (Schmaltz C 1998). Within this context, results showed that iodide acetate minimized or inhibited HIF-1α protein and CA-IX protein and mRNA expression in glioblastoma cells under long term *in-vitro* hypoxia (Said HM 2007) as well as in other tumor of different origin (Staab A 2007). It has previously shown that CA IX may be a therapeutic target for cancer, since, inhibition of carbonic anhydrase isoenzymes with bacteriostatic or non bacteriostatic sulfonamides e.g. acetazolamide result in either reduced tumor invasiveness or blocked tumor growth, respectively (Svastová E 2004, Nodin C 2005). Furthermore, CA isoenzyme antagonism has been observed to augment the cytotoxic effects of various chemotherapeutic agents, including platinum-based drugs

There is a clear involvement of glucose concentration in the HIF-1α and CA-IX expression regulation, since application of glycolsis inhibitor iodide acetate lead to a minimized expression of both of them in different glioblastoma cell lines (Figure). Accumulation of HIF-1-□ depends on Glucose concentration. Glycolysis inhibitors, when added under hypoxia, lead to a reduced accumulation of HIF-1□. It has also been shown that inhibition of mitochondrial respiration leads to the inhibition of HIF-1α stabilization at low O_2 concentrations [Mateo J 2003]. Interference in the glycolysis path of glioblastomas by iodide acetate can represent a therapeutic alternative in CA-IX involved therapeutic approaches and potentially other HIF-1□ regulated hypoxia induced gene. On the other hand we can use CA-IX status for diagnostic purposes to potentially aid in the selection of patients who might benefit from CA-IX-targeted therapies (2003 Bui MH). Ca9 can represent an optimal target for therapeutic applications in hypoxia related glioblastoma tumours. In glioblastoma inhibition of HIF-1α regulated hypoxia induced genes like Ca9 is accomplished via the functional interference into the tumor cell glycolysis pathaway via IAA and Chetomin. Cancer cell energy metabolism deviates from that of normal tissues by maintaining high glycolytic rates which has also been associated with disease progression in several tumor entities [Brizel DM 2001, Galarraga J1986, Isidoro A 2005]. We and others have recently shown that the hypoxic accumulation of HIF-1α occurs in a cell-type-specific manner [Said

HM 2007, Staab 2007] and is strongly dependent on glucose availability [2005 Kwon SJ, Sobhanifar S 2005, Vordermark D 2005]. Glucose metabolism modulation investigation using the glycolysis inhibitors iodoacetate (IAA) or 2-deoxyglucose (2 - DG), affects the hypoxic accumulation of HIF-1α and to characterize the mechanism of glucose-dependent HIF-1α regulation had been accomplished. The hypoxic accumulation of HIF-1α depends strongly on the availability of glucose [2005 Kwon SJ, Vordermark 2005]. Recent work has shown that that there is strong evidence that HIF-1 regulates glucose metabolism and maintenance of tumor growth [Griffiths JR 2002, Yasuda S 2004].

One explanation of this effect is increased oxygen availability for prolyl hydroxylation of HIF-1α when mitochondrial oxygen consumption is reduced such that hypoxia is not recognized by prolyl hydroxylases [Hagen T 2003].

Glycolysis inhibitors, when added under hypoxia, lead to a reduced accumulation of HIF-1α. The regulation of HIF-1α by inhibition of glycolysis is independent of the activation by prolyl hydroxylases in HT1080 cells. Furthermore, pyruvate was not able to increase hypoxic HIF-1α levels when glycolytic inhibitors were added to HT1080 cells, suggesting that the lack of pyruvate is not the reason for the reduced accumulation of HIF-1α under hypoxic conditions when glycolysis was inhibited. In contrast to the report by Lu et al. we found no evidence for a key role of pyruvate as a glycolytic metabolite promoting HIF-1α accumulation [Lu H 2002].

To further investigate the mechanism by which the availability of glucose or glucose metabolites interacts with HIF-1α, we performed real-time RT-PCR to quantify the mRNA expression of the HIF-1α gene in cells under normoxia or hypoxia treated with IAA or 2-DG. We did not observe any significant changes in HIF-1α gene expression profiles after incubation of HT1080 cells with IAA or 2-DG. This finding corresponds to previous reports showing that hypoxia inhibits mRNA translation by suppressing multiple key regulators [Liu L 2004, Liu L2006] and limited nutrient availability can lead to drastically reduced protein synthesis [Faulhammer F 2005].

We therefore presume that glucose levels affect the expression of HIF-1α on a translational level or by phosphorylation instead of transcriptional regulation. A likely explanation for the reduced hypoxic accumulation of HIF-1α after inhibition of glycolysis, as compared to full glucose availability, is the glucose dependence of mRNA translation.

The interaction of glycolysis and the HIF-1 pathway may well explain in part the effects of glycolysis inhibitors shown in preclinical and clinical studies where such agents have increased the efficacy in chemotherapy protocols and after radiation treatment [Maher JC 2004, Varshney R 2005]. One can speculate that this effect depends on a reduced intratumoral accumulation of HIF-1α and thereby reduced expression of HIF-1-regulated genes. Previous publications have shown that glucose deprivation leads to an activation of multiple signal transduction pathways, changes in gene expression and induction of oxidative stress which mediate glucose-deprivation-induced cytotoxicity and metabolic oxidative stress in human cancer cells [Yun H 2005, Ahmad IM 2005].

Modulation of glycolysis reduces the hypoxic accumulation of HIF-1α protein in human tumor cells through a translational or post-translational process. Therefore, manipulation of tumor glucose levels represents a potential approach to therapeutically target HIF-1α. A clear involvement of glucose availability in the hypoxic HIF-1a and CA IX expression in malignant glioma cells exist since application of the glycolysis inhibitor iodoacetate led to a sharply reduced expression of both proteins and CA9 mRNA in all cell lines tested. Most previous reports have focused on the effects of HIF-1 on glucose metabolism, rather than vice versa: Glycolytic enzymes are induced by hypoxia and lactate production by glycolysis is a major cause of the acidic extracellular pH of tumors [Semenza GL 1994].

Suboptimal oxygen availability switches on cellular metabolism to anaerobic pathways for ATP production, which occurs through pyruvate transformation to lactic acid via the catalytic activity of lactate dehydrogenase 5 [Holbrook JJ 2002, Harris RA 1975]. Because intracellular acidosis triggers apoptosis blocking, increased glycolytic activity by down regulating HIF-1a may reduce apoptosis of hypoxic tumor cells [Schmaltz C1998]. We could previously show in non-brain tumor cell lines that the hypoxic accumulation of HIF-1a and expression of CA IX in vitro depend on the glucose concentration in the medium [Vordermark D 2005, Vordermark D 2005].

Glycolysis inhibitors, when added under hypoxia, led to a reduced accumulation of HIF-1α via a translational or post-translational effect [Staab A 2007]. Interference with the glycolysis of malignant gliomas by iodide acetate may therefore represent a therapeutic approach in targeting HIF-1a or CA IX. HIF-1 inhibition has been shown to slow tumor growth in in-vitro and in-vivo tumor models [Kung AL 2004, Welsh S 2004] and to act synergistically with other treatment modalities such as radiotherapy [Moeller BJ 2004].

In human fibrosarcoma cell line that HIF-1 targeting with chetomin (150 nM) suppresses the transcriptional response to hypoxia and reduces hypoxic radioresistance *in vitro*. This is, to our knowledge, the first report of increased radiosensitivity of hypoxic cells in vitro in response to chetomin. in a human fibrosarcoma cell line that HIF-1 targeting with chetomin (150 nM) suppresses the transcriptional response to hypoxia and reduces hypoxic radioresistance in vitro (Staab A 2007). Experimental conditions now chosen were based on our previous observation that a near-maximal HIF-1α expression occurs at 12 h of hypoxia at an oxygen concentration of 0.1% O_2, which represents a level of hypoxia that is frequently observed in solid tumors and radiobiologically relevant [Vordermark D 2004]. At the dose level of 150 nM, chetomin exhibited a maximum specific effect on HRE-regulated.

Potential Role of Chemical Inhibitors in Human Brain Cancer Treatment

Most anticancer drugs are transported by either active transport or passive diffusion into cells, where they frequently undergo further metabolism (Stubbs M 2000).

It is well known that Carbonic anhydrase isoform IX (CA IX) is highly over expressed in many types of cancer. Its expression, which is regulated by the HIF-1α (Wykoff CC 2000, Said HM 2007) transcription factor, is induced by hypoxia and correlates with a poor response to classical anti cancer therapeutic approaches like chemo- and radiotherapies (Said HM 2007). This chemo- and radio resistance occur due to the CA IX contribution to the tumor environment acidification by efficiently catalyzing the hydration of carbon dioxide to bicarbonate and protons leading to metastatic phenotypes acquisition and chemoresistance to weakly basic anticancer drugs (Supuran CT 2000). Among them are CA-IX-selective inhibitors, which can be inhibited via potent inhibitors derived from acetazolamide, benzenesulfonamides and ethoxzolamide which have been shown to inhibit the growth of several tumor cells *in vitro* and *in vivo* (Supuran CT 2006), (Supuran CT 2007). These drugs are pH sensitive. Therefore it is suggested that their cytotoxic activity depend on both intracellular pH (pHi) and pHe (CT-2008). Targeting CA IX with such specific CA IX inhibitors (Pastorekova S 2004), or also antibodies (Chrastina A 2003) should contribute, on one hand, to the enhancing action of weakly basic drugs and on the other hand, to reduce the acquisition of metastatic phenotypes by controlling the pH imbalance in the tumor cells. (Thiry A, 2008). Selective CA IX inhibitors could prove useful for elucidating the role of CA IX in hypoxic cancers, for controlling the pH imbalance in tumor cells and for developing diagnostic or therapeutic applications for tumor management. Ca9 specific enzymatic inhibition activity by specific inhibitors belonging to the group of sulphonamides like indisulam, reverts these processes, establishing a clear-cut role for CA IX in tumorigenesis. (Thiry A, 2008). Practically, CA inhibitors have been previously shown to elicit synergistic effects when used in combination with other chemotherapeutics agents in animal models (Teicher BA 1993). The antiproliferative effect of CA inhibitors might also be due to their effect on other CA isoforms such as CA II or CA V, which provide the bicarbonate substrate for cell growth in carboxylation reactions involved in lipogenesis, nucleotide biosynthesis and gluconeogenesis, among others, thereby limiting the unrestrained proliferation of the tumor cells (Scozzafava, A 2006), (Supuran CT 2007) and (Supuran CT 2003).

Inhibition of this enzymatic activity by specific inhibitors, such as the sulfonamide indisulam reverses these processes, establishing a clear-cut role for CA IX in tumorigenesis. Thus, selective CA IX inhibitors could prove useful for elucidating the role of CA IX in hypoxic cancers, for controlling the pH imbalance in tumor cells and for developing diagnostic or therapeutic applications for tumor management. Indeed, fluorescent inhibitors and membrane-impermeable sulfonamides have recently been used as proof-of-concept tools, demonstrating that CA IX is an interesting target for anticancer drug development. The Research of these CAIX inhibitors is undergoing continuous development. One of the mean reasons for that is in order to reach a high selectivity of these drugs to avoid any side effects by other CA isozymes inhibition and avoiding them to play their physiological roles (Thiry A, 2006).

Glucose Metabolism in Human Cancer Cells

Cellular glucose metabolism may occur either aerobically or anaerobically. In aerobic metabolism, glucose is converted to CO_2 and H_2O via the tricarboxylic acid (TCA) cycle with the generation of about 36 moles of ATP per mole of glucose consumed. In anaerobic glycolysis, glucose is metabolized to lactic acid, producing 2 moles each of ATP and H+ ions per mole of glucose [Stryer L, 1988]. For fundamental thermodynamic reasons [Pfeifer T 2001], the efficiency of aerobic metabolism is achieved at the cost of decreased maximum rate, and ATP production by the respiratory pathway rapidly saturates at high levels of glucose or limited oxygen supply. In the lower-yield anaerobic pathway, more of the energy from glucose degradation is used to drive the reaction, allowing a greater maximum rate of metabolism. The net ATP production rate of the anaerobic pathway, in the presence of adequate glucose, can be similar to that of the aerobic route despite the relative inefficiency.

Malignant brain tumors from either humans or animal models lack metabolic flexibility, in contrast to normal brain that oxidizes glucose as well as ketone bodies for energy. They are largely dependent on glucose for energy [Seyfried TN 2003, Mangiardi JR 1990]. Rhodes CG 1983, Nagamatsu S 1996, Roslin M 2003, Floridi A 1989, Galarraga J 1986, Mies G 1990, .

Oudard S 1997]. Enhanced glycolysis produces excess lactic acid that can return to the tumor as glucose through the Cori cycle [Tisdale MJ 1997].

Normal mammalian cells under physiological conditions utilize high-yield aerobic glucose metabolism, but can adapt to periods of hypoxia by elevating the anaerobic pathway, provided the transition to hypoxia is gradual and allows for induction of response mechanisms such as HIF. The energy cost of this transition is substantial, as the output of ATP per mole of glucose is reduced by over 90%. To compensate this decreased efficiency, glycolytic flux must increase several-fold. Warburg [WARBURG O 1930] first demonstrated tumour glucose metabolism alteration. Transformed cells *in vivo* and *in vitro* typically rely on anaerobic pathways to generate ATP from glucose even in the presence of abundant oxygen. A rough correlation between malignancy degree and glycolytic rate has long been noted [Burk D 1967]. The decreased efficiency of anaerobic metabolism is compensated by increased glucose, flux, maintaining energy production sufficiently in excess of basal metabolic demands to allow for cellular proliferation.

Metabolic Control Analysis in Human Brain Tumors

Metabolic control analysis evaluates the degree of flux in metabolic pathways and can be used to analyze and treat complex diseases [Veech RL 2004, Greene AE 2003]. The approach is based on findings that compensatory genetic and biochemical pathways regulate the tumor cells phenotype and bioenergetic potential [Veech RL 2004, Greene AE 2003 and Strohman R 2002]. As rate-controlling enzymatic steps in biochemical pathways are dependent on the physiological system metabolic environment, the management of disease phenotype depends more on the flux of the entire system than on the expression of any specific gene or enzyme alone [Strohman R 2002, Kacser H 1981, and Greenspan RJ 2001]. Complex disease phenotypes can be managed through self-organizing networks that display system wide dynamics involving glycolysis and respiration. Global manipulations of these metabolic networks can restore orderly adaptive behavior to widely disordered states involving complex gene-environmental interactions [Strohman R 2002, Kacser H 1981, Greenspan RJ 2001, Seyfried TN 2003, Seyfried TN 2005].

GLYCOLYTIC REGULATION IN HUMAN BRAIN TUMORS

Involvement of Glucose Availability in Hypoxia Induced Gene Expression

Glycolytic enzymes are induced by hypoxia and lactate production by glycolysis is a major cause of the acidic extracellular pH of tumors [Semenza GL 1994]. Suboptimal oxygen availability switches on cellular metabolism to anaerobic pathways for ATP production, which occurs through pyruvate transformation to lactic acid via the catalytic activity of lactate dehydrogenase 5 [Harris RA 1975, Holbrook JJ 2002]. Because intracellular acidosis triggers apoptosis blocking, increased glycolytic activity by down regulating HIF-1a may reduce apoptosis of hypoxic tumor cells [Schmaltz C 1998]. We could previously show in non-brain tumor cell lines that the hypoxic accumulation of HIF-1a and expression of CA IX in vitro depend on the glucose concentration in the medium [Vordermark 2005, Vordermark D, Kraft P 2005]. Glycolysis inhibitors, when added under hypoxia, led to a reduced accumulation of HIF-1α via a translational or post-translational effect [Staab A 2007]. Interference with the glycolysis of malignant gliomas by iodide acetate may therefore represent a therapeutic approach alternative. In glioblastoma there is a clear involvement of glucose availability in hypoxic HIF-1α and CA IX expression in malignant glioma cells since application of the glycolysis inhibitor iodoacetate led to a sharply reduced expression of both proteins and CA9 mRNA in all cell lines tested. Most previous reports have focused on the effects of HIF-1 on glucose metabolism, rather than vice versa.

HYPOXIA INDUCED HIF-1 GENE REGULATION IN HUMAN GLIOBLASTOMA

Hypoxia Induced Ca9 Expression in Human Brain Tumors Cells

Endogenous hypoxia markers are genes or gene products that are specifically up-regulated under hypoxic conditions. Tumor hypoxia has been recognized to confer resistance to anticancer therapy since the evolvement of this branch of cancer therapy and its fundamental role in tumorigenesis has been established. Hypoxia-inducible factor HIF–1α has been identified as an important transcription factor that mediates the cellular response to hypoxia, promoting both cellular survival and apoptosis under different conditions, and has been extensively studied as an endogenous hypoxia marker and its mechanism of accumulation under hypoxia is well understood (Harris AL 2002, Semenza GL 2003).

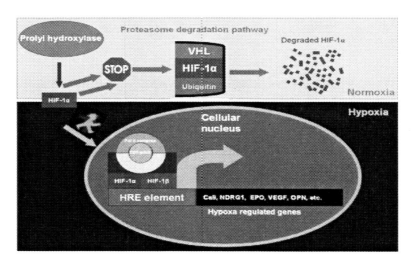

Figure1. HIF-1α Induced regulation of hypoxia induced genes figure. Under normoxia, HIF-1α is rapidly degraded via the *von Hippel – Lindau tumour suppressor gene product* (pVHL) – mediated ubiquitin proteasome pathway. When the tumor environment develop to hypoxic aeration conditionc, HIF-1α subunit becomes stable and interacts with coactivators of which its transcription machinery is consisted such as p300 / CBP to modulate the transcriptional activity of numerous hypoxia inducible genes, like carbonic anhydrase 9 (Ca9), OPN, NDRG1, EPO and VEGF and about 60 other hypoxia induced genes.

Ca9 that is regulated by HIF-1α (Figure 1) has been shown to be induced in a wide range of malignant cells, *in – vitro* (Wykoff CC 2000), in a high degree of expression that overlaps with pimonidazole (Olive PL 2001, Beasley NJ 2001).

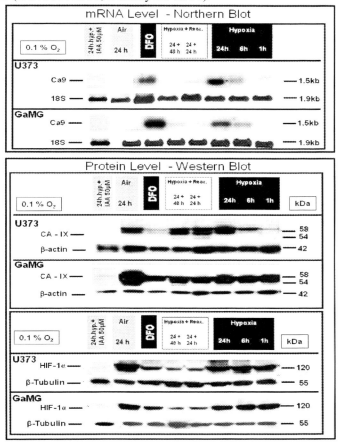

Figure 2. Ca9 and HIF-1α gene expression in response to hypoxia in human brain tumor. Cells *in vitro* => Upper panels: Comparative Northern blot analysis of CA9 mRNA expression under in vitro hypoxia and reoxygenation in the human malignant glioma cell lines U373 and GaMG. Treatment with 100 μM DFO under aerobic conditions served as a positive control, 50 μM IAA was used as a glycolysis inhibitor. Representative Northern blots of CA9 mRNA with 18S as a loading control.

Lower panels: A-Comparative Western blot analysis of CA IX protein expression under *in vitro* hypoxia and reoxygenation in wholecell lysates of the human malignant glioma cell lines U373 and GaMG. Treatment with 100 μM DFO under aerobic conditions served as a positive control, 50 μM IAA was used as a glycolysis inhibitor. Representative Western blots of CA IX protein with β-actin as a loading control.

B-Comparative Western blot analysis of HIF-1a protein expression under *in vitro* hypoxia and reoxygenation in nuclear extracts of the human malignant glioma cell lines U373 and GaMG. Treatment with 100 μM DFO under aerobic conditions served as a positive control, 50 μM IAA was used as a glycolysis inhibitor. Representative Western blots of HIF-1a protein with β-tubulin as a loading control.

Also, Ca9 has been shown to be over expressed in many tumors being a common feature of cancer cells required for tumor progression. It may contribute to tumor microenviroment for maintaining extracellular acidic pH and helping cancer cells to grow (Ivanov S 2001).

Most studies of tumor hypoxia have been based on direct pO_2 measurements using oxygen microelectrodes (Evans SM 2000). However there are limitations due to the invasive nature of the procedure. Hypoxia marker drugs, such as nitromidazole derivatives (e.g., EF5 and pimonidazole), also have been used to detect hypoxia in tumor samples; however, the requirement of prior administration restricts their clinical use to prospective studies (Kaanders JH 2002, Brown JM 2002).

Pimonidazole hydrochloride was selected as the hypoxia marker because of its high water solubility, chemical stability, efficient tumor uptake, and low toxicity. 2000 mg/m^2 of pimonidazole hydrochloride, 1-[(2-hydroxy-3-piperidinyl) propyl]-2-nitroimidazole hydrochloride (Hypoxyprobe) in 100 ml normal saline i.v. over 20 min is the maximum tolerated dose (Kennedy AS 1997) on patients.

The *in-vitro* data presented suggest that hypoxia may contribute to increased levels CA-IX expression in gliomas, *in - vitro*. Western and northern blot analysis revealed a difference between four cell lines in expression level under the various O_2 conditions but with almost a similar tendency in its expression behaviour. One of the factors of these differences together with the different response to reoxygenation could be explained by the genetic background of the cell lines investigated (Said HM, 2007) as it might indirectly influence at least their expression degree.

Also a difference appeared in the expression tendency between CA-IX protein and corresponding Ca9 mRNA. One of the reasons might be different posttranscriptional processing cause some difference between CA9 mRNA and CA-IX protein levels under coressponding conditions or that CA-IX protein level posttranscriptionally regulates a Ca9 mRNA (Bishop JM, 1987, Prendergast G C1989).

But, because CA IX is relatively stable because of the strong basal expression with differences in inter-glial CA-IX expression and a high stability during hypoxia / reoxygenation cycles (Swinson DE 2003, Giatromanolaki A 2001), therefore, when applicable *in-vivo*, we can say that CA IX expression status may be a reliable marker for glial tumor aggressiveness prediction associated with tumor hypoxia, so that, it can be detected in routine via clinical biopsies without the need for invasive procedure or prior drug administration.

Tumor cells and their survival and propagation can be further enhanced by genomic changes such as loss of apoptotic potential. These new cell variants have advantages over less adapted cells in a hypoxic microenvironment and expand through clonal selection becoming the dominant cell type in most cases. These variants further intensify hypoxia, establishing through clonal selection, often becoming the dominant cell type. Further intensification of hypoxia, establishing a vicious circle of hypoxia, malignant progression, and treatment resistance is the consequence (Kim SJ 2004), Glycolytic enzymes are induced by hypoxia (Semenza GL1994). The demonstration that an extracellular CA is up-regulated by microenvironmental tumor hypoxia has potentially important implications for understanding the regulation of tumor pH and the response to hypoxia. It has been widely held that lactate production by glycolysis is a major cause of the acidic extracellular pH of tumors. The hypoxic tumor environment favours the intensification of anaerobic metabolic pathways in cancer cells. Suboptimal oxygen availability switches on cellular metabolism to anaerobic pathways for ATP production, which occurs through pyruvate transformation to lactic acid via the catalytic activity of lactate dehydrogenase 5 (Holbrook JJ 1975).

Role of VEGF in Human Brain Tumors under Hypoxic Conditions

VEGF was originally discovered as a VPF, a protein secreted by tumour cells that potently stimulates ascites formation and vascular leak [Senger DR 1983]. Elevated levels of circulating VEGF provide a predictive measure of the progression of cancer and metastasis in certain cancers [Kuroi, K 2001]. In malignant gliomas, rapid cellular proliferation results in hypoxic conditions within the tumor. The release of humoral factors that promote angiogenesis, such as vascular endothelial growth factor (VEGF), seem to play a particularly important role in the process of neovascularization in malignant gliomas [Plate KH 1992, Kurimoto M1996].

The VEGF family of growth factors is unique, as it comprises the only angiogenic factor that also potently induces vascular leak. Although VEGF-induced angiogenesis is often accompanied by a vascular permeability response, VEGF-induced vascular leak is not required for angiogenesis [Eliceiri B 1999].

Angiogenesis is associated with expression of hypoxia-inducible factor HIF-1α and vascular endothelial growth factor (VEGF) in perinecrotic pseudopalisading glioma cells [Fisher, Zagzag 2005]. A powerful hypoxia-induced mitogen for endothelial cell growth is vascular endothelial growth factor (VEGF), which plays a critical role in the development of tumor vessels [Yancopoulos GD 2000]. VEGF expression is stimulated by hypoxia regulation and oncogenic mutations. Inhibiting tumor angiogenesis provides an opportunity for therapy [Schlaeppi JM 1999]. One of the key molecules responsible for the regulation of angiogenesis is vascular endothelial growth factor (VEGF), which is an endothelial cell-specific mitogen and survival factor. VEGF also stimulates vascular permeability and recruits progenitor endothelial cells from bone marrow. Clinical observations have demonstrated that VEGF status is significantly correlated with neovascularization grade and prognosis in various types of solid tumors. It has also been shown that VEGF status is predictive of the resistance to various treatments, including radiotherapy, chemotherapy and hormonal therapy. Similarly, VEGF expression level in the tumor tissue was a significant predictor of relapse-free survival and overall survival in node-negative breast cancer patients treated with loco-regional radiotherapy [Linderholm B1999]. Important limiting factor in the growth rate of a tumor is its blood supply and that by interrupting new vessel formation; tumor growth can be effectively arrested. With the identification of various pro- and antiangiogenic factors and their signalling mechanisms, a better understanding of the molecular basis of angiogenesis has emerged [Davis GE 1995, Ingber DE 1995, Jang YC 1999, Plate KH 1992]. Cancer mortality has changed little over the past forty years, mainly because of our failure to develop curative chemotherapy for the common solid cancers. The way forward is to carry out extensive phase I and II clinical trials of the many new types of anticancer agent that have become available as a result of increased knowledge about cancer cells and how they differ from normal tissues. Tumor growth could be abrogated by inhibiting angiogenesis represented a major departure from the then prevalent concept of targeting tumor cells directly as a means of preventing their growth [1971Folkman J]. Different approaches to study VEGF by the several study groups were performed. Importantly, hypoxia has been thought of as a primary trigger that tips the balance toward angiogenesis, as it will increase HIF1 activity and hence VEGF levels [Laderoute KR 2000, Mazure NM 1996, Diaz-Gonzalez JA2005]. In tumour lines expressed VEGF at low levels under normoxia, but several hours of hypoxia significantly increased VEGF expression *in vitro*. In contrast to Holash's theory, [Haroon ZA and his coworkers] did not observe vascular stasis before angiogenesis onset, but angiogenesis was accelerated when HIF1α was upregulated. They defined a physiological m called the 'acceleration model', where they proposed that HIF1α upregulation accelerates tumour angiogenesis, as opposed to its having a role in the initiation stages [Haroon ZA 2000]. VEGF upregulation is a trigger for initiation of angiogenesis from dormant metastases. Hypoxia, on the other hand will increase HIF1 activity to upregulate VEGF while downregulating thrombospondin, to create a pro-angiogenic environment [Laderoute KR 2000]. Some metastatic tumours replace normal parenchymal cells with tumour cells thereby co-opting normal vasculature. For example, human breast tumours that have metastasized to liver show this phenctype. They have been reported to exhibit little evidence for hypoxia (indicated by expression of the endogenous hypoxia marker protein carbonic anhydrase IX) and express low levels of VEGF [Stessels, F 2004, Colpaert CG 2003]. Hepatic metastases of colorectal cancer, by contrast, show high levels of carbonic anhydrase IX and increased VEGF and clearly exhibit angiogenesis [Stessels, F 2004]. VEGFR-1 antagonists and a tyrosine kinase inhibitor of VEGFR-2 forced a reversion of both radiation refractory tumor models to a radiation-sensitive phenotype. These findings suggest that the high VEGF expression might define a radio-resistant phenotype [Geng L 2001].

Hypoxia Induced OPN Expression in Human Brain Tumors Cells

Hypoxia regulated expression of OPN has been shown in several occasion [Said HM 2005, Said HM 2006, Said HM, Staab A 2007, Vordermark D 2006, Bache M 2006]. Several previous reports have identified links between cancer outcomes and the level of HIF-1a protein or the expression of one or two individual genes that are induced by hypoxia, such as Carbonic Anhydrase IX [Said HM 2007, Vordermark D 2004, Vordermark D 2006]. OPN was displayed a high level of cancer tissue expression specificity due to the favour expression in human (GBM) when compared to (LGA) based on the relative mRNA expression of hypoxia-related genes data. Regulation of OPN, mRNA and protein expression as a response to the hypoxic development in the tumor cell enviroment *in vitro* and *in vivo* represent an absolute phenomenon in human glioblastoma as a cell-specific post-transcriptionally regulated event. Further, the phenotype of combined OPN and CA9 overexpression represent a clear phenotype that is associated with GBM that also appears at a lower frequency in LGA. CA9 expression in GBM occurs at a high frequency both on protein and mRNA level as is the case for OPN, rendering OPN and CA9 as optimal diagnostic markers or targets for tumor-specific treatment approaches. Therapeutic strategies for treatment of human astrocytic tumors involving OPN, CA9 and to a certain extent EPO as target molecule represent potential approaches in conjunction with tumor hypoxia in the human brain. Also we have finally to mention that Understanding of the prognostic value of the gene expression patterns we have identified and to develop a small panel of well characterized markers that can be rapidly analyzed in clinical laboratories and that It will be important to understand what specific hypoxia-driven biological processes underlie the phenotypic differences between tumors in the high hypoxia response group and those in the low-hypoxia response group.

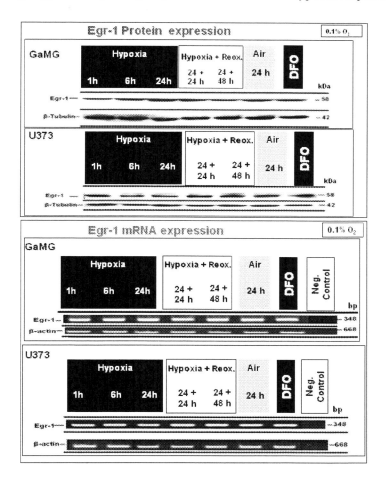

Figure 3. Egr-1 gene-expression as a response to the hypoxic development in human brain tumor cells. Upper panels: Regulation of Epidermal growth factor-1 (Egr-1) expression at the protein level *in vitro* in human GBM cell lines exposed to hypoxic (0.1% O_2) conditions for 1h, 6 h or 24h.

Protein laysates subjected to 24h under normoxia or to treatment with desferroxamine (100μM) served as negative and positive control, respectively

Lower panels: Examination of hypoxia-inducible regulation of epidermal growth factor-1 (Egr-1) gene expression at the mRNA level (semiquantitative RT-PCR) *in vitro* in human GBM cell lines (hypoxia time course experiments at O_2 concentration of 0.1%. GBM cell lines exposed to hypoxic (0.1% O_2) conditions for 1h, 6 h or 24h. Total mRNA from cells subjected to 24h under normoxia or to treatment with desferroxamine (100μM) served as negative and positive control, respectively. RT-PCR did not reveal any regulatory event under different oxygenation, hypoxia and reoxygenation conditions. Bar graphs show band intensities after densitometric evaluation and normalisation to β-actin expression as it is known from previous experiments. Results from a single representative experiment for each the protein and the mRNA expression level analysis out of three experiments.

Hypoxia Induced Epo Expression in Human Brain Tumors Cells

Erythropoietin (Epo) has been well characterized as a renal glycoprotein hormone that promotes erythrocytic progenitors survival, proliferation, and differentiation of hemopoietic tissues. Recombinant human Epo (rHuEpo) and related compounds have proved most useful for treatment of the anemia associated with chronic renal failure and, more restrictedly, certain types of nonrenal anemias [**Molineux G** 2003, **Heidenreich S** 1991]. It has been shown in the research work of one group that 81% of human lung carcinoma tissues possessed Epo-binding sites as detected by use of biotinylated rHuEpo. Epo-R transcripts and Epo-R protein were subsequently demonstrated in human renal carcinoma [Westenfelder C 2000]. tumors of the cervix and other organs of the female reproductive tract [2003 Acs G, Yasuda Y 2001, Yasuda Y 2002] and in various specimens of common pediatric tumors such as neuroblastomas, brain tumors, hepatoblastomas, and Wilms' tumors [Batra 2003]. By immunohistochemistry, Epo-R has been shown to be expressed in breast carcinoma [Acs G 2002, Arcasoy MO 2002, Hengartner MO 1994] and in vestibular schwannoma [Dillard DG 2001].

The role of Epo in tumor therapy needs to be further explored. Anemia-associated tissue hypoxia promotes angiogenesis, growth, and metastasis of tumors [Shannon AM 2003, Vaupel P 2004].

Since rHuEpo was introduced as a drug for treatment of renal anemia almost 20 years ago, several groups of investigators have carefully studied whether Epo can induce or promote tumor growth. Clinically, no evidence has been reported so far indicating that the erythrocytic growth factor Epo directly stimulates tumor cell proliferation. In addition, an elegant study in transgenic mice transfected with a construct that linked the human Epo gene to an erythroid-specific regulatory element has shown that the continuous stimulation of erythropoiesis leads to erythrocytosis but not to erythroleukemia [Madan A 2003] However, there is at least one case report of Epodependent leukemic transformation of myelodysplastic syndrome (MDS) to acute monoblastic leukemia (AML) [Bunworasate U 2001]. A careful examination has shown Epo-R expression on leukemia cells in 60% of patients with all French – American – British types of AML and in 29% of acute lymphoblastic leukemia (ALL) cases [Takeshita A 2002].

In vitro a proliferative response to Epo was observed in 16% of patients. Patients with both Epo-R expression and in vitro response to Epo had shorter remission duration than those without Epo-R [Takeshita A 2002]. Thus, close observation for leukemic transformation is necessary in patients with MDS on rHuEpo therapy.

Further, The mRNA expression levels for the other individual genes in patient tumor samples (GBM and LGA) were determined for EPO, OPN, CA9, VEGF (Figure 4). OPN mRNA was found uniformly upregulated in GBM, compared to normal brain and to LGA. CA9 exhibited a strong upregulation in GBM in about half of the tumor specimens (7/15 greater induction than the highest seen in (LGA); EPO was overexpressed in GBM as compared to normal brain, but not significantly so compared to LGA, due to rather strong expression in some LGA samples. VEGF expression was over 2-fold of normal brain in 2/15 (LGA) and 7/15 (GBM), resulting in a significant overexpression in GBM vs. LGA while on the experiments examining the tumor on protein level (Figure 5) we could find that all these genes where clearly upreglated as well as HIF-1α.

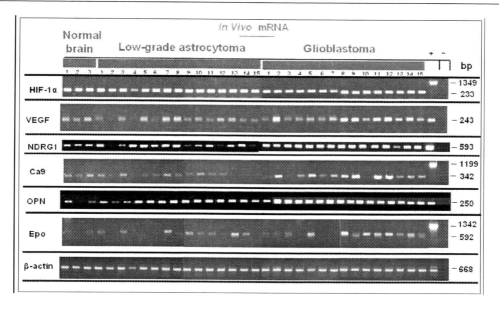

Figure 4. Hypoxia induced genes mRNA expression in correlation with grading of human brain tumors. Hypoxia induced genes mRNA expression in vivo in human GBM and LGA tumor samples. Expression of carbonic anhydrase IX (CA IX), osteopontin (OPN), erythropoietin (Epo), vascular endothelial growth factor (VEGF), N Myc- downregulated gene 1 NDRG1 and hypoxia-inducible factor-1a (HIF-1a) protein in a representative semi quatitative human tumor samples of low-grade astrocytoma (LGA) and glioblastoma (GBM). GaMG protein lysates subjected to 24 h under normoxia or to treatment with desferroxamine (100 μM) served as negative and positive control, respectively.

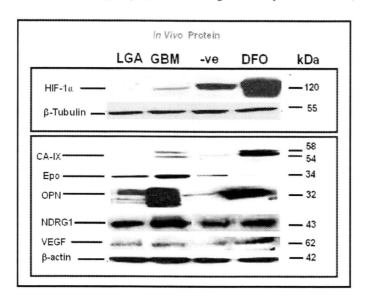

Figure 5. Hypoxia induced genes protein expression in correlation with grading of human brain tumors. Expression of carbonic anhydrase IX (CA IX), osteopontin (OPN), erythropoietin (Epo), vascular endothelial growth factor (VEGF), N Myc- downregulated gene 1 NDRG1 and hypoxia-inducible factor-1a (HIF-1a) protein in a Western blot of representative human tumor samples of low-grade astrocytoma (LGA) and glioblastoma (GBM). GaMG protein lysates subjected to 24 h under normoxia or to treatment with desferroxamine (100 μM) served as negative and positive control, respectively.

Hypoxia Induced NDRG1 Expression in Human Brain Tumor Cells

Hypoxia is a factor playing an important role within the solid tumor microenvironment. It significantly influences the behaviour of tumor cells via activation of genes encoding proteins involved in adaptation to hypoxic stress. Also, it plays an important role in tumor progression. It selects for cells with enhanced glycolytic activity, causing production of large amounts of lactic acid, one of the most common features of tumor cells (Warburg effect). As an important phenomenon, it attracts a lot of attention owing to its significant correlation with the tumor progression, treatment result and the overall prognosis of disease [Brown JM 2000, Kallio PJ 1997]. Tumor tissue growth requires a sufficient supply of oxygen and nutrients. However, proliferating tumor cells quickly overgrow the diffusion distance of the oxygen from the nearest blood vessel (100 -150 μm), leading to a tumor vasculature that is highly irregular and tortuous, with arteriovenous shunts, blind ends, and incomplete endothelial linings. This has an effect on blood flow, which is less efficient than in normal tissues [Richard·DE 1999, Guppy M 2002]. Tumor expansion is characterized by rapid growth of cancer cells when tumors establish themselves in host tissues of organs. Rapid growth of tumor is accompanying alterations in the cancer cell microenvironment, caused by an inability of local vasculature to supply enough oxygen and nutrients to the rapidly dividing tumor cells [Qu X 2002]. This makes hypoxia one common feature of solid tumors [Angst E 2006]. NDRG1 is a member of the N – myc downregulated gene (NDRG) family. *NDRG1* (also known as *Drg1, RTP, Rit42, PROXY-1*, and *Cap43*) was identified as a gene up-regulated during cellular differentiation [van Belzen N 1997, Bandyopadhyay S 1999Piquemal D 2003].

It is induced by hypoxia [Salnikow K 2003, Greijer AE 2005]. HIF-1 as a transcription factor plays a major role in the regulation of hypoxia-responsive genes [Lachat P 2002, Chen B 2006, Sibold S 2007] and is also involved in the transcriptional regulation of the *NDRG1* gene [Han YH 2007, Cangul H 2004], together with other transcription factors. In this relation it is of interest to investigate the expression of NDRG1 protein in human cancer [Stein S 2004]. This gene is necessary for p53-mediated apoptosis and regulated by PTEN (phosphatase and tensin homologue). In several cancers, it was suggested to be a tumor suppressor gene [Ando T 2006].

In several experimental analysis for the activity of hypoxia induced genes, in collected two groups of tumor specimens from human patients, one group consisted of patients with low-grade astrocytoma while the other one was comprised of patients suffering from glioblastoma, We found that *in vivo*, mRNA expression of HIF-1· was similar in tumor specimens from patients with low-grade astrocytoma (LGA) or glioblastoma (GBM) with a group of normal brain tissues samples as a control group (Figure 4). A tumor-grade association of NDRG1 mRNA expression was exhibited *in vivo*. No increase in NDRG1 expression was shown in low-grade astrocytoma While an increase of at least 2-fold in NDRG1 expression was shown in 10/15 patients in glioblastoma. NDRG1 protein (Figure 5) is also higher expressed in GBM when compared to (LGA)

Regulation via Other Hypoxia Gene Regulators

Early growth response factor 1 (Egr-1) is a transcription factor that triggers transcription of downstream genes within 15 - 30 min of various stimulations [Akutagawa O 2008].

In several publications [Ellen T 2008, Zhang P 2007] it has been shown that the transcription factor Egr-1 is regulated via hypoxia, and hypothesized to be responsible for the hypoxia induced regulation of N-myc downregulated gene 1 (NDRG1) in human tumours cells. HIF-1α is a transcription factor consisted of two HIF-1 are basic-helix-loop-helix proteins containing a PAS domain subunits [1995 Wang GL].

In normoxia, the von Hippel-Lindau tumour suppressor (pVHL), which is the recognition component of an E3 ubiquitin ligase complex, targets HIF-1α [Iwai K 1999, Lisztwan J 1999], leading to its ubiquitylation and consequent proteasomal degradation [Lisztwan J 1999, Cockman ME 2000, Kamura T 2000, Ohh M 2000, Tanimoto K2000].

HIF-1α is responsible of the regulation of several hypoxia induced genes. These genes are expressed rapidly through specific promoter activation by binding to the so called Hypoxia responsive element (HRE) and by that; they mediate cell growth and angiogenesis [Dachs GU 1995, Melillo G1997]. Due to HRE positioning in the distal promoter region, HIF-1 is acting as a transcriptional enhancer, as hypothesized in a similar gene expression model [Wang GL1995]. In hypoxia, the α/β heterodimer binds to the core pentanucleotide sequence (RCGTG) in the hypoxia response elements (HREs) of target genes. HIF-β subunits are non-oxygen responsive nuclear proteins that also have other roles in transcription [2000 Gu YZ].

In contrast, the HIF-α subunits are highly inducible by hypoxia responsive element (HRE) bound by nuclear HIF-1α in human glioblastoma cells *in vitro* under different oxygenation conditions, Also, the clear enhanced binding of nuclear extracts from glioblastoma cell samples exposed to extreme hypoxic conditions confirms the HIF-1 western results [Said HM 2008, Said HM 2009] and the NDRG1 regulation by HIF-1 α [Said H 2006, Said HM 2007].

Our findings demonstrate that EGR-1 is not up-regulated in response to the extreme hypoxic (0.1 %O_2) or even reoxygenative conditions after hypoxia in human glioblastoma. Therefore, HIF-1α is still one of the promising targets for new therapeutic strategies in cancer research, especially therapeutic modulation of the adaptive hypoxic response. At the same time we believe based on the data that resulted from the research work of the different research groups worldwide, that Egr-1 Could not be a new target for therapeutic modulation of the adaptive hypoxic response, at least in human glioblastoma.

CONCLUSION

Hypoxia significantly influences the behaviour of human tumor cells via activation of genes involved in the adaptation to hypoxic stress, representing an important indicator of cancer prognosis and is associated with aggressive growth, metastasis, and poor response to treatment and with malignant progression.

In malignant glioma therapy, the main aim, as with all cancers, is to either eradicate the tumor or convert it into a controlled, quiescent chronic disease. Angiogenesis and hypoxia induced, HIF-1α regulated genes inhibition remains the main parts of therapeutic approaches in human oncology. It is well known that cancer cell metabolism can be perturbed specifically at the level of glycolysis leading to interesting therapeutic activities in cancer that can be displayed. This functional characteristic was applied as proof-of-concept tools, demonstrating that CA IX and also its main regulator HIF-1α represent interesting targets for anticancer drug development. The differences between different types of brain tumors and brain tumor cell lines regarding the response of the hypoxia induced genes CA9, EPO, OPN, VEGF, and NDRG1 to hypoxia and reoxygenation which was observed here can, in part, be explained by the genetic background of the cell lines investigated which may indirectly influence their degree of expression. Glycolytic inhibitors, when added in controlled doeses under hypoxia, lead to a reduced accumulation of HIF-1α and can function as indirect inhibitors of hypoxia genes like OPN, EPO, VEGF, NDRG1 and CA9 beside other direct genes inhibitor like sulphonamide derivates or Chetomin and other tools likes siRNA rendering them as optimal tools for the development of optimized therapeutic in human cancer treatment especially in human brain cancer treatment.

ACKNOWLEDGMENTS

The authors would like to thank Astrid Katzer, Stefanie Gerngras and Siglinde Kühnel for technical assistance during the different stages of this analysis. The author would like to thank The University of Würzburg, Medical Faculty, Department of Radiation Oncology the Deutsche Forschungsgemeinschaft (VO 871/2-3) to DV and by IZKF Würzburg (B25) to CH and GHV for financing this research. Also, the authors would like to acknowledge the efforts & contributions made by the different research groups in tumor hypoxia hypoxia signalling and regulation.

REFERENCES

Acs, G., Zhang, P. J., Rebbeck, T. R., Acs, P. & Verma, A. (2002). Immunohistochemical expression of erythropoietin and erythropoietin receptor in breast carcinoma. *Cancer*, 95, 969–981.

Acs, G., Zhang, P. J., McGrath, C. M., Acs, P., McBroom, J., Mohyeldin, A., Liu, S., Lu, H. & Verma, A. (2003). Hypoxia-inducible erythropoietin signaling in squamous dysplasia and squamous cell carcinoma of the uterine cervix and its potential role in cervical carcinogenesis and tumor progression. *Am J Pathol.*, 162, 1789–1806.

Aebersold, D. M., Burri, P., Beer, K. T. et al. (2001). Expression of hypoxia-inducible factor-1α: a novel predictive and prognostic parameter in the radiotherapy of oropharyngeal cancer. *Cancer Res.*, 61, 2911–6.

Ahmad IM, Aykin - Burns N, Sim JE, et al, (2005) Mitochondrial O2 and H2O2 mediate glucose deprivation-induced cytotoxicity and oxidative stress in human cancer cells. J Biol Chem; 280: 4254 - 63.

Akutagawa, O., Nishi, H., Kyo, S., Terauchi, F., Yamazawa, K., Higuma, C., Inoue, M. & Isaka, K. (2008) Early growth response-1 mediates downregulation of telomerase in cervical cancer. Cancer Sci., 99(7), 1401-6.

Alabovskii, V. V, Khamburov, V. V & Vinokurov, A. A, (2004). Some mechanisms of adenosine protective effect in the "calcium paradox". Ross. Fiziol. Zh. Im. I. M. Sechenova, 90(7), 889-901.

Ando, T., Ishiguro, H., Kimura, M. et al. (2006). Decreased expression of NDRG1 is correlated with tumor progression and poor prognosis in patients with esophageal squamous cell carcinoma. Dis. Esophagus, 19, 454–458.

Angst, E., Sibold, S., Tiffon, C. et al. (2006). Cellular differentiation determines the expression of the Hypoxia - inducible protein NDRG1 in pancreatic cancer. *Br. J. Cancer*, 95, 307-13.

Arcasoy, M. O., Amin, K., Karayal, A. F., Chou, S. C., Raleigh, J. A., Varia, M. A. & Haroon, Z. A. (2002). Functional significance of erythropoietin receptor expression in breast cancer. Lab Invest., 82, 911–918.

Bache, M., Reddemann, R., Said, H. M. et. al. (2006). Immunohistochemical detection of osteopontin in advanced head-and-neck cancer: prognostic role and correlation with oxygen electrode measurements, hypoxia-inducible-factor-1alpha-related markers, and hemoglobin levels. *Int J Radiat Oncol Biol Phys.*, 66(5),1481-7.

Bandyopadhyay, S., Pai, S. K., Gross, S. C., et al. (2003). The Drg-1 gene suppresses tumor metastasis in prostate cancer. Cancer Res, 63, 1731–6.

Batra, S., Perelman, N., Luck, L. R., Shimada, H. & Malik, P. (2003). Pediatric tumor cells express erythropoietin and a functional erythropoietin receptor that promotes angiogenesis and tumor cell survival. Lab Invest, 83, 1477–1487.

Birner, P., Schindl, M., Obermair, A. et al. (2001). Expression of hypoxia-inducible factor-1α in epithelial ovarian tumors: its impact on prognosis and on response to chemotherapy. *Clin Cancer Res.*, 7, 1661–8.

Bos, R., van der Groep, P., Greijer, A. E. et al. (2003). Levels of hypoxia-inducible factor- 1α independently predict prognosis in patients with lymph node negative breast carcinoma. Cancer, 97, 1573–81.

Brizel, D. M., Schroeder, T., Scher, R. L. et al. (2001). Elevated tumor lactate concentrations predict for an increased risk of metastases in head-and-neck cancer. *Int J Radiat Oncol Biol Phys.*, 51, 349–53.

Brizel, D. M., Scully, S. P., Harrelson, J. M., Layfield, L. J., Bean, J. M., Prosnitz, L. R. & Dewhirst, M. W. (1996). Tumor oxygenation predicts for the likelihood of distant metastases in human soft tissue sarcoma. Cancer Res., 56, 941-943.

Brown, J. M. (2000). Exploiting the hypoxic cancer cell: mechanisms and therapeutic strategies. Mol. Med. Today, 6, 157–162.

Brown JM, QT Le, (2002), Tumor hypoxia is important in radiotherapy, but how should we measure it?, Int. J Radiat. Oncol. Biol. Phys 54 (5): 1299 -1301

Brown LM, Cowen RL, Debray C, et al. (2006), Reversing hypoxic cell chemoresistance in vitro using genetic and small molecule approaches targeting hypoxia inducible factor. Mol Pharmacol; 69: 411-8.

Bunn, H. F. & Poyton, R. O. (1996). Oxygen sensing and molecular adaptation to Hypoxia. Physiol. Rev., 76, 839–885.

Bunworasate, U., Amouk, H., Mindeman, H., O'Loughlin, K. L., Sait, S. N. J., Barcos, M., Stewart, C. C. & Baer, M. R. (2001). Erythropoietindependent transformation of myelodysplastic syndrome to acute monoblastic leukemia. *Blood*, 98, 3492–3494.

Burk, D., Woods, M. & Hunter, J. (1967). On the significance of glycolysis for cancer growth, with special reference to Morris rat hepatomas. *J Natl Cancer Inst.*, 38, 839–63.

Beasley NJ, Wykoff CC, Watson PH, Leek R, Turley H, Gatter K, Pastorek J Cox GJ, Ratcliffe P, Harris AL (2001), Carbonic anhydrase IX, an endogenous hypoxia marker, expression in head and neck squamous cell carcinoma and its relationship to hypoxia, necrosis, and microvessel density, *Cancer Res.* 61(13):5262-7.

Bui MH, Seligson D, Han KR, Pantuck AJ, Dorey FJ, Huang Y, Horvath S, (2003), Carbonic anhydrase IX is an independent predictor of survival inadvanced renal clear cell carcinoma: implications for prognosis and therapy. *Clin. Cancer Res.* 9(2):802-11.

Bishop JM (1987), The molecular genetics of cancer, Science 235(4786):305-11.

Colpaert, C. G. et al. (2003). Cutaneous breast cancer deposits show distinct growth patterns with different degrees of angiogenesis, hypoxia and fibrin deposition. *Histopathology*, 42, 530–540

Cangul, H. (2004). Hypoxia upregulates the expression of the NDRG1 gene leading to its overexpression in various human cancers. BMC Genet, 5, 27.

Chen, B., Nelson, D. M., Sadovsky, Y. (2006). N - Myc downregulated gene 1 (Ndrg1) modulates the response of term human trophoblasts to hypoxic injury. *J. Biol. Chem.*, 281, 2764 – 2772.

Chrastina A, Pastoreková S, Pastorek J.(2003), Immunotargeting of human cervical carcinoma xenograft expressing CA IX tumor-associated antigen by 125I-labeled M75 monoclonal antibody. Neoplasma. 50 (1): 13 - 21.

Chan, D. A. & Giaccia, A. J. (2007), Hypoxia, gene expression, and metastasis. *Cancer Metastasis Rev.* 26, 333–339

Chomczynski, P. & Sacchi, V. (1987). Single-step method of RNA isolation by acidic guanidinium thiocyanate-phenol-chloroform extraction. *Anal Biochem.*, 162, 156-9.

Clarke, D. D. & Sokoloff, L. (1999). Circulation and energy metabolism in the brain. In G. J. Siegel, B. W. Agranoff, R. W. Albers, S. K. Fisher, & M. D. Uhler (Eds.) Basic Neurochemistry (6th edition, pp. 637-669). New York: Lippincott-Raven.

Cockman, M. E., Masson, N., Mole, D. R., Jaakkola, P., Chang, G. W., Clifford, S. C., Maher, E. R., Pugh, C. W., Ratcliffe, P. J. & Maxwell, P. H. (2000). Hypoxia inducible factor-alpha binding and ubiquitylation by the von Hippel-Lindau tumor suppressor protein. *Journal -of Biological Chemistry*, 275, 25733–25741.

Coles, N. W. & Johnstone, R. M. (1962). Biochem J, 83, 284–291.

Dachs, G. U., Patterson, A. V., Firth, J. D., Ratcliffe, P. J., Townsend, K. M., Stratford, I. J. & Harris, A. L. (1997). Targeting gene expression to hypoxic tumor cells. *Nat Med.*, 3(5), 515-20.

Davis GE, Camarillo CW (1995), Regulation of endothelial cell morphogenesis by integrins, mechanical forces, and matrix guidance pathways. Exp Cell Res 216: 113–123.

Diaz-Gonzalez, J. A., Russell, J., Rouzaut, A., Gil-Bazo, I. & Montuenga, L. (2005). Targeting hypoxia and angiogenesis through HIF-1α inhibition. *Cancer Biol. Ther.* 4, 1055–1062

Dillard, D. G., Venkatraman, G., Cohen, C., Delgaudio, J., Gal, A. A. & Mattox, D. E. (2001). Immunolocalization of erythropoietin and erythropoietin receptor in vestibular schwannoma. Acta Otolaryngol, 121, 149–152.

Ebert, B. L., Firth, J. D. & Ratcliffe, P. J. (1995). Hypoxia and Mitochondrial Inhibitors Regulate Expression of Glucose Transporter-1 via Distinct Cis-acting Sequences. *J. Biol. Chem.*, 270, 29083 –29089.

Ellen, T., Ke, Q., Zhang, P. & Costa, M. (2008). NDRG1, a Growth and Cancer Related Gene: Regulation of Gene Expression and Function in Normal and Disease States. Carcinogenesis, 29(1), 2-8.

Eliceiri BP, Paul R, Schwartzberg PL, Hood JD, Leng J, Cheresh DA (1999). Selective requirement for Src kinases during VEGF-induced angiogenesis and vascular permeability. Mol. Cell 4, 915--924

Erler JT, Bennewith KL, Nicolau M, Dornhöfer N, Kong C, Le QT, Chi JT, Jeffrey SS, Giaccia AJ.(2006). Lysyl oxidase is essential for hypoxiainduced metastasis. *Nature*, 440, 1222–1226

Evans, S. M. & Koch, C. J. (2003). Prognostic significance of tumor oxygenation in humans. *Cancer Lett.*, 195, 1–16.

Evans SM, Hahn S, Pook DR, Jenkins WT, Chalian AA, Zhang P, Stevens C, Weber R, Weinstein G, Benjamin I, Mirza N, Morgan M, Rubin S, McKenna WG, Lord EM, Koch CJ, (2000), Detection of hypoxia in human squamous cell carcinoma by EF5 binding, *Cancer Res*. 60: 2018–2024.

Fandrey, J. (1995). Hypoxia-inducible gene expression, Respir. Physiol., 101, 1–10.

Faulhammer F, Konrad G, Brankatschk B, Tahirovic S, Knödler A, Mayinger P (2005), Cell growth–dependent coordination of lipid signaling and glycosylation is mediated byinteractions between Sac1p and D pm1p. J Cell Biol. 168: 185-91.

Folkman J (1971): Tumor angiogenesis: therapeutic implications. N Engl J Med 285: 1182–1186

Floridi, A., Paggi, M. G. & Fanciulli, M. (1989). Modulation of glycolysis in neuroepithelial tumors. *J Neurosurg Sci.*, 33, 55-64.

Galarraga, J., Loreck, D. J., Graham, J. F., DeLaPaz, R. L., Smith, B. H., Hallgren, D. & Cummins, C. J. (1986). Glucose metabolism in human gliomas: correspondence of in situ and in vitro metabolic rates and altered energy metabolism. *Metab Brain Dis.*, 1, 279-291.

Geng L, Donnelly E, McMahon G, Lin PC, Sierra- Rivera E, Oshinka H, Hallahan DE (2001), Inhibition of vascular endothelial growth factor receptor signalling leads to reversal of tumor resistance to radiotherapy. *Cancer Res*. 61:2413-2419.

Giatromanolaki, A., Koukourakis, M., Sivridis, E. et al. (2001) Relation of hypoxia inducible factor 1α and 2α in operable non-small celllung cancer to angiogenic molecular profile of tumors and survival. *Br J Cancer*, 85, 881–90.

Galarraga J, Loreck DJ, Graham JF, DeLaPaz RL, Smith BH, Hallgren D, Cummins CJ (1986) Glucose metabolism in human gliomas: correspondence of in situ and in vitro metabolic rates and altered energy metabolism. *Metab Brain Dis*.1: 279 - 91.

Greene, A. E., Todorova, M. T. & Seyfried, T. N. (2003). Perspectives on the metabolic management of epilepsy through dietary reduction ofglucose and elevation of ketone bodies. J Neurochem, 86, 529-537.

Greenspan, R. J. (2001). The flexible genome. Nat Rev Genet, 2, 383-387.

Greijer, A. E., van der Groep, P., Kemming, D. et al. (2005). Up-regulation of gene expression by hypoxia is mediated predominantly by hypoxia-inducible factor 1 (HIF-1). *J. Pathol.*, 206, 291–304.

Griffiths JR, McSheehy PM, Robinson SP, Troy H, Chung YL, Leek RD, Williams KJ, Stratford IJ, Harris AL, Stubbs M. (2002), Metabolic changes detected by in vivo magnetic resonance studies of HEPA-1 wild-type tumors and tumors deficient in hypoxia-inducible factor-1beta (HIF-1beta): evidence of an anabolic role for the HIF-1 pathway. *Cancer Res.*; 62: 688 – 95.

Grumann, T., Arab, A., Bode, C. et al. (2006). Reoxygenation of human coronary smooth muscle cells suppresses HIF-1alpha gene expression and augments radiation-induced growth delay and apoptosis. *Strahlenther Onkol.*, 182, 16–21.

Gu, Y. Z., Hogenesch, J. B. & Bradfield, C. A. (2000). The PAS superfamily: sensors of Environmental and developmental signals. *Ann. Rev Pharmacol Toxicol.*, 40, 519–561.

Guppy, M. (2002) The hypoxic core: a possible answer to the cancer paradox. *Biochem. Biophys. Res. Commun.*, 299, 676 – 80.

Hagen, T., Taylor, C.T., Lam, F. et al. (2003). Redistribution of intracellular oxygen in hypoxia by nitric oxide: effect on HIF1alpha. Science, 302, 1975–8.

Han, Y. H., Xia, L., Song, L. P. et al. (2007). Comparative proteomic analysis of hypoxia-treated and untreated human leukemic U937 cells. Proteomics, 6, 3262–3274.

Harris, R. A., Bowker-Kinley, M. M., Hyang, B. & Wu, P. (2002). Regulation of the activity of the pyruvate dehydrogenase complex. Adv Enzyme Regul, 42, 249–259.

Haroon, Z. A., Raleigh, J. A., Greenberg, C. S. & Dewhirst, M. W, (2000), Early wound healing exhibits cytokine surge without evidence of hypoxia. *Ann. Surg.* 231, 137–147

Holbrook JJ, Liljas A, Steindel SJ, Rossman MG (1975), Lactate dehydrogenase. In: Boyer PD (eds) The enzymes. Volume 11, 3rd ed. Academic Press, NY, pp 191–292

Hagen T, Taylor CT, Lam F, et al. (2003), Redistribution of intracellular oxygen in hypoxia by nitric oxide: effect on HIF1alpha. Science 302: 1975 - 8.

Harris RA, Bowker - Kinley MM, Hyang B, Wu P (2002), Regulation of the activity of the pyruvate dehydrogenase complex. *Adv Enzyme Regul.*, 42 :249– 59.

Holbrook JJ, Liljas A, Steindel SJ, Rossman MG, (1975), Lactate dehydrogenase. In: Boyer PD, editor. The enzymes. Volume 11, 3rd ed. NY: Academic Press;.p.191 – 292.

Hedeskov, C. J. (1968). *Biochem J.*, 110, 373–380.

Heidenreich, S., Rahn, K. H. & Zidek, W. (1991). Direct vasopressor effect of recombinant human erythropoietin on renal resistance vessels. Kidney Int, 39, 259–265.

Hengartner, M. O. & Horvitz, H. R. (1994). C. elegans cell survival gene ced-9 encodes a functional homolog of the mammalian proto-oncogene bcl-2. Cell, 76, 665–676.

Hilvo, M., Rafajova, M., Pastorekova, S., Pastorek, J. & Parkkila, S. (2004). Expression of carbonic anhydrase IX in mouse tissues. *J Histochem. Cytochem.*; 52, 1313–22.

Höckel, M., Knoop, C., Schlenger, K., et al. (1993). Intratumoral pO2 predicts survival in advanced cancer of the uterine cervix. *Radiother Oncol.*, 26, 45–50.

Höckel, M., Schlenger, K., Aral, B. et al. (1996). Association between tumor hypoxia and malignant progression inadvanced cancer of the uterine cervix. *Cancer Res.*, 56, 4509–15.

Höckel, M. & Vaupel, P. (2001). Tumor hypoxia: definitions and current clinical, biologic, and molecular aspects. J Natl Cancer Inst, 93, 266–76.

Holbrook, J. J., Liljas, A., Steindel, S. J. & Rossman, M. G. (1975). Lactate dehydrogenase. In P. D. Boyer (Eds.) The enzymes (3rd edition, pp. 191–292). NY: Academic Press.

Huang, L. E., Arany, Z., Livingston, D. M. & Bunn, H. F. (1996). Activation of Hypoxia-inducible Transcription Factor Depends Primarily upon Redox-sensitive Stabilization of Its α Subunit, J. Biol. Chem., 271, 32253-32259.

Isidoro, A., Casado, E., Redondo, A. et al. (2005) Breast carcinomas fulfill the Warburg hypothesis and provide metabolic markers of cancer prognosis. *Carcinogenesis*, 26, 2095–104.

Ivanov, S., Liao, S. Y., Ivanova, A., Danilkovich-Miagkova, A., Tarasova, N., Weirich, G., Merrill, M. J., Proescholdt, M. A., Oldfield, E. H., Lee, J., Zavada, J., Waheed, A., Sly, W., Lerman, M. I., Stanbridge, E.J. (2001). Expression of hypoxia-inducible cell-surface transmembrane carbonic anhydrases in human cancer. *Am. J. Pathol.*, 158, 905 - 919.

Iwai, K., Yamanaka, K., Kamura, T., et al. (1999). Identification of the von Hippellindau tumor-suppressor protein as part of an active E3 ubiquitin ligase complex. *PNAS*, 96, 12436–12441.

Ingber DE, Prusty D, Sun Z, Betensky H, Wang N (1995), Cell shape, cytoskeletal mechanics, and cell cycle control in angiogenesis. *J Biomech.* 28: 1471–1484

Isidoro A, Casado E, Redondo A, Acebo P, Espinosa E, Alonso AM, Cejas P, Hardisson D, Fresno Vara JA, Belda-Iniesta C, González-Barón M, Cuezva JM. (2005) Breast carcinomas fulfill the Warburg hypothesis and provide metabolic markers of cancer prognosis. Carcinogenesis 26: 2095–2104.

Kacser, H., Burns, J. A. (1981). The molecular basis of dominance. *Genetics*, 97, 639 -666.

Jang YC, Arumugam S, Gibran NS, Isik FF (1999), Role of alpha V integrins and angiogenesis during wound repair. *Wound Repair Regen.* 7: 375–380.

Kallio, P. J., Pongratz, I., Gradin, K., McGuire, J. & Poellinger, L. (1997). Activation of hypoxia-inducible factor 1α: Posttranscriptional regulation and conformational change by recruitment of the Arnt transcription factor. PNAS, 94, 5667-5672.

Kaanders JH, Wijffels KI, Marres HA, Ljungkvist AS, Pop LA, van den Hoogen FJ, de Wilde PC, Bussink J, Raleigh JA, van der Kogel AJ (2002), Pimonidazole binding and tumor vascularity predict for treatment outcome in head and neck cancer, Cancer Res. 62: 7066–7074

Kamura, T., Sato, S., Iwai, K., Czyzyk-Krzeska, M., Conaway, R. C. & Conaway, J. W. (2000). Activation of HIF1alpha ubiquitination by a reconstituted von Hippel-Lindau (VHL) tumor suppressor complex. PNAS, 97, 10430–10435.

Kim, S. J., Rabbani, Z. N., Vollmer, R. T., Schreiber, E. G., Oosterwijk, E., Dewhirst, M. W., Vujaskovic, Z. & Kelley, M. J. (2004). Carbonic anhydrase IX in early-stage non small cell lung cancer. Clin Cancer Res, 10, 7925-33.

Knisely, J., Rockwell, S. & Knisely, J. (2002). The importance of hypoxia in the brain tumor, *Neuroimaging Clin. N. Amer.*, 12, S25–S35.

Koukourakis, M. I., Bentzen, S. M., Giatromanolaki, A., Wilson, G. D., Daley, F. M., Saunders, M. I., Dische, S., Sivridis, E., Harris, A. L. (2006). Endogenous markers of two separate hypoxia response pathways (hypoxia inducible factor 2 alpha and carbonic anhydrase 9) are associated with radiotherapy failure in head and neck cancer patients recruited in the CHART randomized trial. J. Clin. Oncol., 24(5), 727-35.

Kurimoto M, Endo S, Hirashima Y, Nishijima M, Takaku A (2001). Elevated plasma basic fibroblast growth factor in brain tumor patients. Neurol Med Chir (Tokyo) 36: 865–868; 869, 1996.

Kuroi, K. & Toi, M. Circulating angiogenesis regulators in cancer patients. *Int. J. Biol. Markers*, 16, 5 -26

Kung AL, Zabludoff SD, France DS, Friedmann SJ, Tanner EA, Vieira A, Cornell-Kennon S, Lee J, Wang B, Wang J, Memmert K, Naegeli HU, Petersen F, Eck MJ, Bair KW, Wood AW, Livingston DM: Small molecule blockade of transcriptional coactivation of the hypoxia-inducible factor pathway. *Cancer Cell*, 2004, 6: 33 – 43

Kwon SJ, Lee YJ. Effect of low glutamine/glucose on hypoxia-induced elevation of hypoxia-inducible factor-1alpha in human pancreatic cancer MiaPaCa-2 and human prostatic cancer DU-145 cells. Clin Cancer Res 2005; 11: 4694 - 4700.

Lachat, P., Shaw, P., Gebhard, S., et al. (2002). Expression of NDRG1, a differentiation-related gene, in human tissues. Histochem Cell. Biol, 118, 399–408.

Lee, J. W., Bae, S. H., Jeong, J. W. et al. (2004). Hypoxia-inducible factor (HIF-1) alpha: its protein stability and biological functions. Exp Mol Med, 36, 1–12.

Laderoute, K. R. et al. (2000) Opposing effects of hypoxia on expression of the angiogenic inhibitor thrombospondin 1 and the angiogenic inducer vascular endothelial growth factor. *Clin. Cancer Res.* 6, 2941–2950

Lisztwan, J., Imbert, G., Wirbelauer, C., Gstaiger, M. & Krek, W. (1999). The von Hippel-Lindau tumor suppressor protein is a component of an E3 ubiquitin-protein ligase activity. *Genes & Development*, 13, 1822–1833.

Linderholm B, Tavelin B, Grankvist K, Henriksson R (1999), Does vascular endothelial growth factor (VEGF) predict local relapse and survival in radiotherapy-treated node-negative breast cancer? Br J Cancer 81:727-732

Lin X, Zhang F, Bradbury CM, et al. (2003) 2-Deoxy-D-glucose-induced cytotoxicity and radiosensitization in tumor cells is mediated via disruptions in thiol metabolism. *Cancer Res*.;63:3413–17.

Liu L, Cash TP, Jones RG, et al. (2006), Hypoxia-induced energy stress regulates mRNA translation and cell growth. Mol Cell. 21:521–31.

Liu L, Simon C. (2004), Regulation of transcription and translation by hypoxia. *Cancer Biol Ther*.;3: 492 - 7.

Lu H, Forbes RA, Verma A. (2002), Hypoxia-inducible factor 1 activation by aerobic glycolysis implicates the Warburg effect in carcinogenesis. *J Biol Chem*., 277: 23111-5.

Madan, A., Lin, C., Wang, Z. & Curtin, P. T. (2003). Autocrine stimulation by erythropoietin in transgenic mice results in erythroid proliferation without neoplastic transformation. Blood Cells Mol Dis, 30, 82–89.

Mangiardi, J. R. & Yodice, P. (1990). Metabolism of the malignant astrocytoma. *Neurosurgery*, 26, 1-19.

Mayer, R., Hamilton-Farrell, M. R., van der Kleij, A. J. et al. (2005). Hyperbaric oxygen and radiotherapy. *Strahlenther Onkol.*, 181, 113–23.

Maher JC, Krishan A, Lampidis TJ. (2004) Greater cell cycle inhibition and cytotoxicity induced by 2 deoxy-D-glucose in tumor cells treated under hypoxic vs aerobic conditions. *Cancer Chemother Pharmacol*.;53: 116 - 22.

Mateo J, Garcia-Lecea M, Cadenas S, et al. (2003), Regulation of hypoxia-inducible factor-1alpha by nitric oxide through mitochondria-dependent and -independent pathways. Biochem J;376:537-44.

Moeller BJ, Cao Y, Li CY, Dewhirst MW (2004), Radiation activates HIF-1 to regulate vascular radiosensitivity in tumors: role of reoxygenation, free radicals, and stress granules. *Cancer Cell*, 5: 429 – 441

Mazure, N. M., Chen, E. Y., Yeh, P., Laderoute, K. R. & Giaccia, A. J (1996). Oncogenic transformation and hypoxia synergistically act to modulate vascular endothelial growth factor expression. *Cancer Res.* 56, 3436–3440

Macheda ML, Rogers S, Best JD, (2005), Molecular and cellular regulation of glucosetransporter (GLUT) proteins in cancer, J. Cell. Physiol, 202:654–62.

Melillo, G., Musso, T., Sica, A., Taylor, L. S., Cox, G. W. & Varesio, L. (1995). A hypoxia-responsive element mediates a novel pathway of activation of the inducible nitric oxide synthase promoter. *J Exp Med.*, 182(6), 1683-93.

Mies, G., Paschen, W., Ebhardt, G. & Hossmann, K. A. (1990). Relationship between of blood flow, glucose metabolism, protein synthesis, glucose and ATP content in experimentally-induced glioma (RG1 2.2) of rat brain. *J Neurooncol.*, 9, 17-28.

Molineux, G. (2003). Biology of erythropoietin. In: G. Molineux, M. A. Foote, & S. G. Elliot (Eds.), Erythropoietins and erythropoiesis. (pp. 113-133). Basel: Birkhäuser.

Molls, M., Stadler, P., Becker, A., et al. (1998). Relevance of oxygen in radiation oncology. Mechanisms of action, correlation to low hemoglobin levels. *Strahlenther Onkol.*, 174, Suppl: 13–6.

Nagamatsu, S., Nakamichi, Y., Inoue, N., Inoue, M., Nishino, H. & Sawa, H. (1996). Rat C6 glioma cell growth is related to glucose transport and metabolism. *Biochem J.*, 319 (Pt 2), 477-482.

Nodin, C., Nilsson, M. & Blomstrand, F. (2005). Gap junction blockage limits intercellular spreading of astrocytic apoptosis induced by metabolic depression. *Journal of Neurochemistry*, 94(4), 1111-23.

Nordsmark, M., Bentzen, S. M., Rudat, V. et al. (2005). Prognostic value of tumor oxygenation in 397 head and neck tumors after primary radiation therapy. An international multi-center study. Radiother Oncol, 77, 18 – 24.

Ohh, M., Park, C. W., Ivan, M., Hoffman, M. A., Kim, T. Y., Huang, L. E., Pavletich, N., Chau, V. & Kaelin, W. G. (2000). Ubiquitination of hypoxia-inducible factor requires direct binding to the beta-domain of the von Hippel-Lindau protein. *Nature Cell Biology*, 2, 423–427.

Opavsky, R., Pastoreková, S., Zelník, V., Gibadulinová, A., Stanbridge, E. J., Závada, J., Kettmann, R. & Pastorek, J. (1996). Human MN/CA9 gene, a novel member of the carbonic anhydrase family: structure and exon to protein domain relationship. *Genomics*, 33, 480-487.

Oudard, S., Boitier, E., Miccoli, L., Rousset, S., Dutrillaux, B. & Poupon, M. F. (1997). Gliomas are driven by glycolysis: putative roles of hexokinase, oxidative phosphorylation and mitochondrial ultrastructure. Anticancer Res, 17, 1903-1911.

Overgaard, J. (1989). Sensitization of hypoxic tumour cells – clinical experience, *Int J. Radiat. Biol.*, 56, 801 – 11.

Olive PL, Aquino-Parsons C, MacPhail SH, Liao SY, Raleigh JA, Lerman MI, Stanbridge EJ, (2001), Carbonic anhydrase 9 as an endogenous marker for hypoxic cells in cervical cancer, Cancer Res. 61(24):8924-9.

Parkkila, S., Rajaniemi, H., Parkkila, A. K., Kivelä, J., Waheed, A., Pastoreková, S., Pastorek, J. & Sly, W. S. (2000). Carbonic anhydrase inhibitor suppresses invasion of renal cancer cells in vitro. PNAS, 5, 2220–2224.

Pastorek, J., Pastoreková, S., Callebaut, I., Mornon, J. P., Zelník, V., Opavsky, R., Zatóvicová, M., Liao, S., Portetelle, D., Stanbridge, E. J., Závada, J., Burny, A. & Kettmann, R. (1994). Cloning and characterization of MN, a human tumor- associated protein with a domain homologous to carbonic anhydrase and a putative helix-loop-helix DNA binding segment, Oncogene, 9, 2788- 2888.

Pastoreková, S., Parkkila, S., Parkkila, A. K., Opavsky, R., Zelník, V., Saarnio, J. & Pastorek, J. (1997). Carbonic anhydrase IX, MN/CA IX: analysis of stomach complementary DNA sequence and expression in human and rat alimentary tracts. *Gastroenterology*, 112, 398-408.

Pastorekova, S. & Zavada, J. (2004). Carbonic anhydrase IX (CA IX) as a potential target for cancer therapy. Cancer Ther, 2, 245–62.

Pastorekova S, Casini A, Scozzafava A, Vullo D, Pastorek J, Supuran CT (2004). Carbonic anhydrase inhibitors: the first selective, membrane-impermeant inhibitors targeting the tumor-associated isozyme IX. *Bioorg Med. Chem Lett.* 23; 14(4): 869 - 73.

Prendergast G C, Cole M D (1989), Posttranscriptional regulation of cellular gene expression by the c-myc oncogene, *Mol. Cell Biol.* 9(1): 124–134.

Pfeiffer, T., Schuster, S. & Bonhoeffer, S. (2001). Cooperation and competition in the evolution of ATP-producing pathways. *Science*, 292, 504–7.

Piquemal, D., Joulia, D. & Commes, T. (1999). Transforming growth factor-ß1 is an autocrine mediator of U937 cell growth arrest and differentiation induced by vitamin D3 and retinoids. Biochim. Biophys. Acta, 1450, 364–73.

Plate KH, Breier G, Weich HA, RisauW (1992), Vascular endothelial growth factor is a potential tumour angiogenesis factor in human gliomas in vivo. *Nature*, 359: 845–848

Qu, X. Zhai, Y. Wei, H. et al. (2002). Characterization and expression of three novel differentiation - related genes belong to the human NDRG gene family. *Mol Cell Biochem.*, 229, 35–44.

Reitzer, L. J., Wice, B. M. & Kennell, D. (1979). J Biol Chem, 254, 2669–2676.

Rhodes, C. G., Wise, R. J., Gibbs, J. M., Frackowiak, R. S., Hatazawa, J., Palmer, A. J., Thomas, D. G. & Jones, T. (1983). In vivo disturbance of the oxidative metabolism of glucose in human cerebral gliomas. *Ann Neurol.*, 14, 614-626.

Richard, D. E., Berra, E. & Pouyssegur, J. (1999). Angiogenesis: how a tumor adapts to hypoxia. Biochem. Biophys. Res. Commun., 266, 718-722.

Rohrer Bley, C., Ohlerth, S., Roos, M., et al. (2006). Influence of pretreatment polarographically measured oxygenation levels in spontaneous canine tumors treated with radiation therapy. Strahlenther Onkol, 182, 518 – 24.

Roslin, M., Henriksson, R., Bergstrom, P., Ungerstedt, U. & Bergenheim, A. T. (2003). Baseline levels of glucose metabolites, glutamate and glycerol in malignant glioma assessed by stereotactic microdialysis. *J Neurooncol.*, 61, 151-160.

Rofstad, E. K. (2000).Microenvironment-induced cancer metastasis. *Int. J. Radiat. Biol.* 76, 589–605

Said, H. M., Katzer, A., Flentje, M. & Vordermark, D. (2005) Response of the plasma hypoxia marker osteopontin to in vitro hypoxia in human tumor cells. *Radiother Oncol.*, 76, 200-5.

Said, H. M., Katzer, A., Flentje, M. & Vordermark D. (2006). Response of the plasma hypoxia marker osteopontin to in vitro hypoxia in human tumor cells. Radiother Oncol., Letter to the editor, 78, 230–231.

Said, H. M., Polat, B., Hagemann, C. et al. (2008). Rapid detection of the hypoxia-regulated CA-IX and NDRG1 gene expression in different glioblastoma cells in vitro. Oncology Rep., 20, 413-419.

Said, H. M., Staab, A., Hagemann, C. et. al. (2007). Distinct patterns of hypoxic expression of carbonic anhydrase IX (CA IX) in human malignant glioma cell lines. *J Neurooncol.*, 81, 27-38.

Said, H. M., Stein, S., Hagemann, C. et al. (In Press). Oxygen-dependent regulation of NDRG1 in human glioblastoma cells in vitro and in vivo. Oncology Rep.

Said, H. M., Stein, S., Hagemann, C., Polat, B., Schömig, B., Staab, A., Theobald, M., Flentje, M., Vordermark, D. (2007). NDRG1 regulation as a response to an alternating hypoxic microenviroment in vivo and in vitro in human brain tumors. *FEBS J*, 274 (s1), 281.

Said H, Stein S, Staab A, Katzer A, Flentje M, Vordermark D: NDRG1 is regulated in human glioblastoma in vitro as a consequence to the changing concentrations of the oxygen Microenviroment. *FEBS J.* 273 (s1):345, 2006.

Sakata, K., Someya, M., Nagakura, H. et al. (2006). A clinical study of hypoxia using endogenous hypoxic markers and polarographic oxygen electrodes. Strahlenther Onkol, 182, 511–7.

Salnikow, K., Davidson, T., Zhang, Q. et al. (2003). The involvement of hypoxia-inducibletranscription factor-1-dependent pathway in nickel carcinogenesis. *Cancer Res.*, 63, 3524–3530.

Schmaltz, C., Hardenbergh, P. H., Wells, A. & Fisher, D. E. (1998). Regulation of proliferation—survival decisions during tumor cell hypoxia. *Mol Cell Biol.*, 18, 2845–2854.

Senger, D. R. et al. Tumor cells secrete a vascular permeability factor that promotes accumulation of ascites fluid. *Science*, 219, 983 - 985 (1983).

Semenza, G. L., Roth, P. H., Fang, H.-M. & Wang L. W. (1994). Transcriptional regulation of genes encoding glycolytic enzymes by hypoxia-inducible factor 1. *J Biol Chem.*, 269, 23757–23763.

Semenza GL, (2003), Targeting HIF-1 for cancer therapy, *Nat. Rev. Cancer*, 3: 721 –732.

Seyfried, T. N., Mukherjee, P., Adams, E., Mulroony, T. & Abate, L. E. (2005) Metabolic Control of Brain Cancer: Role of Glucose and Ketone Bodies. *Proc Amer Assoc Cancer Res.*, 46, 1147.

Seyfried, T. N., Sanderson, T. M., El-Abbadi, M. M., McGowan, R. & Mukherjee, P. (2003). Role of glucose and ketone bodies in the metabolic control of experimental brain cancer. *Br J Cancer*, 89, 1375-1382.

Shannon, A. M., Bouchier-Hayes, D. J., Condron, C. M. & Toomey, D. (2003). Tumor hypoxia, chemotherapeutic resistance and hypoxia-related therapies. *Cancer Treat Rev.*, 29, 297-307.

Sibold, S., Roh, V., Keogh, A. et al. (2007). Hypoxia increases cytoplasmic expression of NDRG1, but is insufficient for its membrane localization in human hepatocellular carcinoma. *FEBS Lett.*, 581, 989–94.

Sobhanifar, S., Aquino-Parsons, C., Stanbridge, E. J. et al. (2005). Reduced expression of hypoxia-inducible factor-1alpha in perinecrotic regions of solid tumors. *Cancer Res.*, 65, 7259–66.

Stubbs M, McSheehy PM, Griffiths JR, Bashford CL(2000), Causes and consequences of tumour acidity and implications for treatment, *Mol. Med. Today*, 6: 15–19.

Supuran CT, Scozzafava A. (2000). Carbonic anhydrase inhibitors: aromatic sulfonamides and disulfonamides act as efficient tumor growth inhibitors. *J Enzyme Inhib.* 15(6): 597 - 610.

Swinson DE, Jones JL, Richardson D, Wykoff C, Turley H, Pastorek J, Harris AL, O´Byrne KJ, (2003), Carbonic anhydrase IX expression, a novel surrogate marker of tumor hypoxia, is associated with a poor prognosis in non- small-cell lung cancer, *J. Clin. Oncol.* 21: 473–482.

Staab A, Löffler J, Said HM, Katzer A, Beyer M, Polat B, Einsele H, Flentje M, Vordermark D, (2007) Modulation of glucose metabolism inhibits hypoxic accumulation of hypoxia-inducible factor-1alpha (HIF-1alpha). *Strahlenther Onkol.* 183(7):366-73.

Stein, S., Thomas, E. K., Herzog, B. et al. (2004). NDRG1 is necessary for p53-dependent apoptosis. *J. Biol. Chem.*, 279, 48930–48940.

Stessels F, Van den Eynden G, Van der Auwera I, Salgado R, Van den Heuvel E, Harris AL, Jackson DG, Colpaert CG, van Marck EA, Dirix LY, Vermeulen PB (2004). Breast adenocarcinoma liver metastases, in contrast to colorectal cancer liver metastases, display a non-angiogenic growth pattern that preserves the stroma and lacks hypoxia. *Br. J. Cancer*, 90, 1429–1436

Strohman, R. (2002). Maneuvering in the complex path from genotype to phenotype. *Science*, 296, 701-703.

Stryer, L. (1988). Biochemistry (3rd edition, pp. 420–1). New York: Freeman and Company.

Svastová, E., Hulíková, A., Rafajová, M., Zatovicová, M., Gibadulinová, A., Casini, A., Cecchi, A., Scozzafava, A., Supuran, C. T., Pastorek, J., Pastoreková, S. (2004). Hypoxia activates the capacity of tumor-associated carbonic anhydrase IX to acidify extracellular pH, *FEBS Letters*, 577(3), 439–445.

Takeshita, A., Shinjo, K., Naito, K., Ohnishi, K., Higuchi, M. & Ohno, R. (2002). Erythropoietin receptor in myelodysplastic syndrome and leukemia. *Leuk Lymphoma*, 43, 261–264.

Tanimoto, K., Makino, Y., Pereira, T. & Poellinger, L. (2000). Mechanism of regulation of the hypoxia-inducible factor-1 alpha by the von Hippel-Lindau tumor suppressor protein. *EMBO J.*, 19(16), 4298-309.

Toi M, Matsumoto T, Bando H (2001), Vascular endothelial growth factor: its prognostic, predictive, and therapeutic implications. *Lancet Oncol.* 2: 667-673

Teicher BA, Liu SD, Liu JT, Holden SA, Herman TS. (1993), carbonic anhydrase inhibitor as a potential modulator of cancer therapies, *Anticancer Res.* 13:1549 – 1556

Tisdale, M. J. (1997). Biology of cachexia.. *J Natl Cancer Inst.*, 89, 1763-1773.

van Belzen, N. Dinjens, W. N., Diesveld, M. P. et al. (1997). A novel gene which is up-regulated during colon epithelial cell differentiation and down-regulated in colorectal neoplasms. *Lab Invest.*, 77, 85–92.

Vaupel, P., Mayer, A. & Hoeckel, M. (2006) Impact of haemoglobin levels on tumor oxygenation: the higher, the better?. *Strahlenther Onkol.*, 182, 63–71.

Vaupel, P., Mayer, A. & Hoeckel, M. (2004). Tumor hypoxia and malignant progression. *Methods Enzymol*, 381, 335–354.

Varshney R, Dwarakanath B, Jain V. (2005), Radiosensitization by 6-aminonicotinamide and 2-deoxy D glucose in human cancer cells. *Int J Radiat Biol.*; 81: 397 - 408.

Veech, R. L. (2004). The therapeutic implications of ketone bodies: the effects of ketone bodies in pathological conditions: ketosis, ketogenic diet, redox states, insulin resistance, and mitochondrial metabolism. *Prostaglandins Leukot Essent Fatty Acids*, 70, 309-319.

Vordermark, D., Kaffer, A., Riedl, S., Katzer, A. & Flentje, M. (2005). Characterization of carbonic anhydrase IX (CA IX) as an endogenous marker of chronic hypoxia in live human tumor cells. *Int J Radiat Oncol Biol Phys.*, 61, 1197–1207.

Vordermark, D., Katzer, A., Baier, K. et al. (2004). Cell-type-specific association of hypoxia-inducible factor-1alpha (HIF-1α) protein accumulation and radiobiologic tumor hypoxia. *Int J Radiat Oncol Biol Phys.*, 58, 1242–50.

Vordermark, D., Kraft, P., Katzer, A., Bolling, T., Willner, J. & Flentje, M. (2005). Glucose requirement for hypoxic accumulation of hypoxia-inducible factor-1alpha (HIF-1alpha). *Cancer Lett.*, 230, 122–133.

Vordermark, D., Said, H. M., Katzer, A. et. al. (2006). Immunohistochemical detection of osteopontin in advanced head- and-neck cancer: prognostic role and correlation with oxygen electrode measurements, hypoxia-inducible-factor-1alpha-related markers, and hemoglobin levels. *Int J Radiat Oncol Biol Phys.*, 66(5), 1481-7.

Wang, G. L., Jiang, B. H., Rue, E. A. & Semenza, G. L. (1995). Hypoxia-inducible factor 1 is a basic-helix-loop-helix-PAS heterodimer regulated by cellular O2 tension. *PNAS*, 92, 5510-4.

Wang, T., Marquardt, C. & Foker, J. (1976). *Nature*, 261, 702–705.

Warburg, O. (1925). Klin Wochenschr Berl, 4, 534–536.

Warburg O. (1930). The metabolism of tumors, Constable Press.

Westenfelder, C., Baranowski, R. L. (2000). Erythropoietin stimulates proliferation of human renal carcinoma cells. *Kidney Int.*, 58, 647–657.

Welsh S, Williams R, Kirkpatrick L, Paine-Murrieta G, Powis G. (2004), Antitumor activity and pharmacodynamic properties of PX - 478, an inhibitor of hypoxia-inducible factor-1alpha. *Mol Cancer Ther.*, 3: 233 - 244.

Wingo, T., Tu, C., Laipis, P. J., Silverman, D. N. (2001). The catalytic properties of human carbonic anhydrase IX. *Biochem Biophys. Res. Commun.* 288, 666-669.

Wykoff, CC., Beasley, N., Watson, P., Turner, L., Pastorek, J., Wilson, G., Turley, H., Maxwell, P., Pugh, C., Ratcliffe, P. & Harris, A. (2000). Hypoxia-inducible regulation of tumor-associated carbonic anhydrases. *Cancer Res.*, 60, 7075-7083.

Yasuda, Y., Fujita, Y., Masuda, S., Musha, T., Ueda, K., Tanaka, H., Fujita, H., Matsuo, T., Nagao, M., Sasaki, R. & Nakamura, Y. (2002). Erythropoietin is involved in growth and angiogenesis in malignant tumours of female reproductive organs. *Carcinogenesis*, 23, 1797–1805.

Yasuda, Y., Musha, T., Tanaka, H., Fujita, Y., Fujita, H., Utsumi, H., Matsuo, T., Masuda, S., Nagao, M., Sasaki, R. & Nakamura, Y. (2001). Inhibition of erythropoietin signalling destroys xenografts of ovarian and uterine cancers in nude mice. *Br J Cancer*, 84, 836–843.

Yasuda S, Arii S, Mori A, et al. (2004), Hexokinase II and VEGF expression in liver tumors: correlation with hypoxia-inducible factor-1a and its significance. *J Hepatol*; 40: 117–23.

Yun H, Lee M, Kim SS, et al. (2005), Glucose deprivation increases mRNA stability of vascular endothelial growth factor through activation of AMP-activated protein kinase in DU145 prostate carcinoma. *J Biol Chem*; 280: 9963 -72.

Závada, J., Závadová, Z., Pastorek, J., Biesová, Z., Jezek, K. & Velek, J. (2000). Human tumour-associated cell adhesion protein mediating cell adhesion. *Br. J Cancer*, 82, 1808-1813.

Závada, J., Závadová, Z., Pastoreková, S., Ciampor, F., Pastorek, J. & Zelník, V. (1993). Expression of MaTu-MN protein in human tumor cultures and in clinical specimens. *Int. J. Cancer*, 54, 268-274.

Zhang, P., Tchou-Wong, K. M. & Costa, M. (2007). Egr-1 mediates hypoxia-inducible transcription of the NDRG1 gene through an overlapping Egr-1/Sp1 binding site in the promoter. *Cancer Res.*, 67(19), 9125-9133.

In: Neuro-Oncology and Cancer Targeted Therapy
Editor: Lucía M. Gutiérrez pp.99-108
ISBN 978-1-61668-708-3
© 2010 Nova Science Publishers, Inc.

Chapter 3

GENETICS OF RARE PEDIATRIC BRAIN TUMORS OF CHILDHOOD

Elvis Terci Valera[*], María Sol Brassesco[†] and Luiz Gonzaga Tone*

University of São Paulo, Brazil.

ABSTRACT

Brain cancers are the most common solid tumors affecting children and adolescents. According to the last World Health Organization (WHO) classification of tumors of the central nervous system (CNS), more than one hundred different histological subtypes can primarily arise in the brain or spine. Cytogenetic and molecular information about these tumors is very heterogeneous and usually revised and pooled data about this topic are only available for the most prevalent subtypes. Although the molecular pathways involved in the initiation or progression of rare tumors may provide important evidence about the genetic mechanisms of tumorigenesis, the literature lacks systematic reviews of this topic. This chapter aims to gather and review recent information about conventional and molecular genetic findings for rare (1% or less) pediatric CNS tumors.

Keywords: Cytogenetics; brain cancer; rare tumors; children.

INTRODUCTION

Cancer in children is a rare event. Among the various tissues and organs that may potentially give rise to childhood solid tumor, the central nervous system (CNS) is the most frequent site of origin. According to the last revision of the World Health Organization

---

[*] Address for correspondence: Elvis Terci Valera, MD, PhD, Hospital das Clínicas da Faculdade de Medicina de Ribeirão Preto – Universidade de São Paulo. Departamento de Puericultura e Pediatria., Av. Bandeirantes, 3900 – Bairro Monte Alegre, CEP 14049-900. Ribeirão Preto – SP, Brazil., Tel: 55 16 36022772, Fax: 55 16 36022700, email: etvalera@hcrp.fmrp.usp.br

[†] Brassesco, MS and Valera ET contributed equally.

(WHO) classification of tumors of the CNS, there are more than one hundred different histological subtypes that can primarily arise in the brain or spine (Louis *et al.*, 2007). Genetic information about the less prevalent subtypes of CNS tumors, particularly in children and adolescents, is very scarce. The molecular pathways involved in the initiation or progression of rare tumors are of great interest since they can provide important evidence about the genetic mechanisms of tumorigenesis and insights about the diagnosis and treatment of these growths. In this chapter, we pooled and described recent information about the genetic and molecular findings regarding rare pediatric CNS tumors.

1. ASTROCYTIC TUMORS

I. Pleomorphic Xanthoastrocytoma

Pleomorphic astrocytomas (PXA) were initially described by Kepes *et al.* in 1979. These are rare grade II tumors that typically occur in children and young adults in superficial cerebral locations. Since PXA account for less than 1% of all astrocytic tumors and are very rare, few genetic studies have been performed on them and, as a result, the molecular pathways associated with their pathogenesis are still poorly understood.

Early studies have shown that PXA lack loss of heterozygosity (LOH) at 1p or 19q and only rarely present LOH involving 10q (Paulus *et al.*, 1996). Other reports have demonstrated that genes such as *CDK4*, *MDM2*, or *EGFR* are not amplified in these tumors (Kaulich *et al.*, 2002), suggesting that the genetic events that underlie PXA formation and progression might differ significantly from those typically associated with the diffusely infiltrating astrocytic and oligodendroglial gliomas.

MDM2 protein hyperexpression (Matsumoto *et al.*, 2004) and *P53* mutations have been described (Louis, 1994; Nasuha *et al.*, 2003); however, in most cases the results appear to be inconclusive due to the reduced sampling.

Cytogenetically, Yin *et al*, (2002) showed by comparative genome hybridization (CGH) gain of chromosome 7 and loss of 8p in two of three cases studied. Further studies by CGH characterized 50 PXA and found the most common imbalance to be loss of chromosome 9 in 50% of tumors, while other chromosomal imbalances including losses of chromosomes 8, 17, 18, 22 and gains of chromosomes X, 4, 5, 7, 9q, 19 and 20 were restricted to less than 20% of the tumors (Weber *et al.*, 2007). Array-CGH performed by the same group identified a critical region at 9p21.3 which contains the *CDKN2A/p14ARF* and *CDKN2B* loci (Weber *et al.*, 2007), disagreeing with previous results on 62 PXA that had previously shown that those genes did not reveal any homozygous deletion, mutation, promoter hypermethylation, or complete loss of mRNA expression (Kaulich *et al.*, 2002).

More recently, Grau *et al.* (2009) demonstrated another specific subchromosomal instability profile for PXA tumor samples. These authors showed that primary and relapsed tumors presented subtelomeric duplication at 3pter, 14qter and 19pter; and deletion at 4qter, 6qter, 9qter, 17pter, 18qter and 21qter, suggesting that the candidate gene(s) located in these regions may play a role in the development of PXA.

II. Giant Cell Glioblastoma

Giant cell glioblastoma (GCG) is a rare histological variant of glioblastoma that displays bizarre and multinucleated giant cells. This lesion accounts for less than 5% of all glioblastomas. Most GCG evolve rapidly but there are more recent reports on this variant that indicate a more indolent clinical course (Kozak & Moody, 2009). These lesions frequently carry *TP53* mutations (Louis *et al.*, 2007). Other genetic features of pediatric glioblastomas are poorly defined and some of the most characteristic genetic alterations present in their adult counterparts, such as *EGFR* amplification and *PTEN* mutations, are uncommon in the pediatric setting (Rood *et al.*, 2005). To date, only a handful of studies investigating the molecular biology of childhood GCG have been performed, mainly because of the difficulty in obtaining a large enough series of samples. High frequencies of *TP53* mutations have been found in adult and pediatric GCG (Peraud *et al.*, 1999). Cytogenetic studies have been seldom reported. Bigner *et al.* (1985) studied the chromosomes of a giant cell glioblastoma from an 11-year-old girl which was found to be near haploid and to include two copies of chromosomes 1, 7 or 7p+, and 18. More recently, Dahlback *et al.* (2009) reported a case of GCG from an 18-year-old boy with a karyotype consisting of 46 to 51 chromosomes, with tetraploidy of chromosomes 7 and 12 and structural rearrangements involving chromosomes 13 and 15 as the most common aberrations. Our group has also obtained clinical and cytogenetic findings for two children with GCG. The first case was an HIV-positive (vertical transmission) 16 year-old female who presented multiple heterogeneous tumors in the frontal lobes. The other case was of a 7-year-old female with a large mass within the left temporal lobe. The cytogenetic analysis of cultured tumor cells from case #1 showed a normal karyotype (46,XX). Conversely, the analysis of chromosome metaphase spreads from case #2 showed cytogenetic heterogeneity, with structural and numerical aberrations. No normal cells were found. The composite karyotype was denoted as 45-48, X, -X [3], -6[3], -10[3], -13[3], -15[3], -22[3], +mar [9], [cp20] (Figure 1). These observations reinforce the heterogenous genetic background usually present in this rare histological variant of glioblastoma.

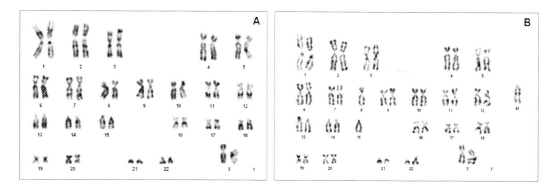

Figure 1. Cytogenetic analysis of GCG cultured cells. A) 46, XX normal karyotype from *patient 1*; B) GTG-banded metaphase from *patient 2* showing a 45, XX, -8, -15, +mar karyotype.

III. Oligoastrocytoma (WHO Grade II)

Oligoastrocytomas (OA) correspond to WHO grade II lesions that usually occur in middle-aged individuals (35-45 years) (Sarkar *et al.*, 2009) and are very rarely observed in the pediatric population. OA usually present as diffusely infiltrative lesions in cerebral hemispheres and, at histopathology, are composed of two distinct neoplastic cell types similar to tumor cells observed in oligodendrogliomas and grade II astrocytomas (Louis *et al.*, 2007). As a result, the genetic features observed in OA resemble those of oligodendrogliomas and astrocytomas. About 60% of OA present simultaneous deletion of 1p and 19q (Reddy, 2008) and 50% present *TP53* mutations, although these characteristics are mutually exclusive (Okamoto *et al.*, 2004). However, in children this tumor is extremely rare and to date there are no genetic reports available in this setting.

IV. Atypical Choroid Plexus Papilloma

Choroid plexus tumors are rare CNS lesions that arise from the intraventricular choroid plexus epithelium. These lesions are graded according to their histopathological characteristics as WHO grade I choroid plexus papilloma (CPP), grade II atypical CPP and the aggressive grade III choroid plexus carcinoma (Louis *et al.*, 2007). As atypical CPP is a relative newly described and rare entity, little is known about the genetic background involved in the pathogenesis and progression of this subgroup. To date, only three cases have been reported, revealing no consistent aberrations. Abnormal numerical changes with gains in chromosomes 7, 12 and 20 were reported by Bhattacharjee *et al.* (1997). More recently, our group described an atypical CCP occurring in the posterior fossa of a 16 year-old male with gains of genetic material from almost all chromosomes (Brassesco *et al.*, 2009a). A complementary study of the tumor showed chromosome numbers ranging from 38 to 123, and revealed that polyploidy was associated with dicentric chromosomes in 70% of cells (Figure 2) (Valera *et al.*, 2009). Alternatively, a second case occurring in the fourth ventricle of a 9-month-old male showed a normal chromosome complement by GTG-banding and CGH (Brassesco *et al.*, 2009b).

V. Astroblastoma

Astroblastomas (AB) are rare WHO non-graded CNS lesions with uncertain biological behavior that present as circumscribed, vasocentric glial neoplasms (Louis *et al.*, 2007). The number of cases of AB studied so far is very small. The first cytogenetic analysis performed in AB from a 15-year-old girl revealed an abnormal hypodiploid karyotype with 45 chromosomes and monosomies of chromosomes 10, 21, and 22 and two marker chromosomes (Jay *et al.*, 1993). Later CGH studies performed on a series of 7 patients (mean age 14 years) showed gains of chromosome arm 20q (4/7 tumors) and chromosome 19 (3/7). Interestingly, these gains occurred simultaneously in three cases, pointing to the possibility of a typical cytogenetic profile for AB in addition to their distinctive clinicopathologic features (Brat *et al.*, 2000).

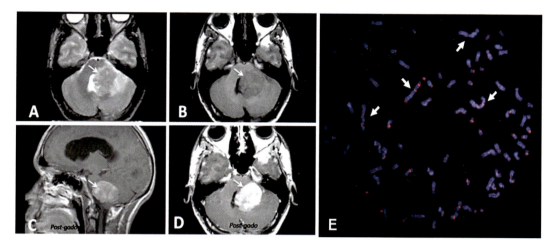

Figure 2. Atypical choroid plexus papilloma in a 16-year-old male. A) Brain MRI with a T2-weighted axial image, B) T1- weighted axial pre-contrast, C) and D) Sagittal and axial post-contrast T1-w images, respectively. The arrows point at the choroid plexus papilloma. E) Hypertriploid metaphase showing dicentric and tricentric chromosomes. The white arrows indicate centromeres (in red) detected by FISH with alphoid DNA.

VI. Choroid Glioma of the Third Ventricle (WHO grade II)

Very few cases of Choroid Glioma of the Third Ventricle (CGTV) have been reported in children and adolescents. To date, there are still no reports on the genetic features of CGTV in children. In the literature only a small series of 4 adult cases has been analyzed by CGH, although no chromosomal imbalances were detected. Furthermore, additional molecular genetic analyses performed on the same samples also failed to detect any aberrations of *TP53* or *CDKN2A* tumor suppressor genes or amplification of the *EGFR*, *CDK4*, and *MDM2* proto-oncogenes (Reinfenberger *et al.*, 1999).

VII. Angiocentric Glioma (WHO grade I)

Angiocentric gliomas (ACG) are slow-growing epileptogenic lesions that primarily affect children and adolescents (Louis *et al.*, 2007). Little is known about the genetic pathways involved in ACG development and progression. To date, only a single study has provided some information about this rare tumor although the results were found to be heterogeneous. While CGH showed chromosomal loss of bands 6q24-q25 in one adult ACG, high-resolution screen by array-CGH identified a copy number gain of 2 adjacent clones from chromosomal band 11p11.2 in two pediatric samples (Preusser *et al.*, 2007).

2. NEURONAL AND MIXED NEURONAL-GLIAL TUMORS

I. Desmoplastic Infantile Astrocytoma and Ganglioglioma (WHO grade I)

Desmoplastic infantile astrocytomas and gangliogliomas (DIAG) are low-grade large cystic tumors that arise in the supratentorial regions (Louis *et al.*, 2007) and display an excellent long-term outcome when total surgical resection is feasible. Only a limited number of cases have been screened for genetic alterations. CGH studies on typical DIAG have shown loss of 8p22-pter in one case and gain of 13q21 in another (Kross *et al.*, 2002). More recently, conventional cytogenetic studies were performed by Cerdá-Nicolás *et al.* (2006) but no clonal aberrations were found. *TP53* mutations are also absent in DIAG (Louis *et al.*, 1992; Kross *et al.*, 2002).

II. Papillary Glioneural Tumors (WHO grade I)

Papillary glioneural tumors (PGNT) are usually circumscribed cerebral lesions that show and indolent clinical course, although late biological progression of malignancy has been described more recently (Javahery *et al.*, 2009). Still, there is no known genetic signature for PGNT. Fluorescent *in situ* hybridization studies have failed to detect any loss of heterozygosity at 1p (Tanaka *et al*, 2005) or 19q (Edgar & Rosenbaum, 2007). Lately, Faria *et al.* (2008) reported a tumor in a 9-year-old girl characterized by gains and structural aberrations involving chromosome 7 with breakpoints at 7p22. By using CGH, the same authors observed a high-level amplification region at 7p14~q12. However, the involvement of this chromosome in PGNT needs further studies.

III. Central Neurocytoma and Extraventricular Neurocytoma

Central neurocytoma (CN) and extraventricular neurocytoma (EN) are WHO grade II neuronal neoplasms that have a peak of incidence in early adulthood. The molecular pathogenesis of CN and EN remains largely unknown. Genetic alterations have been reported such as gain of chromosome 7 in 30% of patients (Taruscio *et al.*, 1997) and gain of chromosomes 2p, 10q, 18q in 40% of the samples analyzed by CGH (Yin *et al.*, 2000). LOH of loci 1p and 19q has been found in some neurocytomas; however, these losses were random and no clear-cut common deletion site was delineated as a diagnostic feature differentiating this entity from oligodendrogliomas (Tong et al., 2000). Unfortunately, although the age of the patients in these studies ranged from 17 to 51 years, the authors did not specify which results corresponded to pediatric patients. Conversely, Jay *et al.* (1999) showed by G-banding and fluorescent in situ hybridization a complex karyotype with a near diploid complement (45-48 chromosomes) with three additional copies of 1q involved in rearrangements with chromosomes 4 and 7, for a neurocytoma in an 11-year-old boy. Absence of 1p and 19q deletions was also demonstrated in an 18-year-old boy with a neurocytoma in the left ventricule (Fujisawa *et al.*, 2002).

3. TUMORS OF THE PINEAL REGION

I. Pineocytoma (WHO grade I)

Pineocytoma (PC) is a pineal parenchymal neoplasm primarily composed of mature-appearing pineocytes (Louis *et al.*, 2007). These are well-circumscribed lesions on the pineal topography with very limited potential to metastasize. Until now, cytogenetic and molecular data on PC have been sparse and inconclusive. For adult PC, numerical alterations involving chromosomes X, 5, 8, 11, 14, and 22, and structural alterations of chromosomes 1, 3, 12, and 22 were described for a 29-years-old woman (Rainho *et al.*, 1992). Alternatively, further studies by CGH were unable to detect any gains or losses in three adult PC (Rickert *et al.*, 2001). There are still no data on genetic alterations for PC in children.

II. Papillary Tumor of the Pineal Region

Papillary tumor of the pineal region (PTPR) is a very rare neuroepithelial tumor of the pineal site, with the few cases reported to date having been observed in the age range from 5 to 66 years (Louis *et al.*, 2007). Nevertheless, PTPR has been most frequently observed in adolescents. Currently, there is a single study about the genetic alterations occurring in PTPR. Hasselblatt and co-workers (2006) demonstrated losses of chromosome 10 (4/5 cases) and 22q (3/5 cases) as well as gains of chromosomes 4 (4/5 cases), 8 (3/5 cases), 9 (3/5 cases) and 12 (3/5 cases) by CGH. However, the age of the patients was not detailed by the authors.

ACKNOWLEDGMENTS

We are grateful to Prof. Antonio Carlos dos Santos for the MRI images presented in Figure 2.

REFERENCES

Bhattacharjee, MB; Armstrong, DD; Vogel, H; Cooley, LD. Cytogenetic analysis of 120 primary pediatric brain tumors and literature review. *Cancer Genet Cytogenet*, 1997, 97(1):39-53.

Bigner, SH; Mark, J; Schuld, SC; Eng, LF; Bigner, DD. A serially transplantable human giant cell glioblastoma that maintains a near haploid stem line. *Cancer Genet. Cytogenet*, 1985, 18: 141-154.

Brassesco, MS; Valera, ET; Neder, L; Castro-Gamero, AM; Arruda, D; Machado, HR; Sakamoto-Hojo, ET; Tone, LG. Polyploidy in atypical grade II choroid plexus papilloma of the posterior fossa. *Neuropathology*, 2009, 29(3):293-298 (a).

Brassesco, MS; Valera, ET; Becker, AP; Oliveira, RS; Scrideli, CA; Machado, HR; Tone LG. Grade II atypical choroid plexus papilloma with normal karyotype. *Childs Nerv Syst*, 2009, 25(12):1623-1626 (b).

Brat, DJ; Hirose, Y; Cohen, KJ; Feuerstein, BG; Burger, PC. Astroblastoma: clinicopathologic features and chromosomal abnormalities defined by comparative genomic hybridization. *Brain Pathol*, 2000, 10(3):342-52.

Cerdá-Nicolás, M; Lopez-Gines, C; Gil-Benso, R; Donat, J; Fernandez-Delgado, R; Pellin, A; Lopez-Guerrero, JA; Roldan, P; Barbera, J. Desmoplastic infantile ganglioglioma. Morphological, immunohistochemical and genetic features. *Histopathology*, 2006, 48(5):617-621.

Dahlback, HS; Brandal, P; Meling, TR; Gorunova, L; Scheie, D; Heim, S. Genomic aberrations in 80 cases of primary glioblastoma multiforme: Pathogenetic heterogeneity and putative cytogenetic pathways. *Genes Chromosomes Cancer*, 2009,48(10):908-924.

Edgar, MA; Rosenblum, MK. Mixed glioneuronal tumors: recently described entities. *Arch Pathol Lab Med*, 2007, 131(2):228-233.

Faria, C; Miguéns, J; Antunes, JL; Barroso, C; Pimentel, J; Martins, Mdo, C; Moura-Nunes, V; Roque L. Genetic alterations in a papillary glioneuronal tumor. *J Neurosurg Pediatr*, 2008, 1(1):99-102.

Fujisawa, H; Marukawa, K; Hasegawa, M; Tohma, Y; Hayashi, Y; Uchiyama, N; Tachibana, O; Yamashita, J. Genetic differences between neurocytoma and dysembryoplastic neuroepithelial tumor and oligodendroglial tumors. *J Neurosurg*, 2002, 97(6):1350-1355.

Hasselblatt, M; Blümcke, I; Jeibmann, A; Rickert, CH; Jouvet, A; van de Nes, JA; Grau, E; Balaguer, J; Canete, A; Martinez, F; Orellana, C; *et al.* Subtelomeric analysis of pediatric astrocytoma: subchromosomal instability is a distinctive feature of pleomorphic xanthoastrocytoma. *J Neurooncol*, 2009, 93:175-182.

Kuchelmeister, K; Brunn, A; Fevre-Montange, M; Paulus, W. Immunohistochemical profile and chromosomal imbalances in papillary tumours of the pineal region. *Neuropathol Appl Neurobiol*, 2006, 32(3):278-283.

Javahery, RJ; Davidson, L; Fangusaro, J; Finlay, JL; Gonzalez-Gomez, I; McComb, JG. Aggressive variant of a papillary glioneuronal tumor. Report of 2 cases. *J Neurosurg Pediatr*, 2009, 3(1):46-52.

Jay, V; Edwards, V; Hoving, E; Rutka, J; Becker, L; Zielenska, M; Teshima I. Central neurocytoma: morphological, flow cytometric, polymerase chain reaction, fluorescence in situ hybridization, and karyotypic analyses. Case report. *J Neurosurg*, 1999, 90(2):348-354.

Jay, V; Edwards, V; Squire, J; Rutka, J. Astroblastoma: report of a case with ultrastructural, cell kinetic, and cytogenetic analysis. *Pediatr Pathol*, 1993, 13(3):323-332.

Kaulich, K; Blaschke, B; Nümann, A; von Deimling, A; Wiestler, OD; Weber, RG; Reifenberger G. Genetic alterations commonly found in diffusely infiltrating cerebral gliomas are rare or absent in pleomorphic xanthoastrocytomas. *J Neuropathol Exp Neurol*, 2002, 61(12):1092-1099.

Kepes, JJ; Rubinstein, LJ; Eng, LF. Pleomorphic xanthoastrocytoma: a distinctive meningocerebral glioma of young subjects with relatively favorable prognosis. A study of 12 cases. *Cancer*, 1979 44(5):1839-1852.

Kozak, KR; Moody, JS. Giant cell glioblastoma: a glioblastoma subtype with distinct epidemiology and superior prognosis. *Neuro Oncol*, 2009, 11(6):833-841.

Kros, JM; Delwel, EJ; de Jong, TH; Tanghe, HL; van Run PR; Vissers K; Alers JC. Desmoplastic infantile astrocytoma and ganglioglioma: a search for genomic characteristics. *Acta Neuropathd*, 2002, 104:144-148.

Louis, DN. The p53 gene and protein in human brain tumors. *J Neuropathol Exp Neurol*, 1994, 53:11–21.

Louis, DN; Deimling, A; Dickersin, GR; Dooling, EC; Seizinger, BR. Desmoplastic cerebral astrocytomas of infancy: a histopathologic, immunohistochemical, ultrastructural, and molecular genetic study. *Hum Pathol*, 1992, 23:1402–1409.

Louis, DN; Ohgaki, H; Wiestler, OD; Cavenee, WK (Eds): WHO classification of tumours of the central nervous system. Lyon: IARC; 2007.

Matsumoto, K; Suzuki, SO; Fukuiand, M; Iwaki T. Accumulation of MDM2 in pleomorphic xanthoastrocytomas. *Pathology International*, 2004, 54: 387-391.

Nasuha, NA; Daud, AH; Ghazali, MM; Yusoff, AAM; *et al.*, Molecular Genetic Analysis of Anaplastic Pleomorphic Xanthoastrocytoma. *Asian Journal of Surgery*, 2003, 26 (2):120-126.

Okamoto, Y; Di Patre, PL; Burkhard, C; Horstmann, S; Jourde, B; Fahey, M; Schuler, D; Probst-Hensch, NM; Yasargil, MG; Yonekawa, Y; Lutolf, UM; Kleihues, P; Ohgaki, H. Population-based study on incidence, survival rates, and genetic alterations of low-grade diffuse astrocytomas and oligodendrogliomas. *Acta Neuropathol*, 2004, 108:49-56.

Paulus, W; Lisle, DK; Tonn, JC; Wolf, HK; Roggendorf, W; Reeves, SA; Louis, DN; Molecular genetic alterations in pleomorphic xanthoastrocytoma. *Acta Neuropathol*, 1996, 91(3):293-297.

Peraud, A; Watanabe, K; Schwechheimer, K; Yonekawa, Y; Kleihues, P; Ohgaki, H; Genetic profile of the giant cell glioblastoma. *Lab Invest*, 1999, 79:123-129.

Preusser, M; Hoischen, A ; Novak, K ; Czech, T ; Prayer, D *et al*. Angiocentric glioma: report of clinico-pathologic and genetic findings in 8 cases. *Am J Surg Pathol*, 2007, 31(11):1709-18.

Rainho, CA; Rogatto, SR; de Moraes, LC; Barbieri-Neto, J. Cytogenetic study of a pineocytoma. *Cancer Genet Cytogenet*, 1992, 64(2):127-132.

Reddy, KS. Assessment of 1p/19q deletions by fluorescence in situ hybridization in gliomas. *Cancer Genetics and Cytogenetics*, 2008, 184:77-86.

Reifenberger, G; Weber, T; Weber, RG; Wolter, M, Brandis, A; Kuchelmeister, K; Pilz, P; Rwsche, E; Lichter, P; Wiestler, OD. Chordoid glioma of the third ventricle: immunohistochemical and molecular genetic characterization of a novel tumor entity. *Brain Pathol*, 1999, 9:617-626.

Rickert, CH; Simon, R; Bergmann, M; Dockhorn-Dworniczak, B; Paulus, W. Comparative genomic hybridization in pineal parenchymal tumors. *Genes Chromosomes Cancer*, 2001, 30(1):99-104.

Rood, BR; MacDonald, TJ. Pediatric highgrade glioma: molecular genetic clues for innovative therapeutic approaches. *J Neurooncol*, 2005, 75: 267–272.

Sarkar, C; Jain, A; Suri, V. Current concepts in the pathology and genetics of gliomas. *Indian J Cancer*, 2009, 46(2):108-119.

Tanaka, Y; Yokoo, H; Komori, T; *et al*. A distinct pattern of Olig2-positive cellular distribution in papillary glioneuronal tumors: a manifestation of the oligodendroglial phenotype? *Acta Neuropathol,* 2005;110:39–47.

Taruscio, D; Danesi, R; Montaldi, A; Cerasoli, S; Cenacchi, G; Giangaspero, F. Nonrandom gain of chromosome 7 in central neurocytoma: a chromosomal analysis and fluorescence in situ hybridization study. *Virchows Arch*, 1997, 430(1):47-51.

Tong, CY; Ng, HK; Pang, JC; Hu, J; Hui, AB; Poon, WS. Central neurocytomas are genetically distinct from oligodendrogliomas and neuroblastomas. *Histopathology*, 2000, 37(2):160-165.

Valera, ET; Brassesco, MS; Castro-Gamero, AM; Santos, AC; Oliveira, RS; Machado HR; Neder, L; Sakamoto-Hojo, ET; Tone, LG. Multiple dicentric chromosomes behind polyploidy in grade II atypical choroid plexus papilloma: a complementary cytogenetic evaluation. *Neuropathology*, 2009, 29(2):200-202.

Weber, RG; Hoischen, A; Ehrler, M; Zipper, P; Kaulich, K; et al. Frequent loss of chromosome 9, homozygous CDKN2A/p14ARF/CDKN2B deletion and low TSC1 mRNA expression in pleomorphic xanthoastrocytomas. *Oncogene*, 2007, 26:1088–1097.

Yin, XL; Hui, AB; Liong, EC; Ding, M; Chang, AR; Ng, HK; Genetic imbalances in pleomorphic xanthoastrocytoma detected by comparative genomic hybridization and literature review. *Cancer Genet Cytogenet*, 2002, 132(1):14-19.

Yin, XL; Pang, JC; Hui, AB; Ng HK. Detection of chromosomal imbalances in central neurocytomas by using comparative genomic hybridization. *J Neurosurg*, 2000, 93(1):77-81.

In: Neuro-Oncology and Cancer Targeted Therapy
Editor: Lucía M. Gutiérrez pp.109-139

ISBN 978-1-61668-708-3
© 2010 Nova Science Publishers, Inc.

Chapter 4

MECHANISMS OF IMMUNE EVASION EXHIBITED BY DIFFERENT RAT GLIOMA CELL LINES

Martin R. Jadus[abc]*, Lara Driggers[a], Neil Hoa[a], Jimmy T.H. Pham[a], Josephine Natividad[a], Christina Delgado[a], Edward W.B. Jeffes[d], Eric Giedzinski[e], Charles Limoli[e], and Lisheng Ge[a]

[a] Pathology and Laboratory Medicine Service
Diagnostic and Molecular Medicine Health Care Group
VA Long Beach Healthcare System 5901 E. 7th Street, Long Beach, CA 90822
[b] Department of Pathology and Laboratory Medicine
University of California, Irvine. Irvine, CA 92697-2695
[c] Neuro-Oncology Program
Chao Comprehensive Cancer Center
University of California, Irvine. Orange, CA 92868
[d] Dermatology Service
VA Long Beach Healthcare System Long Beach, CA 90822
[e] Department of Radiation Oncology
University of California, Irvine
Irvine, CA 92697-2695

This study was funded in part from grants obtained from the Veterans Affairs Medical Center (M.R.J.); the Avon Breast Cancer Foundation via the University of California at Irvine Cancer Research Program (M.R.J.); the American Cancer Society RSG-00-036-04-CNE (C.L.L.).

---

* Address reprint requests to:
Dr. Martin R. Jadus
Box 113 Diagnostics and Molecular Health Care Group
VA Long Beach Healthcare System
5901 E 7th Street, Long Beach, CA, 90822 USA
(562) 826-8000 ext 4079 (562) 826-5623 (fax)
E mail: martin.jadus@va.gov

ABSTRACT

Rat glioma cell lines could be considered the previous work horse of experimental glioma research. At least 9 established glioma cell lines exist and they have been used extensively to study many aspects of glioma biology and potential experimental therapeutics. These glioma cells have been defined as either being immunogenic or non-immunogenic, based upon empirical findings. The mechanisms of this immunogenicity/non-immunogenicity have not been fully elucidated. Traditionally, the major mechanisms by which murine tumors were viewed as being non-immunogenic was: by down-regulating the major histocompatibility complex (MHC) antigens, by lacking tumor specific antigens, or by making molecules that prevent the immune system from properly working. D74 glioma cells only showed low MHC class 1 (RT1-A) expression. Other non-immunogenic gliomas (F98, 36B10 and CNS-1) displayed equivalent levels of RT1-A, as their more immunogenic counterparts (RT2, BT4C, C6, 9L/T9). Human glioma cell lines possess numerous tumor-associated antigens. In contrast, rat tumor-associated antigens are relatively few. A plethora of immunosuppressive molecules are made by glioma cell lines. In this chapter we will examine why established rat glioma cell lines can grow in vivo, despite being considered "immunogenic". The intrinsic properties (lack of MHC molecules, self-defense molecules, production of immunosuppressive cytokines/enzymes, counterattack strategies, growth rates and resistance to cell-mediated killing) of these cells may allow various aspects of rat glioma immunology to be explained and may allow investigators to focus on their favorite mechanism of immune evasion.

INTRODUCTION

Human gliomas, especially glioblastoma multiforme (GBM) are extremely difficult cancers to treat. Observe the times of diagnosis and ultimate demises of high profile Americans stricken with GBM: Gene Siskel (movie critic)-12 months, Robert Novak (political pundit)-13 months, and Edward Kennedy (US Senator),-15 months. Long-term survivors do occur as a result of standard radiation and chemotherapies. Four decades ago, the mean survival of GBM was only 7.5 months [1,2], compared to an average of 16 months with current treatments, thus some incremental progress has been made against this disease. The use of the histone deacetylase inhibitor, temozolomide, has improved survival for many patients diagnosed with high grade gliomas and hence has changed the standard of care to include its use [3]. A cure to this disease will require multiple biological interventions coming from multiple disciplines in order to attack this tumor's vulnerable weak spots.

Immunotherapy using antigen loaded dendritic cells has also generated some clinical excitement in that it has lengthened the time to progression for some of these patients [4-6]. These encouraging results suggest that favorable conditions for successful therapies are attainable. This in turn gives researchers hope that cures under certain circumstances can be obtained, if these precise conditions can be successfully reproduced. However, before human trials can begin, experiments must be performed in laboratory animals to assure the various regulatory agencies that these proposed therapies are safe and potentially effective. In fact, some of the improved human survival over the last three to four decades is undoubtedly due to the therapeutic insights gained by using rat glioma cell lines, attesting to their versatility.

EXPERIMENTAL GLIOMA MODELS

Only a few murine glioma cell lines were known for the last decade: GL26, GL261, and 4C8. The development of transgenic (epidermal growth factor receptor [EGFR], platelet growth factor [PDGF], basic fibroblast growth factor [bFGF], K-Ras) and knock-out (AKT, p53, cyclin-dependent kinase-4 [CDK4], phosphatase and tensin homolog [PTEN]) technologies over the last 10 years has provided the genetic tools not previously used in rat glioma models, and has provided systems that yield significant insight into many aspects of gliomagenesis. To view the currently known and used murine GBM models please visit the Mouse Tumor Biology Database from the Jackson Laboratory (http://tumor.informatics.jax.org/mtbwi/index.do). These genetic approaches permit glioma formation to spontaneously occur without the artificial need to surgically implant homogenous tumor cells. The resultant tumors display a more invasive and heterogeneous phenotype, which is similar to the pathology seen in situ human gliomas. This contrasts to those surgically implanted glioma cells that present as more circumscribed tumors with well-defined margins. The discovery of how to successfully culture "stem-like" cells as neurospheres (i.e., highlighting the need for such growth factors as PDGF, FGF and EGF) for primary gliomas and even for non-cancerous "stem-like cells" has also advanced the understanding of the basics of glioma cell biology.

Certain short nosed canine breeds (brachycephalic breeds: Boxers, English and French Bulldogs, and Boston Terriers) are the most susceptible strains for brain cancers, especially astrocytomas and to a lesser degree GBM. These large-size animals mimic several clinical conditions found within humans [7]. The size of their brains (depending on breed) more closely resemble those of their human counterparts and play important roles in regards to performing established surgical interventions, in developing newer surgical interventions and in defining the pharmacokinetics of cytotoxic drugs. The University of Minnesota has instituted a program to treat dogs suffering from gliomas to test convection-enhanced delivery of cytotoxic drugs or with **combination gene therapies** (http://www.modianolab.org/studyInfo/Glioma_1-CED.shtml). These animals are valuable in that the successful treatments they receive can be harbingers of future therapies which humans could soon receive.

Nevertheless rat glioma cell lines have long been considered the work horse of basic glioma biology and experimental therapeutics for the last half century. At least 9 established cell lines (9L also known as T9, D74 also known as RG2, F98, RT2, C6, CNS-1, 36B10, BT4C, B28) have been used to study many medical aspects of this cancer. Recently, Barth and Kaur [8,9] reviewed the history and origins of many of these cell lines which provide good references for those unfamiliar with these rat glioma cell lines. This chapter will expand on those reviews and explain several mechanisms whereby these cells can evade the immune system.

THE BASICS OF BRAIN NEURO-ONCO-IMMUNOLOGY

There are normally three major cell types involved in immune responses towards any cancer: the tumor cells, the antigen presenting cell and the effector lymphoid cells (usually T cells) (Figure 1A). As a result of normal cell shedding, exosome release or cell death induction by therapy, antigenic material is released from the cancer cells. This material is internalized by the local antigen presenting cells (APC). Within the APC, these absorbed antigenic precursor proteins are digested via proteosomal cleavage and the antigenic peptides are loaded onto the major histocompatibility complex (MHC) molecules within the endoplasmic reticulum. The most potent antigen presenting cell within the body is the dendritic cell. In the brain, however, the microglial cell fills this role as an APC. It has been estimated that about 15% of the cells in the brain are microglial cells [10]. Microglial cells express intercellular adhesion molecules (ICAM), MHC class I and II antigens and co-stimulatory molecules [11-13]. Therefore, the microglial cells can stimulate immune responses by acting as antigen presenting cells. These cells also produce: interleukin-1, interleukin-6, interleukin-12, tumor necrosis factor (TNF) [14-18]. Microglial cells are directly tumoricidal under experimental conditions [17, 19-22].

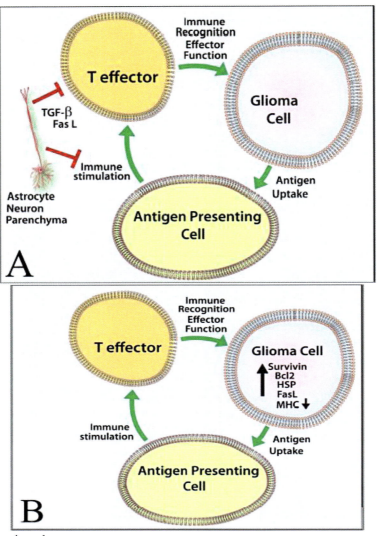

Figure Continued

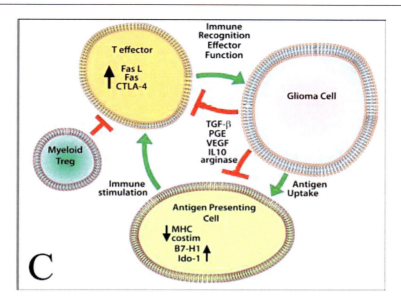

Figure 1. *Basics of glioma immunology.* Panel (A) shows the 3 main cells required for any immune response towards a glioma: the glioma cell, the Antigen Presenting Cell (APC) and the T effecter cells. In addition, the brain parenchyma such as neurons and astrocytes make Transforming Growth Factor-β (TGF- β) and Fas Ligand (Fas L) that can block either APC or T cells. Panel (B) shows that glioma cells make several molecules such as Survivin, Bcl2, heat shock proteins (HSP) or Fas Ligand or have decreased MHC molecules that prevent immune recognition or make the tumor cells harder to kill. Panel (C) shows that the glioma cells can release a number of immunosuppressive molecules (TGF- β, prostaglandins via Cyclooxygenases, VEGF, IL10 and Arginase) that can either inhibit the T cells or APC. These molecules can affect the APC by diminishing the MHC or co-stimulatory molecules needed for proper T cell activation. Or the APC could express inhibitory stimuli like B7-H1 or make Indoleamine 2,3 dioxygenase (Ido-1) that suppress the T cells. Likewise the various inhibitory molecules can activate myeloid suppressor cells or Treg which inhibit the T cells.

Upon APC stimulation of T cells via the correctly peptide loaded MHC and in conjunction with the proper co-stimulatory molecules, these activated lymphoid cells now become the effector cells. These T cells actively seek the tumor cells and begin the killing process upon recognition of the tumor cells. This ability of T cells to selectively destroy tumor cells is perhaps the best advantage that immunotherapy has over surgery, chemotherapy and radiotherapy. These latter three treatments usually cause unintentional collateral damage to normal tissue. If this damage occurs in critical regions of the brain like the brain-stem, pons and other regions that regulate motor skills/life sustaining control centers, the patients die immediately. Thus, many radiation oncologists and neurosurgeons are reluctant to carry out such treatments.

The brain has been considered as an "immunoprivileged site", ever since the time of Peter Medawar [23] in the late 1940's. Since the brain controls many vital physiological responses, it was thought that strong immune responses that damage key neurons could be incompatible with life. Thus, the immune system must be tightly controlled to prevent this deadly possibility. Two molecules (fas ligand and transforming growth factor-β) are believed to make the brain an immunoprivileged site by inhibiting either the APC or the effector lymphocytes [24,25]). Normal parenchymal cells like neurons, glia cells make these immunosuppressive molecules. Thus, any immune response towards brain cancers must first overcome these natural regulatory pathways.

THE REALITIES OF BRAIN CANCER IMMUNOLOGY

The major anti-tumor immune response is thought to be mediated largely through the actions of cytolytic lymphocytes (CD8-positive CTL, NK, NKT). These lymphocytes kill tumor cells by releasing tumor necrosis factor (TNF), lymphotoxin, granzymes and perforin. Additionally these cytolytic effector cells can use cell-surface molecules like fas ligand, membrane-bound TNF or tumor necrosis factor (TNF)-related apoptosis-inducing ligand (TRAIL) to kill tumor cells. CD4-positive T cells can express fas ligand and directly kill only tumor cells that possess the fas antigen [26]. CD4-positive cells release several cytokines (interleukin-2, interleukin-6, interleukin-7, interferon-γ or tumor necrosis factor/lymphotoxin) that activates NK, microglial [21,22], or γδ T cells [27] which can kill the tumor cells. These Th1-mediated effectors are currently thought to be the most effective anti-cancer immune responses. However, this central paradigm in glioma immunology is being challenged by some very interesting, but still circumstantial, clinical evidence.

In a study involving San Francisco area allergy patients, atopic patients had a lowered risk of developing glioma [28]. Those glioma patients with elevated IgE levels survived nine months longer [28]. Glioma patients also have lower serum IgE levels than non-glioma controls [29]. This atopic relationship was confirmed in a larger meta-analysis compiled from eight independent studies that were previously conducted from 1979 to 2007 using 3,450 glioma patients [30]. Interleukin-4 (IL-4) made by T helper type 2 cells, especially high concentrations, is associated with the production of IgE by B cells. IL-4 and granulocyte-macrophage colony stimulatory factor (GM-CSF, derived from both Th1 and Th2 cells) activated dendritic cells can kill glioma cells [31] either through cell-surface interactions or via the release of nitric oxide. Another type of T helper CD4-positive cell type called Th17 cells can also mediate anti-tumor effects through undefined pathways [32,33]. Th17 cells responding to transforming growth factor- β (TGF-β), interleukin-6 (IL-6) and interleukin-23 (IL-23) release a family of cytokines called interleukin-17. IL-17 is a family of six related cytokines (IL-17A to IL-17F) that have a diverse range of biological effects [34-36]. IL-17 can promote tumor killing and tumor immunity [37]. Thus, many cell types and effector cytokines complicate tumor-host relationships. More research is needed to identify the most effective anti-glioma immunocytes and harness their powers against these deadly brain cancers.

Glioma cells are also not passive players. They do possess multiple defense and survival mechanisms (Figure 1B). Glioma cells, like most other cells, are recognized by T cells via their antigenic peptides presented on the cell surface in the context of MHC molecules. Glioma cells can down-regulate their expression of MHC molecules thereby making themselves harder to be recognized by T cells. CD8 cells recognize MHC class I (HLA-A, B or C in human or RT1-A in rats) molecules, while CD4 T cells recognize MHC class II (HLA-DR, DS in human or RT1-B in rats). Human tumor cells can also express non-conventional MHC class Ib molecules (HLA-E and HLA-G), which inhibit immune responses especially with NK cells [38,39]. In rats, there are non-conventional MHC molecules RT1-E2 (equivalent of the human HLA-G and mouse H-2Qa2[40]), but antibodies towards these rat molecules are not commercially available.

Glioma cells can also synthesize molecules that make themselves resistant to being killed either by drugs, radiation or immunotherapy. Some of these defensive molecules are the heat shock proteins (HSP) and anti-apoptotic genes, such as survivin and Bcl2. Tumor cells also release immunomodulatory molecules such as cytokines and enzymes, which create an environment that prevents proper functioning of APC and effector lymphoid cells (Figure 1C). Thus, glioma cells escape cell death through multiple pathways.

Other tumor infiltrating cells are adversely affecting pro-host and anti-tumor immunity. These cells include the myeloid-derived suppressor cells (MDSC) and T regulatory (T reg) cells. As a result of tumor derived cytokines/enzymes or microenvironmental conditions (hypoxia, oxidative stress, lactic acid, metabolic breakdown products, etc), these inhibitory cells now become active and help the tumor to grow by suppressing the anti-tumor actions of the immune system. For more specific reviews of these cell types see [41-46]. Both of these suppressor cell types have been reported being active within experimental and clinical gliomas [47-52]. Another way these regulatory cells inhibit immune responses is to polarize the infiltrative T cells into becoming less potent anti-tumor effector cells, such as becoming Treg.

Lastly, another aspect of T cell biology, not fully appreciated, is that as T cells become fully activated, different T cell homeostatic mechanisms are induced. It has been speculated that multiple pathways were needed to protect the host from over-active immune responses. As naïve T cells get activated, fas, fas ligand, IL-2 receptors (CD25) and cytolytic T lymphocyte antigen-4 (CTLA-4) are induced. These molecules all feed into pathways that can produce activation-induced cell death (AICD)[53,54]. Fas-fas ligand interactions occur in either juxtacrine or autocrine manners. The lack of IL-2 stimulation on CD25-positive T cells can lead to apoptosis via cytokine starvation. CTLA-4 as it becomes expressed interacts with its ligands, CD80 and CD86, found on the dendritic cells. After this interaction both CD8-positive and CD4-positive cells become inhibited, even though under earlier conditions the same DC stimulated the naive T cells into becoming potent anti-tumor effector cells. The use of the anti-CTLA-4 antibody has allowed more profound and better sustained anti-tumor responses to be achieved [55,56]. Those immune responses have built-in self-regulatory properties that must be inhibited to sustain prolonged immune responses against any tumor. Strategies that overcome these inherent T cell homeostatic pathways must be used in any given therapy to generate better clinical outcomes against cancers.

A number of reviews have been published previously exploring the mechanisms of tumor escape, especially with gliomas [57-59]. In light of these diverse processes, one might examine how the various rat glioma cell lines fit into our current views of immunological escape mechanisms.

IMMUNOGENICITY AND NON-IMMUNOGENICITY

Rodent tumors have classically been described as either being immunogenic or non-immunogenic. The experimental design to demonstrate this property is shown in Figure 2. This description is strictly an empirically defined one. Initially, animals are injected with x-irradiated or killed tumor cells. After waiting a short time, the animals are re-injected with a dose of viable cancer cells. If these cancer cells form a tumor, then the vaccinating cancer cells are considered non-immunogenic, because little or no effective immune response was generated that could reject those recently implanted tumor cells. If the cancer cells failed to form tumors, these cells were considered "immunogenic", since some immunological intervention occurred. It has been assumed that human cancers are "non-immunogenic", because these tumors were observed to grow in adults, who appeared to have normal immunity. As shown in Figure 3, both immunogenic and non-immunogenic rat gliomas can grow as either intracranial tumors (Panels A-C) or subcutaneous tumors (Panel D-F). So the assumption that human gliomas are non-immunogenic tumors is largely speculative, since both types of tumors progressively grew in normally healthy animals. One could even speculate that the human gliomas which responded to various immunotherapies [4-6, 61,62] were in fact originally immunogenic tumors.

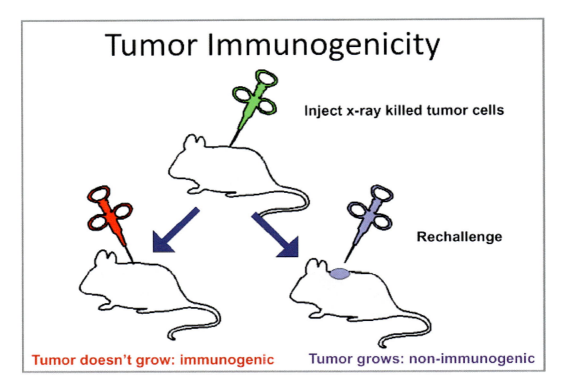

Figure 2. *Tumor Immunogenicity*. To empirically determine immunogenicity, one first injects into animals the killed tumor cells and then wait a period of time. Then one re-challenges the rats with the same tumor cells, except the tumor cells are alive. If the animal fails to form a tumor, then some immune process prevented the tumor cells from growing and these tumor cells are viewed as being immunogenic. If the tumor grows, then the tumor cells were deemed non-immunogenic.

Schreiber [63] showed that tumors induced in immunocompetent mice had a higher incidence of being non-immunogenic tumors, while the tumors derived from immunocomprised mice were more immunogenic. Those studies were done in young mice that have strong immune systems. Immunity peaks around puberty, so these non-immunogenic tumors were selected due to the vitality of their younger immune systems

[64,65]. The majority of oncology patients, especially GBM, are past puberty when the cancers appear (Central Brain Tumor Registry,2008). By age 50, the human thymus has atrophied, and the capacity for T cell production is lost. The thymus from younger individuals is fully capable of generating T cell diversity, which may specifically adapt to the brain tumor-associated antigens; whereas in older people, who lack this adaptive ability, more immunogenic tumor clones could arise and survive. In aged individuals the remaining T cells may be approaching replicative senescence, since their telomeres have significantly shortened due to a lifetime of proliferation towards various related antigens that they encountered. Likewise, the innate immune system also deteriorates with age [66]. The significance of age and immune responses towards human brain cancers has recently been reviewed in Driggers, et al's [67] article. Thus, the concept of immunogenicity/non-immunogenicity may be an artifact and might be dependent upon the patient's age as to when the tumor was isolated. Therefore, studying both non-immunogenic and immunogenic gliomas are reasonable models of either pediatric or geriatric type tumors, respectively. When using young animals, non-immunogenic tumor cells are the most appropriate ones to study, while older animals could use immunogenic gliomas.

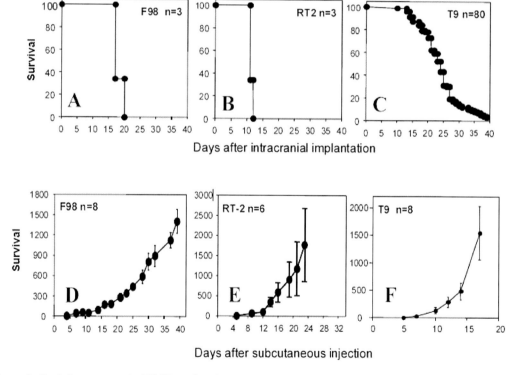

Figure 3. *Both Immunogenic (T9/9L and RT2) and Non-Immunogenic F98 glioma cells will grow in normal rats.* Panels (A-C) show the survival of F344 rats that received 10^4 cells that were surgically implanted into the brain. Panels (D-F) show the growth of these same glioma cells injected subcutaneously into rats.

DECREASED MAJOR HISTO-COMPATIBILITY COMPLEX (MHC) ANTIGEN EXPRESSION

The most common mechanism by which tumor cells become invisible to the immune system is by preventing MHC class I or II expression. These cancer cells are simply not recognized by T cells via their epitope-laden histocompatibility antigens. Figure 4 shows the flow cytometry expression of the glioma cells for the rat MHC class 1, RT1-A, which is the equivalent of the mouse H-2K loci [68]. There is a trend for non-immunogenic glioma cells to have lower RT1-A expression. D74 cells had the lowest amount of this class I MHC molecule. 36B10 and CNS-1 glioma cells also had lower RT1-A levels, too. But BT4C and RT2 cells are considered immunogenic and these cells had equivalent levels as the non-immunogenic, 36B10 and CNS-1 cells. Two cell lines, F98 (non-immunogenic) and T9, also known as 9L, (immunogenic) had roughly equivalent and high levels of RT1-A. The cell line, B28, whose immunogenicity status is not known, had the highest RT1-A expression status of the 9 cell lines tested.

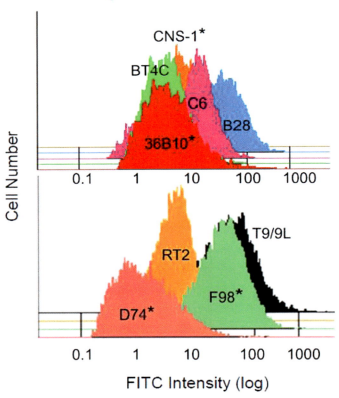

Figure 4. *RT1-A expression on the rat glioma cells.* One half million cells were stained with a monoclonal antibody (Pharmingen) against the public determinants of the rat MHC class I molecule (RT1-A) for 1 hr on ice, washed twice and then labeled with a FITC labeled secondary antibody. These cells were washed twice and then ran on the flow cytometry. The data from ten thousand cells is displayed. The Y-axis shows cell numbers, while the x-axis shows the log fluorescence intensity. The asterisks display the non-immunogenic glioma cells (D74, F98, 36B10, and CNS-1).

CNS-1 gliomas originated from the inbred Lewis rat strain, which is designated as having the RT1-A^l haplotype. T9/9L, RT2, F98 and D74 glioma cells are derived from Fischer 344 (F344) rats. Their haplotype is designated as the "l variant" haplotype, RT1-A^{lv1}, which is closely related to the RT1-A^l haplotype. The BT4C, 36B10 and B28 gliomas are derived from inbred BDX rats (RT1-A^{dv1}). C6 gliomas arose from outbred Wistar rats. Thus studies require the proper use of immunogenetics when designing animal studies.

Due to the out-bred nature of C6 cells, many immunologists would prefer not to use these cells in vivo. Early studies with these cells were difficult to match for the MHC and probably possessed minor histo-compatibility antigens that could augment immunological reactions. These minor histo-compatibility antigens are barriers to organ and bone marrow transplantations, since they elicit T cell and antibody responses that eventually cause transplantation rejection. Minor histo-compatibility antigens are usually polymorphic proteins that are endogenous to those animal strains. The male antigen (H-Y) can also be considered a minor histo-compatibility antigen [69] in that these antigens derived from male-derived cells will provoke immune responses within females. Minor histo-compatibility antigens are presented as peptides on the MHC molecules. As a result, upon introduction into MHC compatible strains, these minor histocompatiblity antigens provoke immune responses due to those different endogenous polymorphic peptides. This basic compatibility complication should discourage the use of these C6 glioma cells within most rat breeds. Buetler, et al. [70] used reverse transcriptase-polymerase chain reactions (RT-PCR) followed by sequencing techniques to prove that the RT1-A allele comes from Wistar-Furth strain and possesses the RT1-A^u genotype. Hence to be properly matched at the MHC, one should use RT1-A^u - positive rats, but the minor histocompatibility differences may still complicate the immunogenetics of any tumor-host relationship simply matched at the RT1-A locus. Despite these histo-incompatibilities, C6 cells can grow in many different strains of rats; i.e., wistar [71,72], F344 [73], BDX [74], Sprague-Dawley [75], and even in immune-competent Balb/c mice [76]. Hence some immunosuppressive mechanism(s) are preventing immunological rejection of these C6 gliomas in spite of the strong expression of RT1-A.

C6 glioma cells possess stem-cell like properties [77] a feature that appeals to many investigators who want to study an invasive glioma, as opposed to the well defined margins associated with the use of other glioma cell lines. Current speculation is that gliomas arise out of mutated glial stem cells. Abdullah, et al [78] showed that embryonic stem cells are naturally resistant to CTL-mediated lysis due to the expression of serpin-6. Whether C6 gliomas and the other rat gliomas also express serpin-6 is currently unknown, but the use of host defense mechanisms by gliomas and "stem-like" cells to resist cell-mediated immunity is a strong possibility that should be acknowledged. For these reasons, C6 cells are still used in vivo.

It should be noted that human glioma cell lines commonly used in immunological studies are also derived from an outbred species. So most well-established human tumor cell lines (U87, U118, U251, T98G, D54, LN229, etc) used in pre-clinical models also have the very same limitations as does the rat C6 glioma. Therefore unless one uses patient-derived lymphocytes with the autologous tumor, the same arguments used against C6 are equally applicable to all human immunological studies using the old, well-established human glioma cell lines.

Glioma-Associated Antigens

The lack of RT1-A expression helps explain the non-immunogenicity of the D74 glioma cell line. The low RT1-A expression can perhaps explain the non-immunogenicity of 36B10 and CNS-1 cells. But other processes need to be employed to explain the lack of immune responses towards 36B10 and CNS-1. Human GBM tumor cells derived from adult patients are quite antigenic [79]. Surprisingly, most human glioma cell lines (17 tested, 3 tumors were probably were cross-contaminated in the past: U251, SNB19 and U373) expressed almost all the same tumor antigens to same degree. There were only three tumor antigens (GP100, trp-1 and Tyrosinase) that had variable expression. Interestingly, GBM derived from adult patients are more antigenic than their pediatric counterparts [80], confirming our suspicion about immunogenicity and age (see 6 paragraphs above). A partial list of these potential human glioma tumor antigens found in adult GBM are shown in Table 1. Very few antigens are truly glioma-specific. EGFRvIII is a deletional mutation and was initially thought to be glioma specific, until it was discovered that other tumors, breast and lung, also expressed this same deletion mutation [81]. Most of these tumor antigens are normal host proteins that are over-expressed by the glioma cells. The term, tumor-associated antigens, is therefore a more appropriate term to use rather than tumor antigen. This then raises the question as to whether the expression of glioma-associated antigens can be used to help explain immunogenicity in the rat glioma model.

Despite being used for 30-40 years, relatively little is known of rat tumor-associated antigens, other than the empirical observation that the tumor cells are either immunogenic or non-immunogenic. There is a higher priority for finding human tumor-associated antigens than the rodent ones, since the former can lead to potential therapies, while the latter interests are more academically pursued.

Monoclonal antibodies against rat glioma cells have also been reported [82]. In 2001, Okada and colleagues [83] used a serological based study (SEREX) to identify at least 3 intracellular antigens that were recognized by the serum of rats immunized with interleukin-4 transduced 9L (a.k.a. T9) cells. These antigens were calcylin, a rat homolog of a J6B7 molecule, and mouse Id-associated protein-1 (MIDA1). Pre-immunization of naïve rats with MIDA1 generated effective immunity against the 9L/T9 gliomas. This antigen was only tested with the 9L/T9 cell line, so its expression profile within other glioma cell lines is presently unknown. Also unknown is whether any T cell immunity was generated with MIDA1, or whether this just represented a humoral antibody response with innate immune cells mediating antibody-dependent cell cytotoxicity.

Some in vitro CTL-based immunity against F344-based gliomas was done by Holladay and coworkers [84-86]. Rats immunized against either 9L or RT2 could yield CTLs, if these in vivo primed lymphocytes were secondarily stimulated in vitro with irradiated cells in the presence of interleukin-2 (IL-2) for a week. As a result of this in vitro stimulation/expansion, killer T cells were generated that lysed Cr^{51}-labeled 9L and RT2 glioma cells but not syngeneic F98 or allogeneic C6 cells. Using a similar approach, Shah and Ramsey [87] also showed similar CTL responses. Thus, T cells can recognize RT1-A specific epitopes.

Table 1. Glioma-associated Antigens

Antigens	Description
ABCG	ATP – Binding Cassette Group
Aim2	Antigen Isolated Melanoma-2
Art-1	Antigen Recognized by T cells-1
Art-4	Antigen Recognized by T cells-4
B-cyclin	B-cyclin
CD133	Cluster Designation 133
EGFRvIII	Epidermal Growth Factor Receptor variant III
EphA2	Ephrin Receptor A2
Ezh2	Enhancer of Zeste Homologue 2
Fos11	Fos related Antigen-1
Galt-3	3-galactosyltransferase, polypeptide 3
GnT-V	b1,6-Nacetylglucosaminyltransferase-V
Gp100	melanoma Glycoprotein-100
Her2	Human Epidermal Growth Factor Receptor 2
HNRPL	Heterogeneous Nuclear Ribonucleoprotein L
IL13Rα2	Interleukin-13 Receptor alpha 2
Mage-1	Melanoma Antigen-1
MELK	Maternal Embryonic Leucine Zipper Kinase
MRP-3	Multidrug Resistance Protein-3
NY-Eso-1	New York Esophageal Carcinoma- 1
p53	Protein 53
PRAME	Preferentially expressed Antigen in Melanoma
PTH-rP	Para-Thyroid Hormone- related Protein
Sart-1	Squamous cell carcinoma Antigen Recognized by T cells-1
Sart-2	Squamous cell carcinoma Antigen Recognized by T cells-2
Sart-3	Squamous cell carcinoma Antigen Recognized by T cells-3
SSX-2	Synovial Sarcoma Chromosome Break Point – 2
Sox 11	Transcription Factor
Survivin	Survivin
h-Tert	Telomerase Reverse Transcriptase
Trp-1	Tyrosinase Related Protein-1
Trp-2	Tyrosinase Related Protein-2
Tyrosinase	Tyrosinase
Ube2V	Ubiquitin-conjugated enzyme 2 Variant
Whsc2	Wolf-Hirschhorn syndrome candidate 2 protein
WT-1	Wilm's Tumor Antigen – 1
Ykl-40	Tyrosine (Y) Lysine (K) Leucine (L)– 40 Kda

In our previous studies, we saw that rats were immunized after being injected with T9/9L cells transduced with the membrane form of macrophage colony stimulating factor (mM-CSF). The mechanism through which these mM-CSF transduced cells are killed by monocytes is through a process called paraptosis, which is thought to be the process that leads to necrosis and an inflammatory pathway [88-90]. The splenocytes from these immunized rats weakly proliferated in response to killed tumor lysates derived from T9, 9L (before we discovered T9 and 9L were the same tumor cell line possessing identical DNA contents by propidium iodide staining), RT2 and D74 gliomas, but not in response to syngeneic rat breast (MADB106) or ovarian (NUTU-19) cancer lysates [91]. Rats immunized towards T9 gliomas also resisted the growth of RT2 and F98 gliomas when rechallenged in subcutaneous sites [92]. When the sera from these hyper-immunized rats were tested, we failed to detect any antibodies that could bind to the cell surface of any glioma cell (negative data not published). Thus, we do not believe this anti-tumor immunity was mediated via the antibody dependent cell-mediated cytotoxicity pathway. Adoptive transfer studies showed that T9-specific immunity could be transferred into naïve rats by the CD4-positive fraction of immunized T cells, indicating that antigenic determinants and tumor memory towards different gliomas can be observed in vivo. Consequently, there must be rat glioma-associated antigens that can stimulate effective immunity.

The lack of detection of identifiable rat glioma antigens is largely due to inability to generate primary mature CTLs. One salient point relates to the fact that one-week old IL-2 activated CTLs used in prior work [84-87] are technically not the exact same cells that are isolated directly from the rats. Either some intrinsic defect within the T cell/APC compartment prevents precursor CTLs from fully maturing into functional CTL or some extrinsic inhibitory factor is preventing fully functional CTL from developing in vivo. We favor the former, since an intensive scan of the literature shows no study where functional rat CTLs can be detected using freshly isolated T cells. We can easily detect functional murine CTLs freshly isolated from mice: with graft-versus-host disease [93], vaccinated with a murine Hepa1-6 hepatoma cells or immunized with dendritic cells pulsed with the alternative form of macrophage colony stimulating factor (altM-CSF) [94]. One important ramification for this finding is that there are still unknown anti-tumor effector mechanisms in the rat glioma model that do not involve the direct cytolytic actions of classic cytotoxic T lymphocytes. The identification of this mechanism of anti-tumor immunity may give additional insight into tumor biology that is currently not apparent using the mouse model.

STRATEGIES THAT TUMOR CELLS USE TO EVADE THE IMMUNE SYSTEM

Gliomas, like most cancers, have evolved multiple mechanisms to not only evade normal cell cycle/proliferation regulation, but simultaneously developed escape routes that prevent their destruction by the immune system. These mechanisms include: 1) tumor host cell responses making them harder to kill (Figure 1B); 2) making immunosuppressive cytokines; 3) producing immunosuppressive enzymes (Figure 1C). Both of these latter two pathways can either down-regulate the antigen presenting cells or the immune effector cells.

Defense Molecules

We examined four molecules (Heat Shock Protein [HSP] -70 and -90, Bcl2, and survivin) that tumors could use to avoid either radiation-, chemical-induced or immunological-induced cell death pathways. We used intracellular flow cytometry to quantitate the amount of four representative defensive molecules within the nine rat glioma cell lines (Figure 5). We also tested neurosphere cultures that were isolated from neonatal mouse brains and cultured in N2 media [95], as a control to establish baseline values (red circles at the left of each panel) for what values could be considered biologically significant. This intracellular flow cytometry technique allows us to determine which factor might be the more dominant molecules in an easily comparable process throughout our various analyses.

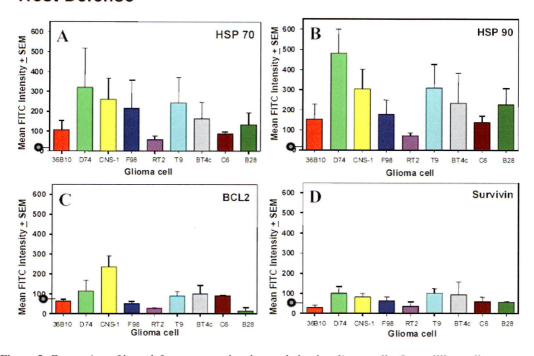

Figure 5. *Expression of host defense type molecules made by the glioma cells.* One million cells were fixed and permeabilized by methanol and then incubated with monoclonal antibodies against HSP70, HSP90, Bcl2 and Survivin for 1 hr. The cells were washed and then incubated with FITC secondary antibodies for 1 hr. After washing, ten thousand cells were analyzed and the mean peak channel was obtained the data for 4-6 runs was obtained and plotted with the SEM. The red circle indicates the values obtained from normal neurospheres.

Heat shock proteins are stress-induced molecules that the cell uses to replace old damaged molecules. These stress-induced elements assist in the correct three-dimensional folding of newly synthesized molecules and are known as chaperones. HSP-90 is the target of clinical trials designed to destabilize this molecule making those treated cancer cells more susceptible to killing to either chemotherapy or radio-therapy [96]. 17-allylamino-17-demethoxygeldanamycin (17-AAG) is a HSP-90 inhibitor that has shown some clinical benefit in human breast cancer trials [97]. In an experimental glioma model [98], 17-AAG has also proved effective. Currently this drug is being used in human GBM trials at Baylor Medical Center. It is thought that HSP molecules (HSP-70, HSP-90 and gp96) assist in peptide loading of the MHC [99,100]. A company, Antigenics Inc., is producing clinical products called "Oncophage", which contains the gp96 derived from the patients' own tumor cells. This product is then used for vaccination purposes to improve immune responses. Phase 1/2 trials for brain cancer are being conducted at the Brain Tumor Research Center at the University of California, San Francisco. However, HSPs are a double-edged sword, where high concentrations of HSP render tumor cells resistant to therapeutic interventions, while these molecules might represent good adjuvants to provoke immune responses once these tumor cells die and release these molecules.

In general, three non-immunogenic tumors (D74, CNS-1 and F98) and 2 immunogenic gliomas (T9 and BT4C) made more HSP-70 (Figure 5A) and HSP-90 (Figure 5B) when compared to normal brain cells cultured as neurospheres. Thus, these 2 molecules can theoretically provide a better defense for the glioma cells against various therapeutic agents.

Two other anti-apoptotic survival genes were examined, Bcl2 and survivin. Bcl2 is the prototypical family member of a series of pro- and anti-apoptotic genes. In human gliomas, these anti-apoptotic family members (Bcl2, Bclx, Bcl2L12, Mcl1) are up-regulated [101,102]. CNS-1 was the best Bcl2 expressing cell lines (Figure 5C). Whether these rat gliomas express the other anti-apoptotic members is unknown due to the paucity of rat specific reagents towards these proteins.

Survivin is another anti-apoptotic molecule that prevents cytochrome c release from the mitochondria, while concurrently inhibiting caspase-9 activation [103]. Survivin also plays a role in cell division involving microtubule-dependent chromosome separation at G2-M phase of the cell cycle [104]. In human [105] and mouse [106] cancer models, survivin, acts as a tumor antigen allowing cytolytic T cells to be generated. Of the rat glioma cell lines tested, none showed any increased survivin protein levels significantly above those levels found within the normal neurosphere cells (Figure 5D). Survivin therefore likely takes on a less important role in mediating rat glioma host defense, as it has been concluded in the murine and human gliomas.

Immunosuppressive Cytokines

For immunosuppressive cytokines, we examined three cytokines: transforming growth factor-β (TGF-β), vascular endothelial growth factor (VEGF) and interleukin-10 (IL-10).

TGF-β was the first identified cytokine to be released by glioma cells that inhibit immune responses [107,108]. Two reviews [109,110] cover the various aspects through which TGF-β mediates it's activities. Figure 6A shows the presence of TGF-β within most of the glioma cells. The immunogenic T9/9L, BT4C and C6 glioma and non-immunogenic 36B10, D74 and CNS-1 cell displayed more TGF-β than the normal neurosphere cells. So TGF-β is important for some, but not of all the rat glioma cells.

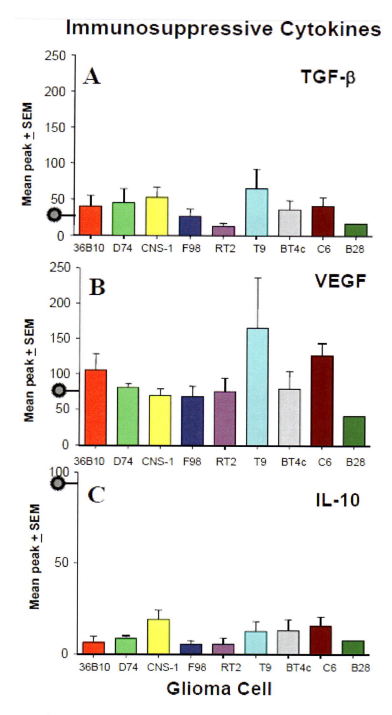

Figure 6. *Expression of immunosuppressive cytokines made by the glioma cells.* One million cells were fixed and permeabilized by methanol and then incubated with monoclonal antibodies against TGF-β, VEGF and IL-10 (R+D Systems) for 1 hr. The cells were washed and then incubated with FITC secondary antibodies for 1 hr. After washing, ten thousand cells were analyzed and the mean peak channel was obtained the data for 4-6 runs was obtained and plotted with the SEM. The red circle on the left y-axis indicates the values obtained from normal neurospheres.

VEGF is known for its pro-angiogenic properties that stimulate new blood vessel formation for the growing tumor, but VEGF also inhibits the antigen presentation functions of APCs [111]. VEGF then shuts down this key immune function thereby allowing the tumor to grow, by preventing T cells from being activated. For VEGF, only T9/9L and C6 cells expressed more of this cytokine than that displayed by the neurosphere cells (Figure 6B). Overall, the glioma and neurosphere cells made more VEGF than TGF-β. We conclude that VEGF probably has a more dominant role than TGF-β, when it comes to suppressing immune responses for most of the rat glioma cells.

Interleukin-10 is also made by gliomas [112] and it modulates APC function and tends to polarize these cells towards a humoral based Th2 response, and away from the cell mediated immune responses that are thought to be more suited for eliminating tumor cells. The rat glioma cells possessed very little fluorescence suggesting that this cytokine is not as prevalent as either VEGF or TGF-β (Figure 6C). In fact the neurosphere cells possessed more intracellular IL-10. This finding could mean that when IL-10 is detected in vivo within rat gliomas, it might be originating from other cell types (macrophages, microglial cells) rather than directly from the glioma cells.

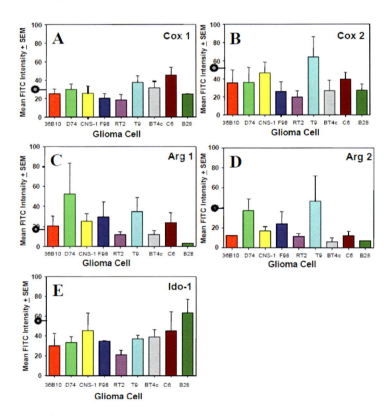

Figure 7. *Expression of immunosuppressive enzymes made by the glioma cells.* One million cells were fixed and permeabilized by methanol and then incubated with either polyclonal antibodies against Cox1, Cox2, Arg1, Arg2 (Santa Cruz Biotechnology) or a monoclonal antibody for Ido-1 (Millepore Corp.) for 1 hr. The cells were washed and then incubated with FITC secondary antibodies for 1 hr. After washing, ten thousand cells were analyzed and the mean peak channel was obtained the data for 4-6 runs was obtained and plotted with the SEM. The red circle on the left y-axis indicates the values obtained from normal neurospheres.

Immunosuppressive Enzymes

Immunosuppressive enzymes provide another way for tumor cells to evade immune responses. In this classification we use the term, immunosuppressive enzyme, to reflect an enzymatic process induced by the glioma cells where the different metabolites are produced which eventually generates an inhibitory condition.

Cyclooxygenase 1 (Cox 1) and 2 (Cox 2) are two related enzymes that convert arachidonic acid into prostaglandins (PG), PGE and PGJ2. Cox 1 is considered a constitutive enzyme, while Cox 2 is supposed to be inducible. PGE can directly inhibit immune responses through several ways [113,114] or help some tumors grow by acting as a potential growth stimulus [115]. Prayson, et al. [116] and Akasaki, et al. [117] showed that cyclooxygenase was made by human gliomas. In Figure 7, Panels A and B, we saw that only a few rat gliomas were making more Cox 1 or Cox 2 than the neurosphere cells. T9 and C6 were making more Cox1, while T9 made more Cox 2 than the other gliomas.

Arginine is amino acid that seems to play a key role in controlling immune responses [118]. Arginine is converted by nitric oxide synthase into nitric oxide and this can polarize T cells DC and macrophages into Type 1 (cell-mediated) pathways. But Arginase is another set of enzymes that catalyze the breakdown of arginine, into ornithine and urea [119]. Arginine is either needed for proper T cell function or one of its breakdown products could directly inhibit T cells. There are 2 forms of arginase. Arginase 1 is a cytoplasmic enzyme, while arginase 2 is a mitochondrial enzyme. PGE can induce macrophages into releasing arginase 1 and help polarize macrophages into a Type 2 (humoral) direction and hence diverting cellular immune responses [120]. Additionally, arginase is produced by myeloid suppressor cells which prevent effective Th1 immune responses through multiple ways [121-123]. D74 cell (Panel C) best expressed Arginase 1; while T9 and D74 cells contained more Arginase 2 (Panel D), but these levels were not considered different from that displayed by the neurosphere cells.

Another enzyme which regulates suppressor cell function is indoleamine 2,3, dioxgenase (Ido-1). Ido-1 is made by T reg [124]. Like arginase, Ido-1 catabolizes another amino acid, tryptophan. Here tryptophan is converted into kynurenine, which limits T cell responses, either because T cells require tryptophan to grow through mid-G1 arrest points or one of its metabolites inhibit T cell-mediated functions[125-127]. Ido-1's role in immune escape mechanisms has been reviewed in Prendergast [124]. Uyttenhove, and colleagues [128] showed that 90% of the human glioblastomas that they examined were positive for Ido-1. Miyazaki, et al. [129] showed that human glioma cell lines produce Ido-1 mRNA. The Ido1 expression was strongly stimulated by IFN-γ. This finding has important significance, because CTLs and NK cells which could be mediating anti-tumor killing, could also inadvertently be stimulating a homeostatic feed-back that in turn inactivates the immune system via the feed-back loop using Ido-1. In our analyses, all the rat giomas were weakly positive for Ido-1 protein expression (Figure 7E). However, the B28 cells had the best expression of Ido-1.

The relatively low intracellular values obtained for the immunosuppressive enzymes (mean channel intensities (MPC) of less than 60) suggest that they could be supplying a constant amount, albeit a low level of these inhibitory molecules. More likely, however, is the possibility that the combination of all these enzymes could collectively interact to stimulate T reg and MSC within the brain. This suggests that even low levels of these molecules may well have dramatic effects in polarizing the various infiltrating cells into immunosuppressive cells.

COUNTERATTACK?

Another mechanism by which tumor cells can shut down immunity may involve the fas ligand (CD95L, Apo-1L, CD178) [130,131] or programmed death ligand-1 (PD-L1) [132]. This proposed pathway has been coined: "counterattack". When CTLs bind to their targeted tumor cells to kill them, if the tumor cells express fas ligand, then the tumor cells can cause the Fas-positive CTLs to die in an apoptotic death. Here the 'hunter' (CTL, NK) can now become the 'hunted' by the tumor cells. Older activated T cells (> 3 days) express more Fas than earlier activated T cells. Human gliomas have been reported to express fas ligand [133-136]. Fas-positive glioma cells after interacting with Fas ligand-positive cells in a juxtracrine manner can also induce Fas-positive glioma cells to produce cytokines, chemokines and angiogenic factors [137]. Certain glioma cells are more resistant to apoptosis induction when exogenous fas ligand is conjugated to fas [133,138], compared to T cells. This asymmetric relationship may favor tumor cell survival. Furthermore, fas ligand can be shed from the tumor cell surface where this soluble form acts as a decoy and inhibits the actions of the cytolytic T cells [139].

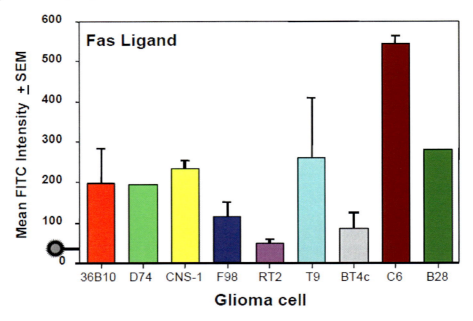

Figure 8. *Fas Ligand expressions on the rat glioma cells.* Here one half million cells were stained with a monoclonal antibody (R+D Systems) against Fas Ligand for 1 hr on ice, washed twice and then labeled with a FITC labeled secondary antibody. These cells were washed twice and then ran on the flow cytometry. The data from ten thousand cells is displayed the mean peak channel was obtained the data for 4-6 runs. The red circle indicates the value obtained from normal neurospheres.

Figure 8 shows that the various rat glioma cells expressed membrane-bound fas ligand on their surfaces with C6 and T9/9L being the best expressing glioma cells.* (we used the anti-Fas ligand antibody from R+D Systems, since some antibodies from other companies including monoclonal antibodies have problems with specificity, [140]. The majority of the other rat glioma cells expressed more fas ligand than that of normal neurosphere cells. Given the current dogma, the expression of fas ligand on glioma cells may be responsible for inhibiting rat host immune responses by T or NK cells.

The concept of counter-attack via a fas ligand and fas pathway as a mechanism of immune escape for tumors has been questioned. Restifo [140] has pointed out some of the problems with this model. Stable transduction of the fas ligand gene into some cells caused enhanced destruction of Fas ligand-positive tumor cells. Some of this destruction of these Fas ligand-positive cells was attributed to the actions of infiltrating neutrophils. Hence these results with fas ligand could also have important theoretical ramifications as possible markers of immunogenicity. Others have shown that upon binding of fas ligand by glioma cells, the interacting T cells can now produce IL-10 [141]. So one must be cognizant that fas ligand could also have two diametrically opposing functions, just as tumor necrosis factor has been discovered to have two distinct roles in cancer: tumor induction and cancer therapy [142,143].

OTHER INTANGIBLE FACTORS THAT GLIOMAS DISPLAY

No discussion of comparative tumor evasion would be complete, without exploring two other aspects of tumor biology that significantly impact of glioma growth, namely cellular doubling times and their susceptibility to immune-mediated killing.

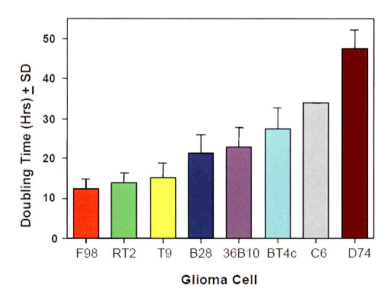

Figure 9. *Doubling times of rat glioma cells.* Five thousand glioma cells were placed in each well of the 24 well plate. The contents of each well (done in duplicates) were sacrificed each day were counted. The doubling time of each cell was calculated by the equation: Number of divisions = ($\log_{10} N1 - \log_{10} N0$)/log 2. N0 is the number of cells found at Day 2 and N1 is the number obtained on Day 4. Population-doubling time hr is calculated by dividing 48 hrs by the number of divisions that were calculated as described by Heidrick and Ryan [148].

Cell division times are critical. If the tumor cells replicate faster than the immune system can kill them, then net tumor growth will occur. Figure 9 compares the doubling times of the glioma cells. This highlights that not all these glioma cell lines grow at the same rate. F98 was the quickest cell to self-replicate itself with a doubling time of 13 hrs. This was followed by RT2 and T9/9L. These faster growing glioma cells might actually be good models of relapsing tumor, where the remaining tumor cells after therapy may correspond to a rapidly proliferating fraction of resistant cells. In contrast, two of the non-immunogenic cells, D74 and CNS-1 had slow doubling times of about 47 and 50 hrs, respectively. Consequently, non-immunogenic tumor cells may not need to depend upon proliferation to the same extent, surviving under slower growth rates and under less aggressive immune attack.

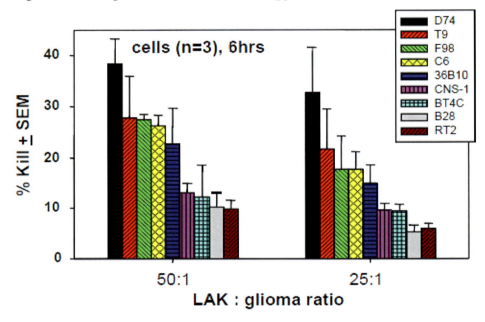

Figure 10. *Lymphokine activated killing of the rat glioma cells.* Rat splenic lymphocytes were cultured in 100 units/ml IL-2 for 3-7 days to become lymphokine activated killer (LAK) cells. These LAK cells were tested against the various rat gliomas at either a 50:1 or 25:1 effectors: target ratio for 6 hrs. The data represents the pooled data from 3 different experiments along with the standard of the errors.

Another important factor is whether these glioma cell lines are equally susceptible to cell-mediated lysis. Since CTL killing is restricted to class 1 MHC restrictions, we used a general cytolytic killer cell, to do comparative studies. LAK cells are thought to be good universal tumor killer cells. Rat LAK cells grown in IL-2 for 3-7 days were used as the effector cells to measure their ability to kill the various glioma cells in 6 hr cytolysis assays. Figure 10 shows the data compiled from 3 different experiments. We found that there were three distinct phenotypes: a hyper-sensitive, a sensitive and a semi-resistant population. D74 was the cell line efficiently eliminated by the LAK cells, >35% lysis at the 50:1 effector:target ratio. LAK cells contain a large fraction of activated NK cells, which effectively recognize and kill those cells that lack conventional MHC molecules. This is likely why that the D74 cells were killed the best in all three assays, due to D74's low RT1-A expression (Figure 3). The second classification was the sensitive target cells, T9, F98, C6 and 36B10. These cells were killed

>25% at the 50:1 LAK:target cell ratio. Finally four cell lines were resistant to LAK killing: CNS-1, BT4C, B28 and RT2 cells, around 12% cytolysis at the 50:1 effector:target ratio. Since LAK, NK and CTLs can kill target cells through perforin and granzymes mediated processes, it might not be surprising that those glioma cells were killed via an osmotic type lytic pathway using perforin with granzymes. Thus, those gliomas that displayed high defensive molecules (HSP, Bcl2) were still killed by the LAK cells. Thus, these last four glioma cells might have some defense pathway that resists the actions of the cell mediated cytolysis. Such molecules could be MHC class1b (RT1-E2) which inactivates NK cells, decay accelerator factor (DAF, CD59) which prevents complement-related proteins like perforin from polymerizing into a membrane attack complex. DAF is known to be made by brain tumors [144,145]. Vitronectin can inactivate perforin [146] and human gliomas can make vitronectin under in vivo conditions [147]. Work is currently in progress to determine which of these scenarios is occurring.

EACH GLIOMA CELL IS UNIQUE IN ITS METHOD OF EVADING IMMUNE RESPONSES

Table 2 summarizes the data into the various mechanisms utilized by the rat gliomas to evade immune responses. When we examined tumor-associated antigen profiles by human glioma cell lines, we were surprised to see how homogenous the different human glioma cells were. In contrast, the rat glioma cell lines appeared more diverse from each other and possessed distinct pathways by which they can avoid immune recognition and continue to grow in its host. The non-immunogenic glioma cells seemed to have multiple processes to escape immunity. In contrast, the immunogenic tumors seemed to have either multiple layers of defense or were just difficult to kill by LAK cell-mediated pathways.

Table 2. Summary of the escape mechanisms used by the rat glioma cells

Non-Immunogenic	Escape Mechanism
D74	Low RT1-A expression, TGF-β, Fas ligand, HSP-70, HSP-90
F98	HSP-70, HSP-90, fast growing cells
36B10	Fas ligand, fast growing
CNS-1	TGF-β, Ido-1, Fas ligand, HSP-70, HSP-90, Bcl2, hard to kill
Immunogenic	
T9/9L	TGF-β, VEGF, Cox, Arg, Fas ligand, HSP-70, HSP-90, fast growing
C6	TGF-β, VEGF, Cox, Ido-1, Fas ligand, fast growing
RT2	fast growing, hard to kill
BT4C	hard to kill
Unknown	
B28	Ido-1, Fas ligand, fast growing, hard to kill

D74 cells possessed little MHC class I expression (Figure 3), so T cells are unlikely to easily recognize these cells. they are therefore able to escape detection by T cells. This may provide one explanation for their survival in the host, despite having one of the slowest measured growth rates (doubling time >46 hrs, Figure 9). Due to the lack of classic MHC class I antigens, the D74 cells were more susceptible to NK/LAK cells (Figure 10) which can recognize those tumor cells displaying lowered amounts of MHC class I antigens. D74 also made TGF-β and expressed fas ligand which could suppress immune responses in any of the responding lymphocytes. In addition, they expressed higher levels of HSP-70 and HSP-90 (Figure 8), which helps replace any damaged proteins due to various therapeutic interventions. Consequently, this cell line might be optimal for studies investigating the HSP90 disruption drug, 17AAG.

F98 cells also made high levels of HSP-70 and HSP-90 (Fig 8), but were not as high as that displayed by the D74 cells. The aggressive characteristics of these cells are likely due to their very fast doubling time. Thus any elicited immune response must be rapidly mobilized at the onset of tumor formation when these tumors are very small, because their rapid growth rate will likely impair any chance of tumor control.

36B10 cells appear to use a lowered MHC class I expression, Fas ligand and a relatively fast doubling time (<20 hrs), to escape immunological containment.

CNS-1 cells could conceivably use at least 7 pathways, second only to T9/9L for varied pathway utilization. CNS-1 made HSP-70, HSP-90 and Bcl2. These last three molecules could explain why these cells were hard to kill by the LAK cells. CNS-1 also made TGF-β, fas ligand and ido-1. Presumably these collective pathways, allow the expansion of these gliomas even under their relatively slow growth rate (>46 hrs).

T9/9L cells also employ multiple mechanisms: HSP-70, HSP-90, TGF-β, VEGF, Cox, Arg, fas ligand and they were the third fastest growing cell line. Thus, if one wants to look at multiple synergistic inhibitory pathways, T9/9L are the best cells to examine. This might also account for why these cells are a favorite of experimental glioma research.

C6 glioma cells were derived from outbred rats. These cells use multiple pathways: Bcl2, TGF-β, VEGF, Cox, Fas ligand (the best of all 9 cell lines examined) and Ido-1 (second best). The collection of these pathways engage multiple defensive strategies that allows for the growth of these cells within various strains of rats and mice [70-75].

RT2 and BT4C cells had the least amount of defensive mechanisms. Their levels of defensive molecules were very low and they were not much different from the phenotype displayed by the normal neurosphere cells. Even though these glioma cells displayed reduced expression of defensive molecules (HSP-70, HSP-90, Bcl2, survivin), both cell lines were surprisingly hard to kill by the LAK cells. We therefore conclude there must be other mechanisms by which these cells resist cell-mediated killing. RT2 did possess one other major escape mechanism in that it had the second shortest doubling time (14 hrs) of all the cells tested.

B28 cells were hard to kill by the LAK cells but had an intermediate doubling time of 20 hrs. These cells also expressed fas ligand and had the highest level of Ido-1. Therefore, we predict that these glioma cells probably will form tumors in vivo, while inducing faster T reg responses as a result of their increased Ido-1 production, when compared to the other glioma cell lines.

CONCLUSION

For years, rat glioma cell lines were the model of choice for experimental neuro-oncology. Their applications as pre-clinical models have lead to many of the clinical therapies that are currently being utilized in human patients. Only recently, these rat models have been surpassed by the various genetic mouse models. However, rat glioma cells still have a lot to offer. At least nine rat glioma cell lines are known. These cell lines are stable cell lines that offer day-to-day consistency. These glioma cells all appear to be truly different in their basic biology. They all form tumors in immunocompetent rats either in brains or other sites. The various rat gliomas had multiple mechanisms whereby they could avoid immune responses. Only D74 cells displayed low levels of RT1-A. While other cells used a variety of either host defense type molecules (HSP-70, HSP-90, Bcl2) or immunosuppressive cytokines (TGF-β, VEGF) or immunosuppressive enzymes (cyclooxgenase, arginase or indoleamine 2, 3 dioxygenase) to inhibit various aspects of effector lymphocyte responses. C6 displayed a high level of Fas Ligand suggesting that a counter-attack pathway is possible. Some cells like F98, RT2 and T9/9L appear to use quicker replication times to over-grow the immune responses. Four cell lines (CNS-1, RT2, BT4C and B28) displayed an unexpected resistance to the actions of cell-mediated killer cells as displayed by LAK cells. Each cell line has its own peculiar traits and may allow researchers to specifically design experiments to their own area of expertise. As a result, researchers will still probably be using these various rat glioma cells for many years to come.

ACKNOWLEDGMENTS

We thank Dr. Carol Kruse (Burnham Institute) for the CNS-1 cells, Dr. William Stallcup (Burnham Institute) for the B28 cells, Dr. Henry Hirschman (Univ. of California, Irvine) for the BT4C cells; Dr. Michael Robbins (Wake Forrest University) for the 36B10 cells. We acknowledge the help of Ms. Susan Holsclaw for her art work presented here. This work was funded in part by the VA Merit Review (M.R.J.), and the Avon Breast cancer fund (via the Chao Comprehensive Cancer Center, UCI) (M.R.J.). The American Cancer Society has funded C.L.L.

REFERENCES

[1] R. Jelsma and P.C. Bucy, *J. Neurosurg.* 27, 388 (1967).
[2] R. Jelsma and P.C. Bucy, *Arch. Neurol.* 20,161 (1967).
[3] M.E. Hegi, A.C. Diserens, and T. Gorlia, *N. Engl. J. Med.* 352, 997 (2005).
[4] J.S. Yu, C.J. Wheeler, P.M. Zeltzer, H. Ying, D.N. Finger, P.K. Lee, W.H. Yong, F. Incardona, R. C. Thompson, M.S. Riedinger, W. Zhang, R.M. Prins and K.L. Black, *Cancer Res.* 61, 842 (2001).
[5] J.S.Yu, G. Liu, H. Ying, W.H. Yong, K.L. Black and C.J. Wheeler, *Cancer Res.* 64, 4973 (2004).

[6] L.M. Liau, R.M. Prins, S.M. Kiertscher, S.K. Odesa, T.J. Kremen, A.J. Giovannone, J.W. Lin, D. J. Chute, P.S. Mischel, T.F. Cloughesy, and M.D. Roth, *Clin. Cancer Res.* 11, 5515 (2005).

[7] M. Candolfi, J. F. Curtin, W. S. Nichols, A.K.M. G. Muhammad, G. D. King, G. E. Pluhar, E. A. McNiel, J. R. Ohlfest, A.B. Freese, P. F. Moore, J. Lerner, P. R. Lowenstein, and M. G. Castro, *J. Neuro Oncol.* 85, 133 (2007).

[8] B. Kaur and R.F. Barth, Rat glioma models for preclinical evaluation of novel therapeutic and diagnostic modalities. *CNS Cancer, Models, Prognostic Factors and Targets.* 10, 181-205 (2009). E. G. Van Meir, Editor Humana Press (Springer), Dr. Beverly Teicher, series Editor

[9] R.F. Barth and B Kaur, *J. Neuro-Oncol.* 94, 299 (2009).

[10] B. Melchior, S.S. Puntambekar, and M.J. Carson, *Neurochem. Int.* 49, 145 (2006).

[11] J. Zielasek, J.J. Archelos, K.V. Toyka, and H.P. Hartung, *Neurosci. Let.* 153, 136 (1993).

[12] R. DeSimone, A. Giampaolo, and B. Giometto, *J. Neuropath. Exp. Neuro.* 54, 175 (1995).

[13] S.C. Lee, W. Liu, P. Roth, D.W. Dickson, J.W. Berman, and C.F. Brosnan, *J. Immunol.* 150, 594 (1993).

[14] M. Righi, L. Mori, and G. DeLibero, *Eur. J. Immunol.* 19, 1443 (1989).

[15] T. Mizuno, M. Sawada, A. Suzumura, and T. Marunouchi, *Brain Res.* 656, 141 (1994).

[16] G. Sebire, D. Emilie, C. Wallon, C. Hery, O. Devergne, J.F. Delfraissy, P. Galanaud, and M. Tardieu, *J. Immunol.* 150, 1517 (1993).

[17] E. Ulvestad, K. Williams, R. Bjerkvig, K. Tiekotter, J. Antel, and A. Matre, *J. Leuko. Biol.* 56, 732 (1994).

[18] R. B. Rock, G. Gekker, S. Hu, W.S. Sheng, M. Cheeran, J.R. Lokensgard, and P.K. Peterson. *Clin. Microbiol. Rev.* 17, 942 (2004).

[19] M.J. Carson, *Glia* 40, 218 (2002).

[20] K. Frei, U. Malipiero, D. Piani, and A. Fontana, *Neuropathol. Appl. Neurobiol.* 20, 206, (1994).

[21] K. Frei, C. Siepl, P. Groscurth, S. Bodmer, C. Schwerdel, and A. Fontana, *Eur. J. Immunol.* 17, 1271 (1987).

[22] J.E. Merrill, L.J. Ignarro, M.P. Sherman, J. Melinek, and T.E. Lane, *J. Immunol.* 151, 2132 (1993).

[23] P.B. Medawar, *Br. J. Exp. Pathol.* 29, 58 (1948).

[24] T.S. Griffith, T. Brunner, S.M. Fletcher, D.R. Green, and T.A. Ferguson, *Science* 270, 1189 (1995).

[25] M.J. Carson, J. M. Doose, B. Melchior, C. D. Schmid, and C. C. Ploix, *Immunol Rev.* 213, 48 (2006).

[26] P. A. Henkart, *Immunity* 1, 343 (1994).

[27] N.L. Bryant, C. Suarez-Cuervo, G.Y. Gillespie, J.M. Markert, L.B. Nabors, S. Meleth, R.D. Lopez, and L.S. Lamb Jr., *Neuro. Oncol.* 11, 357 (2009).

[28] M. Wrensch, J.K Wiencke, J. Wiemels, R. Miike, J. Patoka, M. Moghadassi, A. McMillan, K.T. Kelsey, K. Aldape, K.R. Lamborn, A.T. Parsa, J.D. Sison, and M.D. Prados, *Cancer Res.* 66, 4531 (2006).

[29] J.L. Wiemels, J.K. Wiencke, J. Patoka, M. Moghadassi, T. Chew, A. McMillan, R. Miike, G. Barger, and M. Wrensch, *Cancer Res.* 64, 8468 (2004).

[30] [30] E. Linos, T. Raine, A. Alonso, and D. Michaud, *J. Natl Cancer I.* 99, 1544 (2007).

[31][31] P.M. Schiltz, G.J. Lee, N. Hoa, H. T. Wepsic, R.O. Dillman, and M.R. Jadus, *Cancer Biother. Radio.* 22, 672 (2007).

[32][32] T. Kottke, L. Sanchez-Perez, R. M. Diaz, J. Thompson, H. Chong, K. Harrington, S. K. Calderwood, J. Pulido, N. Georgopoulos, P. Selby, A. Melcher and R. Vile, *Cancer Res.* 67, 1197 (2007).

[33] P. Muranski, A. Boni, P.A. A.L. Cassard, K.R. Irvine, A. Kaiser, C.M. Paulos, D.C. Palmer, C.E. Touloukian, K. Ptak, L.Gattinoni, C. Wrzesinski, K.W. Kerstann, L. Feigenbaum, C.C. Chan, and N.P. Restifo, *Blood* 112, 362 (2008).

[34] T.A. Moseley, D.R. Haudenschild, L. Rose, and A.H. Reddi, *Cytokine Growth F. R.* 14, 155 (2003).

[35] S. Aggarwal and A.L. Gurney, *J. Leuko. Biol.* 71, 1 (2002).

[36] G. Murugaiyan and B. Saha, *J. Immunol.* 183, 4169 (2009)

[37] F. Benchetrit, A. Ciree, V. Vives, G. Warnier, A. Gey, C. Sautès-Fridman, F. Fossiez, N. Haicheur, W.H. Fridman, and E. Tartour, *Blood* 99, 2114 (2002).

[38] H. Wiendl, M. Mitsdoerffer, V. Hofmeister, J. Wischhusen, A. Bornemann, R. Meyermann, E.H. Weiss, A. Melms, and M. Weller, *J. Immunol.* 168, 4772 (2002).

[39] J. Wischhusen, M.A. Friese, M. Mittelbronn, R. Meyermann, and M. Weller, *J. Neuropathol. Exp. Neurol.* 64, 523 (2005).

[40] P Lau, C. Amadou, H. Brun, V. Rouillon, F. McLaren, A.F. Le Rolle, M. Graham, G.W. Butcher, and E. Joly, *BMC Immunol.* 4, 7 (2003).

[41] J. Vila, J.D. Isaacs, and A. E. Anderson, *Curr. Opin. Hematol.* 16, 274 (2009).

[42] H. Jiang and L. Chess, *J. Clin. Invest.* 114, 1198 (2004).

[43] A. Dario. A. Vignali, L.W. Collison, C.J. Workman, Nature Rev. Immunol. 8, 523 (2008).

[44] S. Nagaraj, M. Collazo, C. A. Corzo, J. Youn, M. Ortiz, D. Quiceno, and D. I. Gabrilovich, *Cancer Res.* 69, 7503 (2009).

[45] J.I. Youn, S. Nagaraj, M. Collazo, and D.I. Gabrilovich, *J. Immunol.* 181, 5791 (2008).

[46] X. Xiang, A. Poliakov, C. Liu, Y. Liu, Z.B. Deng, J. Wang, Z. Cheng, S.V. Shah, G.J. Wang, L. Zhang, W.E. Grizzle, J. Mobley, and H.G. Zhang, *Int. J. Cancer.* 124, 2621 (2009).

[47] S. F. Hussain, D. Yang, D. Suki, K. Aldape, E. Grimm, and A. B. Heimberger, *Neuro-Oncol.* 8, 261 (2006).

[48] J.T. Jordan, W. Sun, S.F. Hussain, G. DeAngulo, S.S. Prabhu, and A.B. Heimberger, *Cancer Immunol. Immunother.* 57, 123 (2008).

[49] P. E. Fecci, A. E. Sweeney, P. M. Grossi, S. K. Nair, C. A. Learn, D. A. Mitchell, X. Cui, T. J. Cummings, D. D. Bigner, E. Gilboa and J. H. Sampson, Systemic *Clin. Cancer Res.* 12, 4294 (2006).

[50] A. El Andaloussi and M. S. Lesniak, *Neuro. Oncol.* 8, 234 (2006).

[51] P.E. Fecci, D.A. Mitchell, J.F. Whitesides, W. Xie, A.H. Friedman, G.E. Archer, J.E. Herndon II, D.D. Bigner, G. Dranoff, J.H. Sampson, *Cancer Res.* 66, 3294 (2006).

[52] A.B. Heimberger, M. Abou-Ghazal, C. Reina-Ortiz, *Clin Cancer Res.* 14, 5166 (2006).

[53] D.R. Green, N. Droin, and M. Pinkoski, *Immunol. Rev.* 193, 70 (2003).

[54] S. Maher, D. Toomey, C. Condron, and D. Bouchier-Hayes, *Immunol. Cell Biol.* 80, 131 (2002).

[55] P. Attia, G. Q. Phan, A. V. Maker, M. R. Robinson, M. M. Quezado, J. C. Yang, R. M. Sherry, S. L. Topalian, U. S. Kammula, R. E. Royal, N. P. Restifo, L. R. Haworth, C.

Levy, S. A. Mavroukakis, G. Nichol, M. J. Yellin, and S. A. Rosenberg, *J. Clin. Oncol.* 23, 6043 (2005).

[56] G. Dranoff, *J. Clin. Oncol.* 23, 662 (2005).

[57] G.G. Gomez and C.A. Kruse, *Gene Ther. Mol. Biol.* 10, 133 (2006).

[58] H. Okada, G. Kohanbash, X. Zhu, E.R. Kastenhuber, A. Hoji, R. Ueda, and M. Fujita, *Crit. Rev. Immunol.* 29, 1 (2009).

[59] K.O. Lillehei, *Cancer Control* 10, 138 (2003).

[60] R. Kim, M. Emi, K. Tanabe and K. Arihiro, **Cancer Res.** 66, 5527 (2006).

[61] C.A. Kruse, L. Cepeda, B. Owens, S.D. Johnson, J. Stears, and K.O. Lillehei, Cancer Immunol. *Immunother.* 45, 77 (1997).

[62] Y. Huang, R.L. Hayes, S. Wertheim, E. Arbit, R. Scheff, Crit Rev Onco-Hematol. 39, 17 (2001).

[63] R. D. Schreiber, *Cancer Immun.* 5 (Suppl 1), 1 (2005).

[64] T. Makinodan, M.P. Chang, N. Kinohara, *Exp. Gerontol.* 21, 241.(1986).

[65] R.A. Miller, *Science* 273, 70 (1996).

[66] C.R. Gomez, V. Nomellini, D.E. Faunce, E.J. Kovacs, *Exp. Gerontol.* 43, 718 (2008).

[67] L. Driggers, E.W. Newcomb, J.G. Zhang, N. Hoa, and M.R. Jadus, *J. Neuro-Oncol.* in press 2009.

[68] P. Hurt, L. Walter, R. Sudbrak, S. Klages, I. Müller, T. Shiina, H. Inoko, H. Lehrach, E. Günther, R. Reinhardt, and H. Himmelbauer, *Genome Res.* 14, 631 (2004).

[69] W K. Silvers and S.L. Yang, *Science* 181, 570 (1973).

[70] A. S. Beutler, M.S. Banck, D. Wedekind, and H. J. Hedrich, *Hum. Gene Ther.* 10, 95 (1999).

[71] M. A. Altinoz, E. Ozar, M. Taskin, E. Bozcali, A. Bilir, T. Altug, A. Aydiner, A. Sav, *Pathol. Oncol. Res.* 7, 185 (2001).

[72] B. Badie, J.M. Schartner, A.R. Hagar, S. Prabakaran, T.R. Peebles, B. Bartley, S. Lapsiwala, D. K. Resnick and J. Vorpahl, *Clin. Cancer Res.* 9, 872 (2003).

[73] Y. Luo, J. Rydzewski, R.A. de Graaf, R. Gruetter, M. Garwood, and T. Schleich, *Magn. Reson. Med.* 41, 676 (1999).

[74] J. Trojan, T.R. Johnson, S.D. Rudin, J. Ilan, M.L. Tykocinski ML, and J.J. Ilan, *Science* 259, 94 (1993).

[75] V. Barresi, N. Belluardo, S. Sipione, G. Mudó, E. Cattaneo and D. F. Condorelli, *Cancer Gene Ther.* 10, 396 (2003).

[76] N.W. Bengtson and D.I. H. Linzer, *Mol. Endocrinol.* 14, 1934 (2000).

[77] X. Zheng, G. Shen, X. Yang and W. Liu, Cancer Res. 67, 3691 (2007).

[78] Z. Abdullah, T. Saric, H. Kashkar, N. Baschuk, B. Yazdanpanah, B.K. Fleischmann, J. Hescheler, M. Krönke, and Olaf Utermöhlen, J. Immunol. 178, 3390 (2007).

[79] J.G. Zhang, J. Eguchi, C.A. Kruse, G.G. Gomez, H. Fakhrai, S. Schroter, W. Ma, N. Hoa, B. Minev, C. Delgado H.T. Wepsic, H. Okada and M.R. Jadus, Clin. Cancer Res. 13, 566 (2007).

[80] J.G. Zhang, E. Newcomb, D. Zagzag, C. Kruse, L. Driggers, N. Hoa, and M.R. Jadus, J. Neuro-Oncol. *88, 65 (*2008).

[81] C. J. Wikstrand, L.P. Hale, S. K. Batra, M. L. Hill, P. A. Humphrey, S.N. Kurpad, R.E. McLendon, D. Moscatello, C. N. Pegram, C.J. Reist, S. T. Traweek, A. J. Wong, M.R. Zalutsky and D.D. Bigner, Cancer Res. 55, 3140 (1995).

[82] Y. Lee, C. J. Wikstrand, and D.D. Bigner, *J. Neuroimmunol.* 13, 183 (1986).

[83] H. Okada, J. Attanuci, K.M. Giezeman-Smits, C. Brissette-Storkus, W.K. Fellows, A. Gambotto, I.F. Pollack, K. Pogue-Geile, M.T. Lotze, M.E. Bozik, and W.K. Chambers, *Cancer Res.* 61, 2625 (2001).

[84] F.P. Holladay, G.B. Lopez, M. De, R.A. Morantz, and G.W. Wood, *Neurosurg.* 30, 499 (1992).

[85] F.P. Holladay, R. Choudhuri, T. Heitz, and G.W. Wood, *J. Neurosurg.* 80, 90 (1994).

[86] F.P. Holladay, T. Heitz, Y.L. Chen, M. Chiga, and G.W. Wood, *Neurosurgery.* 31, 528 (1992).

[87] M.R. Shah and W.J. Ramsey, *Cell. Immunol.* 225, 113 (2003).

[88] Y. Chen, T. Douglass, E.W.B. Jeffes Q. Xu, C. Williams, N. Arpajirakul, C. Delgado, M. Kleinman, R. Sanchez, Q. Dan, R.C. Kim,. H.T. Wepsic and M.R. Jadus, *Blood* 100, 1373 (2002).

[89] N. Hoa, J.G. Zhang, C. Delgado, M.P. Myers, L.L. Callahan, G. Vandeusen, Schiltz PM H.T. Wepsic, and M.R. Jadus, *Lab Invest* 87, 115 (2007).

[90] N.T. Hoa, M.P. Myers, J.G. Zhang, C. Delgado, L. Driggers, L.L. Callahan, G. Vandeusen, P.M. Schiltz, H.T. Wepsic, T.G. Douglass, T. Pham, N. Bhakta, L. Ge, and M.R. Jadus, *PLoS One* 4, e4631 (2009).

[91] M. Graf, M.R. Jadus, H.T. Wepsic, J.C. Hiserodt, and G.A. Granger, *J. Immunol.* 163, 5544 (1999).

[92] R. Sanchez, C. Williams, J.L. Daza, Q. Dan, Q. Xu, Y. Chen, C. Delgado, N. Arpajirakul, E.W.B. Jeffes, R.C. Kim, T. Douglass, U. Al Atar, H.T. Wepsic and M.R. Jadus, *Cell Immunol.* 216, 1 (2002).

[93] M.R. Jadus and A.B. Peck, *Transplantation.* 36, 281 (1983).

[94] L. Ge, J.G. Zhang, C.A. Samathanum, C. Delgado, M. Tarbiyat-Boldaji, Q. Dan, N. Hoa, T.V. Nguyen, R. Alipanah, J.T.H. Pham, R. Sanchez, H.T. Wepsic, T.R. Morgan and M.R. Jadus, *Cell. Immunol.* 259, 117 (2009).

[95] J.R. Fike, S. Rosi, and C.L. Limoli, *Semin Radiat Oncol* 19,122 (2009)

[96] K. Camphausen and P.J. Tofilon, *Clin. Cancer Res.* 13, 4326 (2007).

[97] S. Modi, A.T. Stopeck, M.S. Gordon, D. Mendelson, D.B. Solit, R. Bagatell, W. Ma, J. Wheler, N. Rosen, L. Norton, G.F. Cropp, R.G. Johnson, A.L. Hannah, C.A. Hudis, *J. Clin. Oncol.* 25, 5410 (2007).

[98] C.M. Sauvageot, J.L. Weatherbee, S. Kesari, S.E. Winters, J. Barnes, J. Dellagatta, N.R. Ramakrishna, C.D. Stiles, A.L. Kung, M.W. Kieran, P.Y. Wen, *Neuro Oncol.* 11, 109 (2009).

[99] P. Srivastava, *Ann. Rev. Immunol.* 20, 395 (2002).

[100] R. Suto and P.K. Srivastava, *Science* 269, 1585 (1995).

[101] H. Strik, M. Deininger, J. Streffer, E. Grote, J. Wickboldt, J. Dichgans, M. Weller, and R. Meyermann, *J. Neurol. Neurosur. Ps.* 67, 763 (1999).

[102] A. H. Stegh, S. Kesari, J. E. Mahoney, H. T. Jenq, K. L. Forloney, A. Protopopov, D. N. Louis, L. Chin, and R. A. DePinho, *Proc. Natl. Acad. Sci. USA.* 105, 10703 (2008).

[103] D.C. Altieri, *Curr. Opin. Cell Biol.* 18, 609 (2006).

[104] R. H. Stauber, W. Mann, and S. K. Knauer, *Cancer Res.* 67, 5999 (2007).

[105] S.M. Schmidt, K. Schag, and M.R. Muller, *Blood* 102, 571 (2003).

[106] R. Xiang, N. Mizutani, Y. Luo, C. Chiodoni, H. Zhou, M. Mizutani, Y. Ba, J. C. Becker and R. A. Reisfeld, *Cancer Res.* 65, 553 (2005).

[107] D. B. Constam, J. Philipp, U.V. Malipiero, P. TenDijke, M. Schachner, and A. Fontana, *J. Immunol.* 148, 1404 (1992).

[108] T. Roszman, L. Elliott, and W. Brooks, *Immunol. Today*. 12, 370 (1991).

[109] B. Bierie and H.L. Moses, *Nat. Rev. Cancer* 6, 506 (2006).

[110] A.W. Taylor, *J. Leuko Biol.* 85, 29 (2009).

[111] D.I. Gabrilovich, H.L. Chen, K.R. Girgis, H. T. Cunningham, G.M. Meny, S. Nadaf, D. Kavanaugh, and D.P. Carbone, *Nat. Med.* 2, 1096 (1996).

[112] M. Hishii, T. Nitta, H. Ishida, E. Michimasa, A. Kurosu, H. Yagita, K.Sato, and K. Okumura, *Neurosurgery*. 37, 1160 (1995).

[113] R.P. Phipps S.H. Stein, R.L. Roper, *Immunol. Today* 12, 349 (1991).

[114] S. Chattopadhyay, S. Bhattacharyya, B. Saha, J. Chakraborty, S. Mohanty, D. S. Hossain, S. Banerjee, K. Das, G. Sa, T. Das, *PLoS One* 4, e7382 (2009).

[115] R. Pai, B. Soreghan, I. L. Szabo, M. Pavelka, D. Baatar, and A.S. Tarnawski, *Nat. Med.* 8, 289 (2002).

[116] R.A. Prayson, E.A. Castilla, M.A. Vogelbaum, G.H. Barnett, Annals Diag Path 6, 148 (2002).

[117] Y. Akasaki, G. Liu, N. H. C. Chung, M. Ehtesham, K. L. Black, and J. S. Yu, J.Immunol. 173, 4352 (2004).

[118] M. Modolell, I.M. Corraliza, F. Link, G. Soler, and K. Eichmann, Eur. J. Immunol. 25, 1101 (1995).

[119] A. C. Ochoa, A. H. Zea, C. Hernandez and P. C. Rodriguez, Clin. Cancer Res. 13, 721s (2007).

[120] N. Umemura, M. Saio, T. Suwa, Y. Kitoh, J. Bai, K. Nonaka, G. Ouyang, M. Okada, M. Balazs, R. Adany, T. Shibata, and T. Takam, J. Leukoc. Biol. 83, 1136 (2008).

[121] P C. Rodriguez, C.P. Hernandez, D. Quiceno, S.M. Dubinett, J. Zabaleta, J.B. Ochoa, J. Gilbert, and A.C. Ochoa, J Exp Med. 202, 931 (2005).

[122] Y. Liu, J.A. Van Ginderachter, L. Brys, P. De Baetselier, G. Raes, and A.B. Geldhof, J. Immunol. 170, 5064. (2003).

[123] I.M. Corraliza, G. Soler, K. Eichmann, and M. Modolell, Biochem. Biophys. Res. Commun. 206, 667 (1995).

[124] G.C. Prendergast, Oncogene. 27, 3889 (2009).

[125] D.J. Chung, M. Rossi, E. Romano, J. Ghith, J. Yuan, D.H. Munn, and J.W. Young, *Blood* 114, 555 (2009).

[126] M.D. Sharma, D.Y. Hou, Y. Liu, P.A. Koni, R. Metz, P. Chandler, A.L. Mellor, Y. He, and D.H. Munn, *Blood* 113, 61021 (2009).

[127] S. Lob, A. Konigsrainer, D. Zieker, B.L. Brucher, H.G. Rammensee, G. Opelz, P. Terness, *Cancer Immunol. Immunother*. 58, 153 (2008).

[128] C. Uyttenhove, L. Pilotte, I. Théate, V. Stroobant, D. Colau, N. Parmentier, T. Boon and B. J Van den Eynde, *Nat. Med.* 9, 1269 (2003).

[129] T. Miyazaki, K. Moritake, K. Yamada, N. Hara, H. Osago, T. Shibata, Y. Akiyama, and M. Tsuchiya, *J. Neurosurg.* 111, 1 (2008).

[130] J. O'Connell, M. W. Bennett, G. C. O'Sullivan, J. K. Collins, and F. Shanahan, *Nat. Med.* 5:267 (1999).

[131] J. O'Connell, M. W. Bennett, G. C. O'Sullivan, J. K. Collins and F. Shanahan, *Immunol. Today*. 20, 46 (1999).

[132] J.F. Jacobs, A.J. Idema, K.F. Bol, S. Nierkens, O.M. Grauer, P. Wesseling, J.A. Grotenhuis, P.M. Hoogerbrugge, I.J. de Vries, G.J. Adema, *Neuro Oncol.* 11, 394 (2009).
[133] C.D. Riffkin, A. Z. Gray, C.J. Hawkins, C.W. Chow, and D.M. Ashley, *NeuroOncol.* 3, 229 (2001).
[134] A. Rensing-Ehl, K. Frei, R. Flury, B. Matiba, S.M. Mariani, M. Weller, P. Aebischer, P.H. Krammer, and A. Fontana, *Eur. J. Immunol.* 25, 2253 (1995).
[135] P. Saas, P.R. Walker, M. Hahn, A.L. Quiquerez, V. Schnuriger, G. Perrin, L. French, E.G.V. Meir, N. Tribolet, J. Tschopp, and P.Y. Dietrich, *J. Clin. Invest.* 99, 1173 (1997).
[136] M. Weller, P. Kleihues, J. Dichgans, and H. Ohgaki, *Brain Pathol.* 8, 285 (1998).
[137] C. Choi, X. Xu, J.W. Oh, S.J. Lee, G. Y. Gillespie, H. Park, H. Jo, and E.N. Benveniste, *Cancer Res.* 61, 3084 (2001).
[138] J. H. Song, A. Bellail, M.C. L. Tse, V.W. Yong, and C. Hao, *J. Neurosci.* 26, 3299 (2006).
[139] K. Hallermalm, A. De Geer, R. Kiessling, V. Levitsky and J. Levitskaya, Cancer Res. 64, 6775 (2004).
[140] N.P. Restifo, Nature Med. 6, 493 (2000).
[141] B.C. Yang, H.K. Lin, W.S. Hor, J.Y. Hwang, YP. Lin, M.Y. Liu, and Y.J. Wang, J. Immunol. 171, 3947 (2003).
[142] F. R. Balkwill, Am. Assoc. Cancer Res. Educ. Book. 1: 39 (2007).
[143] H. Kulbe, R. Thompson, J.L. Wilson, S. Robinson, T. Hagemann, R. Fatah, D. Gould, A. Ayhan and F.R. Balkwill, Cancer Res. 67, 585 (2007).
[144] S. Chen, T. Caragine, N.K. V. Cheung and S. Tomlinson, Cancer Res 60, 3013, (2000).
[145] A Maenpaa, S Junnikkala, J Hakulinen, T Timonen and S Meri, *Amer J Pathol*, 148, 1139, (1996).
[146] J. Tschopp, D. Masson, S. Schafer, M. Peitsch, K. T. Preissner, *Biochem.* 27, 4103 (1988)
[147] C.L. Gladson, J.N. Wilcox, L. Sanders, G.Y. Gillespie and D.A. Cheresh, *J. Cell Sci* 108, 947 (1995).
[148] M. L. Heidrick and W. L. Ryan, *Cancer Res.* 31, 1313 (1971).

In: Neuro-Oncology and Cancer Targeted Therapy
Editor: Lucía M. Gutiérrez pp.141-160
ISBN 978-1-61668-708-3
© 2010 Nova Science Publishers, Inc.

Chapter 5

BREAKING THE BARRIERS TO TUMOR-TARGETING VIA NANOCARRIER-BASED DRUG DELIVERY TO THE TUMOR MICROENVIRONMENT

Yusuke Doi, Tatsuhiro Ishida and Hiroshi Kiwada*

Department of Pharmacokinetics and Biopharmaceutics, Institute of Health Biosciences,
The University of Tokushima, Tokushima, Japan

ABSTRACT

Nanocarrier-based cancer chemotherapeutics are thought to increase therapeutic efficiency and reduce the side effects of associated chemotherapeutic agents by altering the agents' pharmacokinetics and tissue distribution following intravenous administration. In spite of these favorable properties, nanocarrier-based cancer chemotherapeutics are not always effective because of their heterogeneous intratumoral localization. Accumulation of nanocarriers in solid tumors occurs passively via the highly permeable tumor angiogenic vasculature in a long-circulating property-dependent manner. Accumulation is therefore affected by the heterogeneity of the tumor vascularity and vascular permeability. Homogeneous intratumoral distribution of nanocarriers would improve the efficacy of nanocarrier-based cancer chemotherapeutics in some intractable solid tumors. In this review, we focus on the barriers in the tumor microenvironment that hinder extravasation through the tumor vasculature and penetration of nanocarriers in solid tumors. In addition, we describe and discuss some trials that attempt to manipulate these barriers. Alterations of the tumor microenvironment that relate directly to the intratumoral distribution of nanocarriers may be potential strategies to improve the delivery of nanocarrier-based cancer chemotherapeutics.

---

* Corresponding author: Tatsuhiro Ishida, Ph.D.
Phone: 088-633-7260, Fax: 088-633-7260
E-mail: ishida@ph.tokushima-u.ac.jp

INTRODUCTION

Treatment of tumors with surgery, radiotherapy and chemotherapy has been one of the most progressive fields in medical science. In recent chemotherapy developments, novel anticancer agents, which act differently than conventional anticancer agents, are rapidly being applied in clinical practice. These novel agents are called molecular-targeted or cytostatic agents because they act immunologically, affect gene abnormalities of cancer cells, or are antibodies against cancer cells. Although therapies with these novel agents are effective enough to suppress tumor growth in limited circumstances, conventional chemotherapy is still problematic because of the disproportional relationship between antitumor effects and adverse effects. In current chemotherapy, anticancer agents are easily distributed in the patient's body and indiscriminately reach not only tumors, but also normal organs and tissues. Therefore, the development of a suitable tumor-selective drug delivery system is needed, to avoid the undesirable systemic side effects of anticancer agents. The most effective strategy is to exploit the anatomical and pathophysiological abnormalities of tumor tissue, particularly the tumor vasculature [1]. Nanoparticles such as polymeric micelles and liposomes (Table 1), which have a particle size of 50-200 nm, have been found to effectively accumulate in solid tumors, due to the abnormal features of the tumor microenvironment [2-4]. This characteristic is generally known as the "enhanced permeability and retention (EPR)" effect (Figure 1).

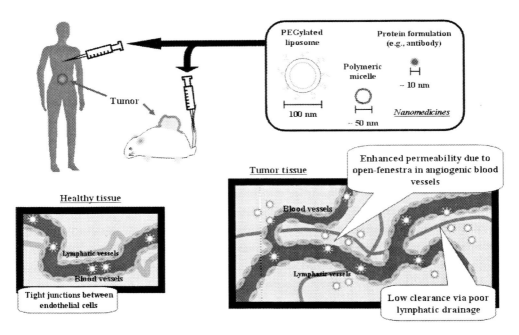

Figure 1. Schematic diagram depicting EPR effect. Angiogenic blood vessels in solid tumor have increased permeability against nanoparticles including PEGylated liposomes, polymeric micelles, and this permeability is attributed to large gap between endothelial cells in vessels. Consequently, PEGylated liposomes remarkably accumulate in solid tumor, due to the so-called "enhanced permeability and retention (EPR) effect."

Table 1. Examples of tumor-targeting nanoparticle

Nanoparticle	Particle	Application	Reference
Protein	≈10 nm	Antibody, cytokine, conjugation with anticancer agents	1, 4, 10, 86
Polymeric micelles	30-80 nm	Composed by block copolymer conjugated with anticancer agents	1, 61
Virus vector	100-150 nm	Transfection of coded target gene via viral replicating system	46, 47, 101
Liposome	100-200 nm	Encapsulation of anticancer agents inside their aqueous phase or phospholipid membrane	1, 6, 10, 16, 61, 67, 98, 99, 102, 104

Tumor localization of nanocarriers after systemic administration is thought to involve three processes (Figure 2-A): distribution through the vascular compartment in solid tumors, transport across the angiogenic vascular wall (extravasation from tumor blood circulation), and diffusion within the tumor interstitium. Various nanocarriers for anticancer agents that benefit from the EPR effect have been developed as drug delivery carriers. However, in spite of some benefits in anticancer drug delivery, nanocarriers (of any design) have not always shown sufficient delivery of associated agents to tumors, and have resulted in insufficient therapeutic effects. The tumor microenvironment, for example, spatial heterogeneity of vascular permeability and/or hypovascularity, may become a barrier to extravasation of nanocarriers from tumor vasculature and their diffusion in the interstitium of solid tumors (Figure 2-B).

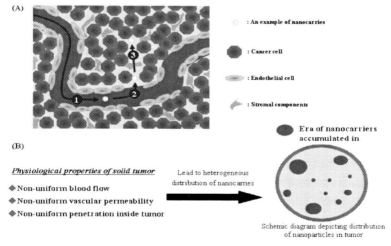

Figure 2. Delivery process of systemically administered nanocarriers to cancer cells in solid tumor and heterogeneous distribution of nanocarriers mediated by tumor heterogeneous microenvironment. (A) Nanocarriers are efficiently accumulated in solid tumor exploiting tumor abnormal microenvironment. Tumor localization of nanoarriers involves following three processes; (1) distribution through vascular compartment, (2) extravasation from tumor blood circulation across the vascular wall, (3) penetration within tumor interstitium. (B) Tumor heterogeneous microenvironment leads to heterogeneous distribution of nanoparticles, resulting in insufficient therapeutic efficacy of EPR effect-based cancer chemotherapy.

This review discusses the barriers to nanoparticle-based delivery in the tumor microenvironment, and how to overcome these barriers by focusing on the three processes for tumor localization of nanocarriers described above.

PROPERTIES AND FEATURES OF THE EPR EFFECT

In certain pathological conditions in which the permeability of tissue vasculature increases, such as inflammation and tumor development, nanocarriers, which are generally excluded from normal tissues, can extravasate from the vasculature and localize in the tumor interstitial space [5]. It is known that vascular remodeling to enable leukocyte extravasation, in response to signals released from infected or inflamed tissues, results in increases in vascular permeability and the localization of nanocarriers in these locations [6,7]. In the case of solid tumors, when tumor cells multiply, cluster together and reach a size of 2–3 mm, angiogenesis begins [8]. This neovasculature differs greatly from that of normal tissues in its microscopic anatomical architecture [9]. For instance, the blood vessels in the tumor are irregular in shape, dilated, leaky or defective, and the endothelial cells are poorly aligned or disorganized with large fenestrations. Such blood vessels, unlike the tight ones in most normal tissues, have gaps as large as 400 nm to 2 μm between adjacent endothelial cells [2,10]. Thus, nanocarriers can extravasate through these gaps into the tumor interstitial space in a size-dependent manner (Figure 1).

Tumor tissues have slow venous return and poor lymphatic drainage [9,11,12,13,14]. Such slow venous return and poor lymphatic clearance in solid tumors leads to their retention of nanocarriers [15]. However, the extravasation of nanocarriers into the tumor interstitium occurs continuously (Figure 1). The impaired lymphatic drainage contributes to the retention of nanocarriers in a solid tumor, and thus large increases in drug concentrations associated with nanocarriers in the tumor (10-fold or more) can be achieved, compared to administration of the same dose of a free drug [16]. However, the nanocarriers are usually localized and heterogeneously distributed in the tumor. Although the factors that result in high concentrations of nanocarriers in one part of the tumor tissue are not yet well understood [17], it seems that the degree of tumor vascularization (hypovascularity in solid tumors; poorly vascularized tumors lead to less nanocarrier accumulation), the degree of angiogenesis (small pre-angiogenic tumors or large necrotic tumors lead to poor or no nanocarrier accumulation), and the size of the pores in the vasculature (cut-off size of tumor vasculature) are critical to the accumulation of nanocarriers in solid tumors. Matsumura et al. [11] used biocompatible plasma proteins when they first reported the concept of the EPR effect, and this concept has been extended to synthetic polymers, to their various conjugates, and to nanocarriers, as well. The characteristics of nanocarriers, such as their size and their resident time in blood circulation (a longer half-life leads to a higher accumulation), are also important to achieve enhanced accumulation of nanocarriers in solid tumors.

Barriers to Accumulation of Nanocarriers in the Tumor Microenvironment

Tumor Vasculature and Blood Flow

To obtain nutrients and oxygen for their growth, and to metastasize to distant organs, tumor cells co-opt host vessels, sprout new vessels from existing ones (angiogenesis), and/or recruit endothelial cells from the bone marrow (postnatal vasculogenesis) [18]. The resulting vasculature in the solid tumor, structurally and functionally abnormal, is leaky, tortuous, dilated and saccular, and has a haphazard pattern of interconnection. These abnormalities contribute to spatial and temporal heterogeneity in tumor blood flow. In addition, solid pressure generated by proliferating tumor cells compresses intratumor blood and lymphatic vessels, which further impairs not only the blood flow but also the lymphatic flow [19]. Such vascular and lymphatic abnormalities in solid tumors are a major cause of the abnormal tumor microenvironment.

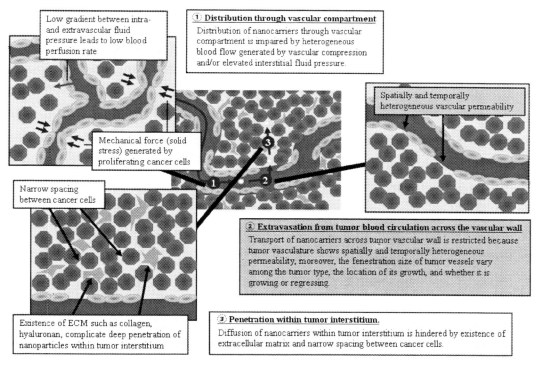

Figure 3. Barriers within tumor interstitium directly affect tumor localization of nanocarriers.

With respect to tumor vascular architecture, the vessel wall structure is very abnormal [20-22]. Large interendothelial junctions, increased numbers of permeable fenestrations, and a lack of normal basement membrane are often found in tumor vessels [23]. In addition, perivascular cells have abnormal morphology and heterogeneous associations with tumor vessels. Consistent with these structural abnormalities in the tumor vessel wall, the vascular permeability of solid tumor vessels relating to the EPR effect is generally higher than that of most normal vessels, resulting in enhanced accumulation of nanocarriers [2-4]. Extravasation of nanocarriers from the bloodstream occurs by diffusion and convection [15]. The diffusion of nanocarriers generally depends on their size, shape, charge, and flexibility during the transvascular transport pathway. However, their extravasation is limited by the cut-off size of the "pores" in the walls of tumor vessels, which vary from 100 nm to 2 μm depending on the tumor type, its growth location, and whether it is growing or regressing [2, 10]. Nanocarriers with a mean diameter of ≈ 200 nm are preferred for tumor targeting carrier systems. The biggest challenge for transvascular transport of nanoparticles in tumors stems from the spatial and temporal heterogeneity in permeability [10,24], which restricts access to some tumor regions (Figure 3).

Blood flow within tumors is heterogeneous because of the abnormal tumor microenvironment. Elevated interstitial fluid pressure—a hallmark of solid tumors—is commonly assumed to compress blood vessels in tumor tissue [25]. In addition, the compressive mechanical force of swiftly proliferating cancer cells causes vessels to compress and collapse, resulting in partial, heterogeneous blood flow in the tumor (Figure 3). These may be the major causes of the heterogeneous blood flow and impaired function of permeable vessels in tumor tissue. This heterogeneous blood flow also causes heterogeneous distribution of free anticancer agents, as well as nanocarriers. As a consequence, following repeated systemic injections, nanocarriers become concentrated in regions where enough has already accumulated [26,27]. However, this means that if tumor vasculature and the blood flow could be made homogeneous, more homogeneous distribution of nanocarriers in tumor tissue could be achieved.

Tumor Substance and Extracellular Matrix

Delivery of anticancer agents to tumor cells associated with nanocarriers requires their transport from the blood stream to the tumor interstium, and then diffusion through the tumor interstitium. Diffusion of nanoparticles through the tumor interstitium occurs largely via passive diffusion through the tumor extracellular space [28,29]. However, as described above, low convective diffusion occurs in the tumor interstitium because of elevated interstitial fluid pressure as a consequence of increased vascular permeability and the absence of functional lymphatics [30,31], as well as the mechanical compression generated by proliferating tumor cells [19]. In addition, the diffusion of nanocarriers in the tumor interstium is affected by the extracellular matrix (ECM) composition and by its geometry [32-34] (Figure 3). Compared with normal tissues, the tumor interstitium is characterized by an altered ECM and an increased number of fibroblasts that extensively synthesize growth factors, chemokines and adhesion molecules [31]. Thus, it is vital to identify the ECM constituents and characteristics that restrict diffusion of nanocarriers in order to design more suitable nanocarrier chemotherapeutics delivery systems. It is well known that the ECM varies greatly among tumors in both amount and composition [35]. Tumor-associated ECM is composed mainly of type 1 collagen, glycosaminoglycans such as hyaluronan, and proteoglycans such as decorin and glycol protein [36,37], and these ECM components form a complex structured gel.

It has been reported that resistance to interstitial flow is strongly linked to glycosaminoglycans, and especially hyaluronan, in the interstitial space of tumors [32,38]. Magzoub et al. [39] indicated that the diffusion of nanoparticles, such as high polymerized-dextran and albumin, was slowed 2- to 10-fold compared with their diffusion in saline. In addition, the diffusion rate depends, of course, on the tumor type, and the size and charge of the nanoparticles [34,40,41]. In oncolytic viral therapy (nanoparticle-based therapy), which is a promising approach to the treatment of certain human malignancies [42,43], the inability of oncolytic viruses to propagate and infect cells distant from the injection site limits their capacity to achieve consistent therapeutic responses [44-46]. McKee et al. [47] indicated that fibrillar collagen also limits virus vector distribution within a melanoma, and thus collagen can be one of the major barriers to nanoparticle transport in the tumor interstium. In addition, Netti et al. [48] showed that there is an inverse correlation between the collagen content of tumors and the diffusion of the proteinic macromolecule, IgG.

Breakthrough to Enhance Extravasation and Subsequent Diffusion of Nanocarriers in Tumors

Increased Blood Flow in Tumors by Relief of Vascular Compression via Alleviation of Mechanical Force

The Concept

Following systemic injection, nanocarriers are transported into tumor tissue via systemic blood flow. Thus, the efficacy of the delivery of nanocarriers to solid tumor is impaired by structural and functional abnormalities in blood and lymphatic vessels. Pedera et al. [19] provided evidence that proliferating cancer cells cause intratumor vessels to compress and collapse. This means that the reduction of such compressive mechanical force and the opening of vessels improve blood perfusion within tumor tissue, resulting in homogeneous intratumoral distribution of nanocarriers.

Diphtheria Toxin Treatment

Arbiser et al. [49] treated tumor-bearing mice with diphtheria toxin, which is much less cytotoxic to mouse cells than to human ones. They found that diphtheria toxin treatment caused cellular death (apoptosis) in human-tumor xenografts grown in mice, while the treatment showed no effect on murine tumors, normal murine tissue (liver) or murine endothelium. As a consequence, diphtheria toxin treatment led to a greater fraction of blood and lymphatic vessels with an open lumen in human tumors than in murine tumors [50]. Treatment with diphtheria toxin also causes vessels to have a more rounded cross-section in human tumors. Compared with collapsed vessels, open vessels are surrounded by fewer cells, suggesting that the local compressive force has decreased. Vessels associated with smooth-muscle α-actin-expressing cells, or with a prominent collagen IV basement membrane, are more likely to have an open lumen. These results confirm that proliferating tumor cells cause intratumor vessels, particularly those without supportive stromal structures, to collapse, thus leading to impaired blood flow. Tumor-selective cytotoxic therapy, which affects growing vascular endothelial cells, growing smooth muscle cells, and growing tumor cells, may result in more homogeneous blood flow in tumors and thereby enhance the efficient delivery of nanocarrier-based drugs to tumor tissue.

Angiotensin-II (AT-II)-Induced Hypertension

It has been reported that the smooth muscle layer, which plays a vital role in regulating blood pressure and flow, is lost in vasculature in some parts of tumor tissue. In normal blood vessels in normal tissue, angiotensin-II (AT-II), a vascular mediator, causes hypertension (increasing blood pressure and flow rate) via AT-II receptors on vascular smooth muscle cells. However, under these conditions the blood flow volume remains constant in normal tissue because of the existence of smooth muscle actin [12,51,52]. Although in AT-II-induced hypertension, in solid tumor tissue, the tumor blood vessels cannot regulate the blood flow volume because of the absence of the smooth muscle layer. Consequently, blood flow volume in tumor tissue increases 2-6 times in proportion to elevated blood pressure [12]. The induction of the hypertensive state by AT-II is, therefore, expected to augment the EPR effect and, thereby, the delivery of macromolecular drugs. In fact, when the systolic blood pressure was raised from 100 to 150 mmHg using AT-II, 1.3-3.0 fold increases in the accumulation of ^{51}Cr-labeled styrene-co-maleic-acid polymer (SMA) conjugated to neocarzinostatin (NCS), known as SMANCS, or ^{51}Cr-albumin (nano-sized formulations) in tumor tissue were observed [53]. This indicates that, by elevating blood pressure and blood flow in tumors using treatment with AT-II, one could accomplish more effective delivery of anticancer agents, particularly those associated with nanocarriers such as liposomes.

Enhanced Extravasation of Nanoparticles From Tumor Blood Circulation

Inhibition of Transforming Growth Factor-β (TGF-β) Signaling

TGF-β is known as a multifunctional cytokine, which regulates the growth, differentiation, migration, adhesion, and apoptosis of various types of cells. TGF-β binds to 2 different types of serine-threonine kinase receptors, known as type I (TβR-I) and type II (TβR-II) [54-56]. Upon ligand binding, TβR-II transphosphorylates TβR-I, which in turn transmits specific intracellular signals. The type I receptors phosphorylate receptor-activated Smads (R-Smads), and induce complex formation between R-Smads and common-partner Smad (co-Smad). TGF-β inhibits the growth and migration of blood vascular endothelial cells *in vitro*, whereas it induces angiogenesis *in vivo* [57]. Mice lacking certain components related to TGF-β signaling (ex. TGF-β1, TβR-II, or TβR-I) exhibited abnormalities in blood vessels [58-60].

To investigate the mechanisms of the effect of TβR-I inhibitor on the neovasculature, changes in three major components of tumor vasculature, endothelium, pericytes, and basement membrane, were analyzed after administration of TβR-I inhibitor [61]. The areas of vascular endothelial cells that were stained by platelet/endothelial cell adhesion molecule CD31 increased slightly with TβR-I inhibitor treatment. Coverage of the endothelium by pericytes, which were determined to be NG2-positive perivascular cells, was decreased by the TβR-I inhibitor treatment. The functional aspects of the effects of low-dose TβR-I inhibitor were investigated using intravenously administered high-polymeric dextran of 2 MDa with a hydrodynamic diameter of 50 nm [62,63], which is equivalent to the common size of nanocarriers. Although the dextran remained mostly in the intravascular space in the control tumor, as reported previously [63], the use of TβR-I inhibitor resulted in extravasation and a far broader distribution of the dextran around the tumor neovasculature. These findings suggest that low-dose TβR-I inhibitor can maintain blood flow in the tumor vasculature and simultaneously induce extravasation of macromolecules. Recently, the effect of administration of TβR-I inhibitor on doxorubicin (DXR)-containing PEGylated liposome (Doxil) or DXR-containing polymeric micelles was investigated in a xenograft murine model of human BxPC3 cells, which are DXR-sensitive *in vitro* [64]. TβR-I inhibitor co-administered with DXR-containing nanocarriers significantly enhanced intratumoral accumulation of DXR, but when co-administered with free DXR it did not increase the intratumoral DXR accumulation. This suggests that only macromolecules such as nanocarriers benefit from the use of TβR-I inhibitor through enhancement of the EPR effect. Consequently, a strategy in combination with TGF-β signaling could be a breakthrough in chemotherapy delivered by nanocarriers in intractable solid tumors.

Tumor Necrosis Factor (TNF)-α

TNF-α is one of the most thoroughly investigated cytokines. In earlier studies, researchers paid attention to the cytotoxic activity of TNF-α against tumor cells. Later, their attention shifted to an indirect TNF-α-induced anti-tumor effect. This was based on the following observations. Systemic administration of TNF-α caused necrosis in well-established subcutaneous tumors, whereas small tumors in the early stage and intraperitoneal tumors did not respond to TNF-α therapy [65]. TNF-α affected tumor-associated vasculature, not the vascularization of normal tissue [66]. Seynhaeve et al. [67] indicated that the alteration of tumor vasculature caused by TNF-α led to further abnormalities—in particular, vascular permeability in the tumor—and that treatment of low-dose TNF-α in combination with i.v. administration of PEGylated liposome facilitated extravasation of the liposome from blood vessels and more homogeneous distribution in solid tumors. This revealed that treatment with TNF-α not only increases the leakiness of some tumor vessels, but also renders more vessels permeable to nanocarriers such as liposomes 100-200 nm in mean diameter, while leaving the vascular function (e.g., flow) intact. Seynhaeve et al. [67] finally demonstrated an improved tumor response due to a more homogeneous distribution of anticancer drug-containing nanocarriers in the tumor.

Addition of Vascular Endothelial Growth Factor (VEGF)

VEGF, initially referred to as vascular permeability factor (VPF), is considered the central factor in both physiological and pathological angiogenesis [68,69]. Its receptors are predominantly expressed on neovasculature, such as that found in tumors [70,71]. VEGF, a mitogen and survival factor for endothelial cells, has vasoactive properties and is 50,000 times more potent than histamine in increasing permeability [72,73]. Together with angiopoietins, VEGF regulates the interaction of endothelial cells with other endothelial cells, pericytes and basal membranes. Hence, VEGF triggers dissociation of the endothelial cells, resulting in leakage and the generation of edema [73-75]. In fact, morphometric studies showed that chronic VEGF exposure increases the number of transvascular pathways, open junctions, and fenestrations in both tumor and normal vessels [2,76-78]. The exogenous addition of VEGF to hypopermeable vessels could be used to increase transvascular transport of macromolecules, including nanocarriers, in these regions [10].

Inhibition of VEGF Signaling

Many researchers have reported that inhibition of VEGF signaling results in the pruning of tumor vessels and reductions in vascularity [79-83]. In addition, it has been demonstrated that agents that block VEGF signaling can decrease interstitial fluid pressure in tumors [81,82]. Jain and co-workers demonstrated that vessels in tumors treated with VEGF inhibitor are structurally and functionally "normalized" [84,85]. This leads to an assumption that treatment with VEGF inhibitors more efficiently delivers the free-form drug co-administered with them to tumor tissues, despite the fact that treatment diminishes tumor vascularity.

However, the normalization of tumor vessels attenuates the extravasation of nanocarriers into the interstitial space of tumor tissue by pruning abnormal vasculature and rectifying abnormal barrier function [23,85]. Nakahara et al. [86] demonstrated how vascular "normalization" caused by inhibition of VEGF signaling affects the distribution and extravasation of nanoparticles such as antibodies and microspheres. The results in the control tumor showed a distinctive, patchy network of extravasated IgG following i.v. administration. On the other hand, the results in the tumor treated with VEGF inhibitor showed a distribution pattern of IgG similar to that in the control tumor, but in a lower amount of accumulation. The distribution pattern of 50 nm-microspheres in tumor tissues differed from that of IgG; extravasated microspheres accumulated in focal regions, unlike the irregular, patchy network of extravasated IgG. It seems that the movement of microspheres in tumor interstitial space is limited, due to their larger size compared to IgG ($\approx$5 nm). Inhibition of VEGF signaling decreased the overall distribution of IgG and microspheres, in large part, due to reduced tumor vascularity. Hence, vascular "normalization" caused by inhibition of VEGF signaling may diminish the EPR effect in macromolecule-containing nanoparticles, resulting in decreased efficiency of nanoparticle-based therapy.

Nitric Oxide (NO)

NO, synthesized from L-arginine by NO synthase (NOS), is a well-known vasoactive agent that increases vascular permeability in tumors [87-90]. This function of NO was confirmed by the fact that extravasation of Evans blue, which is associated with serum proteins, in tumor tissues was suppressed by NO scavengers and NOS inhibitor. Because of such vasoactivity, NO may increase the EPR effect against nanocarriers by widening the endothelial gaps of tumor-feeding arteries. In one such case, in humans, treatment with the NO-releasing agent isosorbide dinitrate enhanced the opening of the tumor-feeding artery, and more drug entered the tumor [91]. This technique, plus co-treatment with AT-II, further enhanced the site-specific delivery of SMANCS–Lipiodol1 to the tumor [91].

Augmentation of Distribution of Nanocarriers in Tumor Substance

Alteration of Extracellular Matrix (ECM) Composition

Chemotherapeutic agents must extravasate from blood and penetrate through the ECM in the tumor interstitial space to reach cancer cells in a tumor. Drug delivery through the ECM relies on passive diffusive transport [28]. Unfortunately, delivery via passive diffusion becomes less efficient for larger particles such as nanocarriers.

Collagenase treatment efficiently digests collagen in tumor ECM, and was found to increase macromolecule diffusion in tumors [38,92,93]. Digestion of type I collagen by collagenase produced a 2-fold increase in the diffusion of 10 kDa dextran at all tumor depths. Collagenase treatment also increased the diffusion of 500 kDa dextran and albumin 2-fold, but only in superficial tumors. This enhancement of diffusion is similar to the 2-fold increase in IgG diffusion reported in superficial tumors after collagenase treatment [92]. Collagenase treatment also enhanced the diffusion of an oncolytic herpes simplex virus (HSV) in superficial tumors, increasing the area of viral distribution by 3-fold [93]. This indicates that collagen in the interstitial space of tumors plays an important role in regulating the initial distribution of viral vectors in certain fibrous tumors. In control tumors (no treatment with collagen), whereas a smaller tracer (2×106 MW dextran) was distributed relatively uniformly within the tumor, the vast majority of HSV virions (150 nm in diameter) were located only in collagen-poor areas. Furthermore, silica microspheres similar in size to the viral particles, but lacking their ability to bind to cell and matrix proteins, were localized in collagen-poor areas of tumors. This suggests that an effective pore size cutoff exists for the collagen network to allow diffusion of such particles in tumors, and the cutoff size is smaller than the size of these particles (≈ 150 nm).

Decorin, a major ECM, also plays a role as an important determinant of macromolecule diffusion in tumor tissue ECM. Decorin digestion by cathepsin C produced a more substantial increase in the diffusion of 500 kDa dextran deeper in tumor tissue [94], similar to the finding for collagen digestion. Decorin digestion may produce a widening of collagen interfibrillar spaces, as it has been implicated in collagen fibril-fibril interactions [95]. This strongly indicates that decorin is a target to enhance macromolecule diffusion in tumors.

Digestion of hyaluronic acid (HA) by hyaluronidase administration was found to enhance the therapeutic efficacy of antitumor agents associated with nanocarriers [96,97]. Hyaluronidase treatment increased the tumor uptake and improved the distribution of liposomal DXR [98]. Similar to an earlier observation [99], in the control tumors, intact liposomal DXR was observed to remain within the vasculature or interstitial space, very close to the blood vessels. On the other hand, Magzoub et al. [39] recently reported that digestion of hyaluronan slowed macromolecule diffusion in tumor tissue. Hyaluronan polymerizes itself and forms cage-like structures ~15 nm in diameter that contain water-filled spaces, allowing the passage of tracers with a small molecular weight [100]. It is assumed that hyaluronidase treatment results in collapse of the water-swelled cage structures, increasing viscous hindrance [40]. This discrepancy with respect to the consequences of hyaluronidase treatment is not well understood. Further research is needed.

Creation of Void Space in Extravascular-Interstitial Compartments in Tumors

The existence of ECM is not the only barrier to the diffusion of nanocarriers through tumor interstitium. The narrow spacing of ~20 nm between tumor cells also hinders the penetration of most nanoparticles, which are significantly larger than 20 nm. Nagano et al. [101] tested whether the void spaces, enlarged due to tumor cell apoptosis, enhance the initial penetration of microspheres (100 nm) and oncolytic HSV in tumors. Tumor cell apoptosis was induced by treatment with doxycycline-regulated expression of CD8/caspase-8, paclitaxel, or paclitaxel plus tumor necrosis factor–related apoptosis-inducing ligand (TRAIL). Compared with the isolated pattern of HSV infection generally located in the center of the control tumor, the treatment induced an interconnected and diffuse pattern of infection, which extended from one edge of the tumor to the other. In the control tumor, the microspheres were restricted to small areas in the tumor center. By contrast, in the treated tumor, the microspheres were distributed in larger areas and found in the periphery of the tumor. The treatment significantly increased the intratumoral microsphere penetration by 3.3-fold, compared with the control tumor. Overall, these results suggest that induction of apoptosis and the resulting void space enlargement in the tumor facilitate penetration of nanoparticles into the tumor tissue.

Another result showed that paclitaxel tumor priming promoted the interstitial transport of nanoparticles, probably due to perturbation of the tumor structure, i.e., a reduction in tumor cell density leading to greater porosity and lower tortuosity [102]. The *in vitro* observation that tumor priming promoted the penetration of protein-bound drugs in tumor fragments supports these results [103]. In addition, paclitaxel tumor priming also reduced the tumor cell density as a result of cellular death, expanded the microvessel diameter, and increased tumor perfusion. Treatment with cytotoxic anticancer agents may have the potential to promote localization of nanocarriers, though optimization of the dose regimen is difficult. We recently reported that metronomic cyclophosphamide (CPA) dosing via oral administration promoted enhanced accumulation of PEGylated liposomes in solid tumor tissue [104]. This enhancing effect may reflect the transient increase in density of microvessels in the tumor tissues. Anti-angiogenic therapy induced by metronomic CPA dosing caused tumor tissue hypoxia by diminishing blood flow, and the resulting hypoxia and acidification of the surrounding tissue might induce a transient increase in the density of microvessels, creating higher permeability for the PEGylated liposome in the tumor. Alternatively, metronomic CPA dosing might transiently normalize the tumor vasculature and microenvironment. Accompanied by vascular normalization, decreased interstitial fluid pressure would restore the pressure gradient across the blood vessel wall, as well as the tumor interstitium, and thus increase the penetration of sequentially administered CPA into the tumor. As a consequence, adequate CPA levels might be reached in the tumor tissue and lead to an enlargement in the tumor interstitial space, into which PEGylated liposomes could extravasate and diffuse.

CONCLUSION

The therapeutic efficiency of cancer treatment by means of nanocarriers is clearly dependent on effective delivery of the encapsulated anticancer agents into tumors after systemic injection. Effective delivery means not only transport of anticancer agents into the tumor, but also deep and homogeneous diffusion of the agents within tumor tissue following extravasation of nanocarriers into the interstitial space of tumor tissue. However, the effectiveness of delivery is often impaired because of barriers in the tumor microenvironment, as described in this chapter. We conclude that modification and control of the nanocarrier extravasation and diffusion process by alteration of the tumor microenvironment would promote enhanced therapeutic effects of anticancer agents delivered by nanocarrier-based drug delivery systems. Innovations in the strategies used to control the tumor microenvironment may lead to a breakthrough in nanocarrier-based chemotherapy.

ACKNOWLEDGMENTS

We thank Dr. James L. McDonald for his helpful advice in writing the English manuscript. This work was supported in part by a Grant-in-Aid for Young Scientists (A) (21689002), the Ministry of Education, Culture, Sports, Science and Technology, Japan.

REFERENCES

[1] Iyer, A. K., Khaled, G., Fang, J., and Maeda, H. Exploiting the enhanced permeability and retention effect for tumor targeting. *Drug Discov Today, 11:* 812-818, 2006.

[2] Hobbs, S. K., Monsky, W. L., Yuan, F., Roberts, W. G., Griffith, L., Torchilin, V. P., and Jain, R. K. Regulation of transport pathways in tumor vessels: role of tumor type and microenvironment. *Proc Natl Acad Sci U S A, 95:* 4607-4612, 1998.

[3] Gerlowski, L. E. and Jain, R. K. Microvascular permeability of normal and neoplastic tissues. *Microvasc Res, 31:* 288-305, 1986.

[4] Yuan, F., Leunig, M., Berk, D. A., and Jain, R. K. Microvascular permeability of albumin, vascular surface area, and vascular volume measured in human adenocarcinoma LS174T using dorsal chamber in SCID mice. *Microvasc Res, 45:* 269-289, 1993.

[5] Hashizume, H., Baluk, P., Morikawa, S., McLean, J. W., Thurston, G., Roberge, S., Jain, R. K., and McDonald, D. M. Openings between defective endothelial cells explain tumor vessel leakiness. *Am J Pathol, 156:* 1363-1380, 2000.

[6] Schiffelers, R. M., Storm, G., and Bakker-Woudenberg, I. A. Host factors influencing the preferential localization of sterically stabilized liposomes in Klebsiella pneumoniae-infected rat lung tissue. *Pharm Res, 18:* 780-787, 2001.

[7] Edens, H. A., Levi, B. P., Jaye, D. L., Walsh, S., Reaves, T. A., Turner, J. R., Nusrat, A., and Parkos, C. A. Neutrophil transepithelial migration: evidence for sequential, contact-dependent signaling events and enhanced paracellular permeability independent of transjunctional migration. *J Immunol, 169:* 476-486, 2002.

[8] Folkman, J. Angiogenesis in cancer, vascular, rheumatoid and other disease. *Nat Med, 1:* 27-31, 1995.

[9] Skinner, S. A., Tutton, P. J., and O'Brien, P. E. Microvascular architecture of experimental colon tumors in the rat. Cancer Res, *50:* 2411-2417, 1990.

[10] Monsky, W. L., Fukumura, D., Gohongi, T., Ancukiewcz, M., Weich, H. A., Torchilin, V. P., Yuan, F., and Jain, R. K. Augmentation of transvascular transport of macromolecules and nanoparticles in tumors using vascular endothelial growth factor. *Cancer Res, 59:* 4129-4135, 1999.

[11] Matsumura, Y. and Maeda, H. A new concept for macromolecular therapeutics in cancer chemotherapy: mechanism of tumoritropic accumulation of proteins and the antitumor agent smancs. Cancer Res, *46:* 6387-6392, 1986.

[12] Suzuki, M., Hori, K., Abe, I., Saito, S., and Sato, H. A new approach to cancer chemotherapy: selective enhancement of tumor blood flow with angiotensin II. *J Natl Cancer Inst, 67:* 663-669, 1981.

[13] Maeda, H. and Matsumura, Y. Tumoritropic and lymphotropic principles of macromolecular drugs. *Crit Rev Ther Drug Carrier Syst, 6:* 193-210, 1989.

[14] Iwai, K., Maeda, H., and Konno, T. Use of oily contrast medium for selective drug targeting to tumor: enhanced therapeutic effect and X-ray image. *Cancer Res, 44:* 2115-2121, 1984.

[15] Jain, R. K. Transport of molecules across tumor vasculature. *Cancer Metastasis Rev, 6:* 559-593, 1987.

[16] Northfelt, D. W., Martin, F. J., Working, P., Volberding, P. A., Russell, J., Newman, M., Amantea, M. A., and Kaplan, L. D. Doxorubicin encapsulated in liposomes containing surface-bound polyethylene glycol: pharmacokinetics, tumor localization, and safety in patients with AIDS-related Kaposi's sarcoma. *J Clin Pharmacol, 36:* 55-63, 1996.

[17] Netti, P. A., Roberge, S., Boucher, Y., Baxter, L. T., and Jain, R. K. Effect of transvascular fluid exchange on pressure-flow relationship in tumors: a proposed mechanism for tumor blood flow heterogeneity. *Microvasc Res, 52:* 27-46, 1996.

[18] Carmeliet, P. and Jain, R. K. Angiogenesis in cancer and other diseases. *Nature, 407:* 249-257, 2000.

[19] Padera, T. P., Stoll, B. R., Tooredman, J. B., Capen, D., di Tomaso, E., and Jain, R. K. Pathology: cancer cells compress intratumour vessels. *Nature, 427:* 695, 2004.

[20] di Tomaso, E., Capen, D., Haskell, A., Hart, J., Logie, J. J., Jain, R. K., McDonald, D. M., Jones, R., and Munn, L. L. Mosaic tumor vessels: cellular basis and ultrastructure of focal regions lacking endothelial cell markers. Cancer Res, *65:* 5740-5749, 2005.

[21] McDonald, D. M. and Choyke, P. L. Imaging of angiogenesis: from microscope to clinic. *Nat Med, 9:* 713-725, 2003.

[22] Chang, Y. S., di Tomaso, E., McDonald, D. M., Jones, R., Jain, R. K., and Munn, L. L. Mosaic blood vessels in tumors: frequency of cancer cells in contact with flowing blood. *Proc Natl Acad Sci U S A, 97:* 14608-14613, 2000.

[23] Winkler, F., Kozin, S. V., Tong, R. T., Chae, S. S., Booth, M. F., Garkavtsev, I., Xu, L., Hicklin, D. J., Fukumura, D., di Tomaso, E., Munn, L. L., and Jain, R. K. Kinetics of vascular normalization by VEGFR2 blockade governs brain tumor response to radiation: role of oxygenation, angiopoietin-1, and matrix metalloproteinases. *Cancer Cell, 6:* 553-563, 2004.

[24] Yuan, F., Dellian, M., Fukumura, D., Leunig, M., Berk, D. A., Torchilin, V. P., and Jain, R. K. Vascular permeability in a human tumor xenograft: molecular size dependence and cutoff size. Cancer Res, *55:* 3752-3756, 1995.

[25] Boucher, Y. and Jain, R. K. Microvascular pressure is the principal driving force for interstitial hypertension in solid tumors: implications for vascular collapse. *Cancer Res, 52:* 5110-5114, 1992.

[26] Jain, M. G., Hislop, G. T., Howe, G. R., and Ghadirian, P. Plant foods, antioxidants, and prostate cancer risk: findings from case-control studies in Canada. *Nutr Cancer, 34:* 173-184, 1999.

[27] Jain, R. K. Understanding barriers to drug delivery: high resolution in vivo imaging is key. *Clin Cancer Res., 5:* 1605-1606, 1999.

[28] Netti, P. A., Hamberg, L. M., Babich, J. W., Kierstead, D., Graham, W., Hunter, G. J., Wolf, G. L., Fischman, A., Boucher, Y., and Jain, R. K. Enhancement of fluid filtration across tumor vessels: implication for delivery of macromolecules. *Proc Natl Acad Sci U S A, 96:* 3137-3142, 1999.

[29] Banerjee, R. K., Sung, C., Bungay, P. M., Dedrick, R. L., and van Osdol, W. W. Antibody penetration into a spherical prevascular tumor nodule embedded in normal tissue. *Ann Biomed Eng., 30:* 828-839, 2002.

[30] Ribatti, D., Nico, B., Crivellato, E., and Vacca, A. The structure of the vascular network of tumors. *Cancer Lett., 248:* 18-23, 2007.

[31] DiResta, G. R., Lee, J., Healey, J. H., Levchenko, A., Larson, S. M., and Arbit, E. "Artificial lymphatic system": a new approach to reduce interstitial hypertension and increase blood flow, pH and pO2 in solid tumors. *Ann Biomed Eng, 28:* 543-555, 2000.

[32] Levick, J. R. Flow through interstitium and other fibrous matrices. *Q J Exp Physiol, 72:* 409-437, 1987.

[33] Graff, B. A., Bjornaes, I., and Rofstad, E. K. Macromolecule uptake in human melanoma xenografts. relationships to blood supply, vascular density, microvessel permeability and extracellular volume fraction. Eur J Cancer, *36:* 1433-1440, 2000.

[34] Pluen, A., Boucher, Y., Ramanujan, S., McKee, T. D., Gohongi, T., di Tomaso, E., Brown, E. B., Izumi, Y., Campbell, R. B., Berk, D. A., and Jain, R. K. Role of tumor-host interactions in interstitial diffusion of macromolecules: cranial vs. subcutaneous tumors. *Proc Natl Acad Sci U S A, 98:* 4628-4633, 2001.

[35] Ohtani, H. Stromal reaction in cancer tissue: pathophysiologic significance of the expression of matrix-degrading enzymes in relation to matrix turnover and immune/inflammatory reactions. *Pathol Int, 48:* 1-9, 1998.

[36] Alberts, B., Bray, D., Lewis, J., Raff, M., Roberts, K., and Watson, J. Extracellular matrix of animals, 3rd edition, p. 971-995. New York: Garland Publishing, 1994.

[37] Gribbon, P. M., Maroudas, A., Parker, K. H., and Winlove, C. P. Water and solute transport in the extracellular matrix: phygical principles and macromolecular and determinants, Vol. Integration and Reductionism, p. 95-124. London: Portland Press, 1998.

[38] Comper, W. D. and Laurent, T. C. Physiological function of connective tissue polysaccharides. *Physiol Rev, 58:* 255-315, 1978.

[39] Magzoub, M., Jin, S., and Verkman, A. S. Enhanced macromolecule diffusion deep in tumors after enzymatic digestion of extracellular matrix collagen and its associated proteoglycan decorin. Faseb J, *22:* 276-284, 2008.

[40] Alexandrakis, G., Brown, E. B., Tong, R. T., McKee, T. D., Campbell, R. B., Boucher, Y., and Jain, R. K. Two-photon fluorescence correlation microscopy reveals the two-phase nature of transport in tumors. Nat Med, *10:* 203-207, 2004.

[41] Stroh, M., Zimmer, J. P., Duda, D. G., Levchenko, T. S., Cohen, K. S., Brown, E. B., Scadden, D. T., Torchilin, V. P., Bawendi, M. G., Fukumura, D., and Jain, R. K. Quantum dots spectrally distinguish multiple species within the tumor milieu in vivo. *Nat Med, 11:* 678-682, 2005.

[42] Everts, B. and van der Poel, H. G. Replication-selective oncolytic viruses in the treatment of cancer. *Cancer Gene Ther., 12:* 141-161, 2005.

[43] Chiocca, E. A. Oncolytic viruses. *Nat Rev Cancer, 2:* 938-950, 2002.

[44] Ichikawa, T. and Chiocca, E. A. Comparative analyses of transgene delivery and expression in tumors inoculated with a replication-conditional or -defective viral vector. *Cancer Res, 61:* 5336-5339, 2001.

[45] Lee, C. T., Park, K. H., Yanagisawa, K., Adachi, Y., Ohm, J. E., Nadaf, S., Dikov, M. M., Curiel, D. T., and Carbone, D. P. Combination therapy with conditionally replicating adenovirus and replication defective adenovirus. *Cancer Res, 64:* 6660-6665, 2004.

[46] Harrison, D., Sauthoff, H., Heitner, S., Jagirdar, J., Rom, W. N., and Hay, J. G. Wild-type adenovirus decreases tumor xenograft growth, but despite viral persistence

complete tumor responses are rarely achieved--deletion of the viral E1b-19-kD gene increases the viral oncolytic effect. Hum Gene Ther, *12:* 1323-1332, 2001.

[47] McKee, T. D., Grandi, P., Mok, W., Alexandrakis, G., Insin, N., Zimmer, J. P., Bawendi, M. G., Boucher, Y., Breakefield, X. O., and Jain, R. K. Degradation of fibrillar collagen in a human melanoma xenograft improves the efficacy of an oncolytic herpes simplex virus vector. Cancer Res, *66:* 2509-2513, 2006.

[48] Netti, P. A., Berk, D. A., Swartz, M. A., Grodzinsky, A. J., and Jain, R. K. Role of extracellular matrix assembly in interstitial transport in solid tumors. *Cancer Res., 60:* 2497-2503, 2000.

[49] Arbiser, J. L., Raab, G., Rohan, R. M., Paul, S., Hirschi, K., Flynn, E., Price, E. R., Fisher, D. E., Cohen, C., and Klagsbrun, M. Isolation of mouse stromal cells associated with a human tumor using differential diphtheria toxin sensitivity. *Am J Pathol, 155:* 723-729, 1999.

[50] Griffon-Etienne, G., Boucher, Y., Brekken, C., Suit, H. D., and Jain, R. K. Taxane-induced apoptosis decompresses blood vessels and lowers interstitial fluid pressure in solid tumors: clinical implications. *Cancer Res, 59:* 3776-3782, 1999.

[51] Greish, K., Fang, J., Inutsuka, T., Nagamitsu, A., and Maeda, H. Macromolecular therapeutics: advantages and prospects with special emphasis on solid tumour targeting. *Clin Pharmacokinet, 42:* 1089-1105, 2003.

[52] Hori, K., Saito, S., Takahashi, H., Sato, H., Maeda, H., and Sato, Y. Tumor-selective blood flow decrease induced by an angiotensin converting enzyme inhibitor, temocapril hydrochloride. *Jpn J Cancer Res, 91:* 261-269, 2000.

[53] Li, C. J., Miyamoto, Y., Kojima, Y., and Maeda, H. Augmentation of tumour delivery of macromolecular drugs with reduced bone marrow delivery by elevating blood pressure. Br J Cancer, *67:* 975-980, 1993.

[54] Heldin, C. H., Miyazono, K., and ten Dijke, P. TGF-beta signalling from cell membrane to nucleus through SMAD proteins. *Nature, 390:* 465-471, 1997.

[55] Shi, Y. and Massague, J. Mechanisms of TGF-beta signaling from cell membrane to the nucleus. Cell, *113:* 685-700, 2003.

[56] Feng, X. H. and Derynck, R. Specificity and versatility in tgf-beta signaling through Smads. Annu Rev Cell Dev Biol, *21:* 659-693, 2005.

[57] Bertolino, P., Deckers, M., Lebrin, F., and ten Dijke, P. Transforming growth factor-beta signal transduction in angiogenesis and vascular disorders. *Chest, 128:* 585S-590S, 2005.

[58] Dickson, K., Philip, A., Warshawsky, H., O'Connor-McCourt, M., and Bergeron, J. J. Specific binding of endocrine transforming growth factor-beta 1 to vascular endothelium. *J Clin Invest, 95:* 2539-2554, 1995.

[59] Oshima, M., Oshima, H., and Taketo, M. M. TGF-beta receptor type II- deficiency results in defects of yolk sac hematopoiesis and vasculogenesis. *Dev Biol, 179:* 297-302, 1996.

[60] Larsson, J., Goumans, M. J., Sjostrand, L. J., van Rooijen, M. A., Ward, D., Leveen, P., Xu, X., ten Dijke, P., Mummery, C. L., and Karlsson, S. Abnormal angiogenesis but intact hematopoietic potential in TGF-beta type I receptor-deficient mice. *Embo J, 20:* 1663-1673, 2001.

[61] Kano, M. R., Bae, Y., Iwata, C., Morishita, Y., Yashiro, M., Oka, M., Fujii, T., Komuro, A., Kiyono, K., Kaminishi, M., Hirakawa, K., Ouchi, Y., Nishiyama, N.,

Kataoka, K., and Miyazono, K. Improvement of cancer-targeting therapy, using nanocarriers for intractable solid tumors by inhibition of TGF-beta signaling. *Proc Natl Acad Sci U S A, 104:* 3460-3465, 2007.

[62] Kano, M. R., Morishita, Y., Iwata, C., Iwasaka, S., Watabe, T., Ouchi, Y., Miyazono, K., and Miyazawa, K. VEGF-A and FGF-2 synergistically promote neoangiogenesis through enhancement of endogenous PDGF-B-PDGFRbeta signaling. J Cell Sci, *118:* 3759-3768, 2005.

[63] Dreher, M. R., Liu, W., Michelich, C. R., Dewhirst, M. W., Yuan, F., and Chilkoti, A. Tumor vascular permeability, accumulation, and penetration of macromolecular drug carriers. *J Natl Cancer Inst, 98:* 335-344, 2006

[64] Watanabe, N., Tsuji, N., Tsuji, Y., Sasaki, H., Okamoto, T., Akiyama, S., Kobayashi, D., Sato, T., Yamauchi, N., and Niitsu, Y. Endogenous tumor necrosis factor inhibits the cytotoxicity of exogenous tumor necrosis factor and adriamycin in pancreatic carcinoma cells. *Pancreas, 13:* 395-400, 1996.

[65] Manda, T., Shimomura, K., Mukumoto, S., Kobayashi, K., Mizota, T., Hirai, O., Matsumoto, S., Oku, T., Nishigaki, F., Mori, J., and et al. Recombinant human tumor necrosis factor-alpha: evidence of an indirect mode of antitumor activity. Cancer Res, *47:* 3707-3711, 1987.

[66] McIntosh, J. K., Mule, J. J., Travis, W. D., and Rosenberg, S. A. Studies of effects of recombinant human tumor necrosis factor on autochthonous tumor and transplanted normal tissue in mice. *Cancer Res, 50:* 2463-2469, 1990.

[67] Seynhaeve, A. L., Hoving, S., Schipper, D., Vermeulen, C. E., de Wiel-Ambagtsheer, G., van Tiel, S. T., Eggermont, A. M., and Ten Hagen, T. L. Tumor necrosis factor alpha mediates homogeneous distribution of liposomes in murine melanoma that contributes to a better tumor response. *Cancer Res, 67:* 9455-9462, 2007.

[68] Carmeliet, P. VEGF as a key mediator of angiogenesis in cancer. *Oncology, 69 Suppl 3:* 4-10, 2005.

[69] Ferrara, N., Gerber, H. P., and LeCouter, J. The biology of VEGF and its receptors. *Nat Med*, 9: 669-676, 2003.

[70] Brown, L. F., Detmar, M., Claffey, K., Nagy, J. A., Feng, D., Dvorak, A. M., and Dvorak, H. F. Vascular permeability factor/vascular endothelial growth factor: a multifunctional angiogenic cytokine. Exs, *79:* 233-269, 1997.

[71] Ferrara, N. and Davis-Smyth, T. The biology of vascular endothelial growth factor. *Endocr Rev, 18:* 4-25, 1997.

[72] Senger, D. R., Brown, L. F., Claffey, K. P., and Dvorak, H. F. Vascular permeability factor, tumor angiogenesis and stroma generation. Invasion Metastasis, *14:* 385-394, 1994.

[73] Dvorak, H. F., Brown, L. F., Detmar, M., and Dvorak, A. M. Vascular permeability factor/vascular endothelial growth factor, microvascular hyperpermeability, and angiogenesis. *Am J Pathol, 146:* 1029-1039, 1995.

[74] Pal, S., Iruela-Arispe, M. L., Harvey, V. S., Zeng, H., Nagy, J. A., Dvorak, H. F., and Mukhopadhyay, D. Retinoic acid selectively inhibits the vascular permeabilizing effect of VPF/VEGF, an early step in the angiogenic cascade. Microvasc Res, *60:* 112-120, 2000.

[75] Nagy, J. A., Vasile, E., Feng, D., Sundberg, C., Brown, L. F., Detmar, M. J., Lawitts, J. A., Benjamin, L., Tan, X., Manseau, E. J., Dvorak, A. M., and Dvorak, H. F. Vascular

permeability factor/vascular endothelial growth factor induces lymphangiogenesis as well as angiogenesis. *J Exp Med, 196:* 1497-1506, 2002.

[76] Roberts, W. G. and Palade, G. E. Increased microvascular permeability and endothelial fenestration induced by vascular endothelial growth factor. *J Cell Sci, 108 (Pt 6):* 2369-2379, 1995.

[77] Roberts, W. G. and Palade, G. E. Neovasculature induced by vascular endothelial growth factor is fenestrated. *Cancer Res, 57:* 765-772, 1997.

[78] Feng, D., Nagy, J. A., Hipp, J., Dvorak, H. F., and Dvorak, A. M. Vesiculo-vacuolar organelles and the regulation of venule permeability to macromolecules by vascular permeability factor, histamine, and serotonin. *J Exp Med, 183:* 1981-1986, 1996.

[79] Yuan, F., Chen, Y., Dellian, M., Safabakhsh, N., Ferrara, N., and Jain, R. K. Time-dependent vascular regression and permeability changes in established human tumor xenografts induced by an anti-vascular endothelial growth factor/vascular permeability factor antibody. *Proc Natl Acad Sci U S A, 93:* 14765-14770, 1996.

[80] Bergers, G., Song, S., Meyer-Morse, N., Bergsland, E., and Hanahan, D. Benefits of targeting both pericytes and endothelial cells in the tumor vasculature with kinase inhibitors. *J Clin Invest, 111:* 1287-1295, 2003.

[81] Willett, C. G., Boucher, Y., di Tomaso, E., Duda, D. G., Munn, L. L., Tong, R. T., Chung, D. C., Sahani, D. V., Kalva, S. P., Kozin, S. V., Mino, M., Cohen, K. S., Scadden, D. T., Hartford, A. C., Fischman, A. J., Clark, J. W., Ryan, D. P., Zhu, A. X., Blaszkowsky, L. S., Chen, H. X., Shellito, P. C., Lauwers, G. Y., and Jain, R. K. Direct evidence that the VEGF-specific antibody bevacizumab has antivascular effects in human rectal cancer. *Nat Med, 10:* 145-147, 2004.

[82] Tong, R. T., Boucher, Y., Kozin, S. V., Winkler, F., Hicklin, D. J., and Jain, R. K. Vascular normalization by vascular endothelial growth factor receptor 2 blockade induces a pressure gradient across the vasculature and improves drug penetration in tumors. *Cancer Res, 64:* 3731-3736, 2004.

[83] Inai, T., Mancuso, M., Hashizume, H., Baffert, F., Haskell, A., Baluk, P., Hu-Lowe, D. D., Shalinsky, D. R., Thurston, G., Yancopoulos, G. D., and McDonald, D. M. Inhibition of vascular endothelial growth factor (VEGF) signaling in cancer causes loss of endothelial fenestrations, regression of tumor vessels, and appearance of basement membrane ghosts. *Am J Pathol, 165:* 35-52, 2004.

[84] Jain, R. K. Normalizing tumor vasculature with anti-angiogenic therapy: a new paradigm for combination therapy. *Nat Med, 7:* 987-989, 2001.

[85] Jain, R. K. Normalization of tumor vasculature: an emerging concept in antiangiogenic therapy. *Science, 307:* 58-62, 2005.

[86] Nakahara, T., Norberg, S. M., Shalinsky, D. R., Hu-Lowe, D. D., and McDonald, D. M. Effect of inhibition of vascular endothelial growth factor signaling on distribution of extravasated antibodies in tumors. *Cancer Res, 66:* 1434-1445, 2006.

[87] Wu, J., Akaike, T., and Maeda, H. Modulation of enhanced vascular permeability in tumors by a bradykinin antagonist, a cyclooxygenase inhibitor, and a nitric oxide scavenger. Cancer Res, *58:* 159-165, 1998.

[88] Maeda, H., Akaike, T., Wu, J., Noguchi, Y., and Sakata, Y. Bradykinin and nitric oxide in infectious disease and cancer. *Immunopharmacology, 33:* 222-230, 1996.

[89] Maeda, H., Noguchi, Y., Sato, K., and Akaike, T. Enhanced vascular permeability in solid tumor is mediated by nitric oxide and inhibited by both new nitric oxide scavenger and nitric oxide synthase inhibitor. *Jpn J Cancer Res, 85:* 331-334, 1994.

[90] Doi, K., Akaike, T., Horie, H., Noguchi, Y., Fujii, S., Beppu, T., Ogawa, M., and Maeda, H. Excessive production of nitric oxide in rat solid tumor and its implication in rapid tumor growth. *Cancer, 77:* 1598-1604, 1996.

[91] Tanaka, S., Akaike, T., Wu, J., Fang, J., Sawa, T., Ogawa, M., Beppu, T., and Maeda, H. Modulation of tumor-selective vascular blood flow and extravasation by the stable prostaglandin 12 analogue beraprost sodium. *J Drug Target, 11:* 45-52, 2003.

[92] Berk, D. A., Yuan, F., Leunig, M., and Jain, R. K. Fluorescence photobleaching with spatial Fourier analysis: measurement of diffusion in light-scattering media. *Biophys J, 65:* 2428-2436, 1993.

[93] Brown, E. B., Wu, E. S., Zipfel, W., and Webb, W. W. Measurement of molecular diffusion in solution by multiphoton fluorescence photobleaching recovery. *Biophys J, 77:* 2837-2849, 1999.

[94] Koninger, J., Giese, N. A., di Mola, F. F., Berberat, P., Giese, T., Esposito, I., Bachem, M. G., Buchler, M. W., and Friess, H. Overexpressed decorin in pancreatic cancer: potential tumor growth inhibition and attenuation of chemotherapeutic action. *Clin Cancer Res, 10:* 4776-4783, 2004.

[95] Scott, J. E., Dyne, K. M., Thomlinson, A. M., Ritchie, M., Bateman, J., Cetta, G., and Valli, M. Human cells unable to express decoron produced disorganized extracellular matrix lacking "shape modules" (interfibrillar proteoglycan bridges). *Exp Cell Res, 243:* 59-66, 1998.

[96] Beckenlehner, K., Bannke, S., Spruss, T., Bernhardt, G., Schonenberg, H., and Schiess, W. Hyaluronidase enhances the activity of adriamycin in breast cancer models in vitro and in vivo. *J Cancer Res Clin Oncol, 118:* 591-596, 1992.

[97] Smith, K. J., Skelton, H. G., Turiansky, G., and Wagner, K. F. Hyaluronidase enhances the therapeutic effect of vinblastine in intralesional treatment of Kaposi's sarcoma. Military Medical Consortium for the Advancement of Retroviral Research (MMCARR). *J Am Acad Dermatol, 36:* 239-242, 1997.

[98] Eikenes, L., Tari, M., Tufto, I., Bruland, O. S., and de Lange Davies, C. Hyaluronidase induces a transcapillary pressure gradient and improves the distribution and uptake of liposomal doxorubicin (Caelyx) in human osteosarcoma xenografts. Br J Cancer, *93:* 81-88, 2005.

[99] Davies Cde, L., Lundstrom, L. M., Frengen, J., Eikenes, L., Bruland, S. O., Kaalhus, O., Hjelstuen, M. H., and Brekken, C. Radiation improves the distribution and uptake of liposomal doxorubicin (caelyx) in human osteosarcoma xenografts. *Cancer Res, 64:* 547-553, 2004.

[100] Masuda, A., Ushida, K., Koshino, H., Yamashita, K., and Kluge, T. Novel distance dependence of diffusion constants in hyaluronan aqueous solution resulting from its characteristic nano-microstructure. *J Am Chem Soc, 123:* 11468-11471, 2001.

[101] Nagano, S., Perentes, J. Y., Jain, R. K., and Boucher, Y. Cancer cell death enhances the penetration and efficacy of oncolytic herpes simplex virus in tumors. *Cancer Res, 68:* 3795-3802, 2008.

[102] Lu, D., Wientjes, M. G., Lu, Z., and Au, J. L. Tumor priming enhances delivery and efficacy of nanomedicines. *J Pharmacol Exp Ther, 322:* 80-88, 2007.

[103] Jang, S. H., Wientjes, M. G., and Au, J. L. Enhancement of paclitaxel delivery to solid tumors by apoptosis-inducing pretreatment: effect of treatment schedule. *J Pharmacol Exp Ther*, *296:* 1035-1042, 2001.

[104] Ishida, T., Shiraga, E., and Kiwada, H. Synergistic antitumor activity of metronomic dosing of cyclophosphamide in combination with doxorubicin-containing PEGylated liposomes in a murine solid tumor model. *J Control Release*, *134:* 194-200, 2009.

In: Neuro-Oncology and Cancer Targeted Therapy
Editor: Lucía M. Gutiérrez pp.161-182
ISBN: 978-1-61668-708-3
©2010 Nova Science Publishers, Inc.

Chapter 6

TUMOR CHEMODOSIMETRY: THE INTERSECTION OF IMAGING, DRUG DELIVERY VEHICLES AND TARGETED THERAPIES FOR THE IMPROVEMENT OF CANCER TREATMENT

J. Hung[1], R. Daniel[1] and B.L. Viglianti[*,1,2]

[1]St. Joseph Mercy Hospital, Ypsilanti, MI
[2]University of Michigan, Ann Arbor, MI

INTRODUCTION

Effective cancer treatment therapy requires drugs to be delivered to tumor cells at cytotoxic concentrations. The ideal goals for chemotherapy are to identify and modify drug distribution, deliver concentrated effective drug dosages to the tumor and/or predict the tumor effect, a concept termed as chemodosimetry [1]. This concept is analogous to radiation dosimetry, which is used when the radiation dose is administered in a prescribed manner based on calculated radiation intensity and known tissue dependent energy absorption. Radiation dosimetry has been successful in improving cancer therapy outcomes, but chemodosimetry has yet to achieve similar success [1-3]. Current non-targeted chemotherapy regimens require drug concentrations that cause dose limiting systemic side effects. With localized targeted drug delivery, mitigation of these systemic side effects is possible and, in the ideal case, chemodosimetry could be achieved.

Although advancements in current cancer therapy have allowed the development of localized treatment to the tumor via minimally invasive procedures, recent research in phase II/III clinical trials focused on molecular targeting and drug carriers for noninvasive target drug delivery. Most recently, data from preclinical trials have demonstrated the ability to monitor drug delivery in real time with nanoparticles, such as liposomes, drug-loaded polymers, polymersomes, and antibodies. Liposomes are small, self-assembling particles with

---

[*] Corresponding Author: benjamin.viglianti@alumni.duke.edu, Department of Medicine, St. Joseph Mercy Hospital, Ypsilanti, MI 48197, 734-712-3456

diameters <400 nm, comprised of an outer phospholipid bilayer and an aqueous center capable of encapsulating and carrying water-soluble drugs (Figure 1)[4]. Since liposomes are the most mature form of nanoparticles in development, this review will primarily discuss liposomes to exhibit the combination of nanoparticle delivery, imaging, and selected drug deposition in conjunction with the use of local regional hyperthermia.

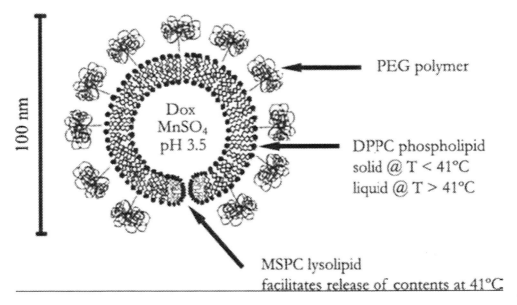

Figure 1. Schematic depiction of a temperature-sensitive liposome containing doxorubicin (Dox) and contrast agent (manganese sulfate, MnSO4). Doxorubicin is actively loaded and retained in temperature-sensitive liposomes by using a pH gradient-driven loading protocol that includes MnSO4. The phospholipid bilayer undergoes a main melting phase transition at 41°C. Lysolipids can form many stable pores at the transition temperature, enabling release of contents (note that only one pore is shown). Polyethylene glycol (PEG) is grafted onto lipids to help liposomes evade immune recognition. DPPC = 1,2 dipalmitoyl- sn -glycerol-3-phosphocholine; MSPC = 1-stearoyl-2-hydroxy- sn -glycero-3-phosphocholine. Reprinted with permission from the Oxford University Press, JNCI [4].

Tumor Physiology

Tumor physiology inhibits adequate drug delivery to the tumor bed, which presents one of the foremost challenges to targeted cancer therapy. Physiologic barriers such as variable vessel structure and permeability, high interstitial fluid pressure, and heterogeneous perfusion all make efficient drug delivery difficult [1,5-15]. Two principle tumor physiological factors influencing adequate drug delivery to the tumor site are perfusion and vessel permeability which allow for extravasation and accumulation of the drug in the peri-vascular space [5,10,15,16]. However, these physical properties within tumors are often heterogeneous and create a variable drug distribution profile [5,10,15]. In general, tumors are highly vascular organs with regions of avascularity and unpredictable vascular anomalies. It should be noted that there are regions in the tumor that have extremely low perfusion and provide a significant barrier to delivery. This chaotic nature of the tumor microvasculature was demonstrated by Dreher et al. (Figure 2)[14]. Another important consideration in effective drug delivery is determined by the tumor vessel permeability. Vessel permeability is a function of solute size, concentration gradient, and the physical property of the vessel barrier, which is dependent on maturity of the vessel. These types of physiologic parameters of the tumor have long hindered drug delivery during traditional cancer chemotherapy.

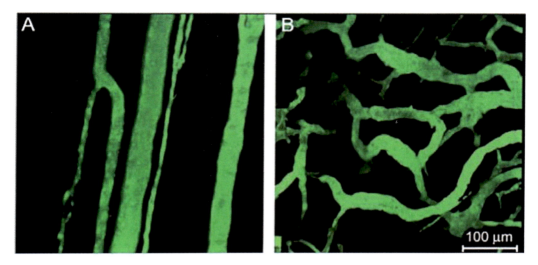

Figure 2. Normal and tumor vasculature. A) Normal vasculature. These vessels are aligned parallel to one another. B) Tumor vasculature. Tumor vessels have a chaotic geometry with vessels that are dilated and have uneven diameters. The vasculature, shown in green, was visualized with fluorescein-labeled 2-MDa dextran administered intravenously and displayed as a transparent projection of about 100 μm of tissue. Scale bar = 100 μm. Reprinted with permission from the Oxford University Press, JNCI [14].

Current Tumor Treatment

Tumor resection with or without adjuvant systemic chemotherapy or radiation therapy has long been the mainstay of care for certain resectable tumors. Unresectable tumors may be treated with alternative treatments including chemoradiation or palliative treatment depending on the extent of the disease. Current evaluation of the tumor tissue drug levels is inferred from serum drug levels or directly through measurement from invasive tissue biopsies [3]. Therapeutic serum levels are often achieved at the cost of debilitating and/or unpalatable systemic side effects that decrease the quality of life for many patients.

Strides to reduce systemic side effects and improve tumor treatment have created a niche for targeted and local tumor treatment options. Localized treatment options currently in practice are utilized for select tumors, such as thyroid radioiodine ablation and minimally invasive procedures, including radiofrequency ablation (RFA) and chemoembolization. Treatments utilizing specific radioactive isotopes targeting a particular tissue bed have been established in practice with thyroid cancer ablation, however more generalized tumor targeting has yet to be fully developed.

Positron emission tomography (PET) and single-photon emission computed tomography (SPECT) imaging are used in oncology management for the detection of tumor or for evaluating for metastatic or recurrent disease. These modalities can also be used for specific delivery of radiolabeled pharmaceuticals, with attached epitopes, that target uptake and can treat selected tissue beds [17]. However, one limitation of utilizing radioablation, PET and SPECT is the ability to identify a tagable substrate. Additionally, radiofrequency ablation is applicable only to specific tissues, and imaging resolution is poor with PET and SPECT.

Minimally invasive techniques currently in practice for local cancer treatment, including RFA and chemoembolization, utilize imaging modalities to physically bypass systemic delivery and directly inject the agent at the tumor bed and/or at a feeding blood vessel. Direct ablation of the tumor or injection of agent through the primary tumor vasculature under direct visualization has been made possible with real-time fluoroscopy, ultrasound, and computed tomography (CT) guidance. RFA causes direct thermal cytotoxic effects by reaching temperatures >55°C [18,19]. However, RFA treatments may have a residual viable rim where cytotoxic temperatures are not reached, resulting in incomplete treatment. Chemoembolization, alternatively, delivers concentrated chemotherapeutic agents directly to the primary vasculature of the tumor bed. This direct injection of chemotherapy is an indirect form of embolization using macroscopic particles to clog the downstream vasculature, thus depriving the tumor and releasing the drug to the tumor bed. Embolization is dependent on accurate identification of the vascular structures that are supplying the tumor in order to occlude the feeding vessels, but if not all tumor dependent vessels are identified or completely occluded, tumor therapy may be suboptimal. Although these techniques allow for visual confirmation of reaching the tumor bed, the challenge of overcoming the barriers of tumor physiology and reassurance of adequate therapeutic drug delivery remain. Thus, localized triggered drug delivery and imaging to ensure delivery are crucial elements for chemodosimetry. Both aspects may be achieved and will be further discussed with liposomal drug delivery below.

OPTIMIZING DRUG DELIVERY

Optimizing drug delivery takes into account several factors: 1) agent size to achieve a desired permeability of the vascular wall while also maintaining a therapeutic plasma circulation time, 2) tumor specific targeting molecules or localized delivery method to only allow accumulation at the tumor, 3) reticuloendothelial system evasion to reduce the rate of clearance and allow more time for tumor targeting, and 4) a method to overcome the barriers of tumor physiology by further increasing the accumulation of drug at the tumor site.

Agent Size

The nanoparticle size of the drug carrier is the simplest modification in constructing a drug carrier vehicle. Choosing the vehicle size has a significant impact on its ability to penetrate the vascular wall and the duration of the drug in circulation. There is an inverse relationship between plasma half-life and permeability. This was shown when Dreher et al. utilized a mouse window chamber model to study a wide range of fluorescently labeled dextran molecules from 3.3 kDa to 2MDa in order to evaluate the characteristics of perfusion and permeability in relation to molecule size (Figure 3) [14,15]. This model permitted the development of imaging the accumulation, distribution, and plasma presence of the nanoparticles in the tumor and normal tissue bed following a systemic injection of the labeled dextrans. Small sized agents were found to permeate further into the perivascular space and readily accumulated there. However the accumulation was short-lived because the molecule was easily washed out due to the short plasma half-life, creating a reversal gradient of the molecule [14]. The opposite was seen for large molecules, which have long plasma half-lives but have difficulty permeating into the peri-vascular space [14]. Thus the optimal intermediate size for vessel permeability into the peri-vascular space was found to be in between at ~70 kDa [14].

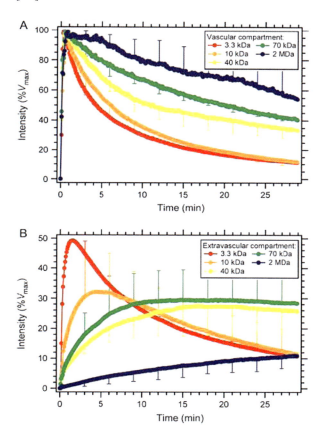

Figure 3. Vascular pharmacokinetics and extravascular accumulation of dextrans with various molecular weights. A) Vascular pharmacokinetics. B) Extravascular accumulation. Zero time corresponds to the time immediately before green fluorescence was detected. Each point on the graph is a separate measurement taken at 5-second intervals that was normalized by the maximum vascular intensity (expressed as %Vmax). The plasma half-life, which is the time at which the vascular fluorescence intensity is equal to half of its maximum value, increased with higher molecular weights (e.g., for 3.3-kDa dextrans, plasma half-life = 3.8 minutes, 95% confidence interval [CI] = 2.5 to 4.2 minutes; and for 70-kDa dextrans, plasma half-life = 19.6 minutes, 95% CI = 18.3 to 21.0 minutes). The initial rate of accumulation in the extravascular compartment, illustrated by the initial slope of the lines in B, increased with the higher permeability of dextrans of low molecular weight. Data are expressed as the means of three experiments. Error bars = 95% CIs (shown at 3-minute intervals). Reprinted with permission from the Oxford University Press, JNCI [14].

Improved drug delivery to the tumor site can also be increased via specific targeted agents, such as antibodies, aptamers, and peptides designed to recognize "overexpressed" tumor epitopes, allowing for specifically designed targeting of the drug to a select location. Other markers especially good for tumor targeting include angiogenic markers due to the increased angiogenesis that is often found with rapidly growing tumors [15,20]. One excellent example of the use of targeted antibodies was found in a study conducted by Sipkins et al., 1998 that targeted a specific angiogenesis marker, the endothelial integrin $\alpha_v\beta_3$, which is often upregulated in tumors [20,21]. In this study, the integrin antibody labeled with gadolinium contrast provided a non-invasive method to identify areas of angiogenesis within the tumor and monitor potential areas of malignant growth (Figure 4) [20]. However, it should be cautioned that these targets may be more ubiquitous, especially in healing tissue from everyday trauma that might occur during the course of treatment. Epitopes, such as the $\alpha_v\beta_3$ antibody, require an extremely specific tumor targeted receptor site as well as an over expression of these receptors over normal tissue. The intricacies and targeted drug delivery with epitopes is an extensive topic beyond the scope of this discussion.

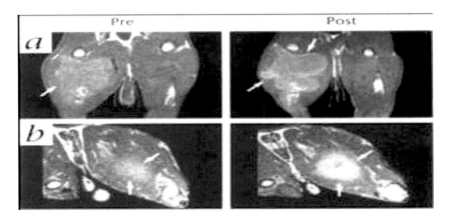

Figure 4. Anti-$\alpha_v\beta_3$ antibody-conjugated paramagnetic liposomes (ACPLs) correlation with T1-weighted MRI signal enhancement of rabbit tumors. Various T1-weighted images showing pre- and 24 hour post-targeted contrast administration showing increased enhancement of tumor sites (as indicated by arrows). a: coronal images of rabbit right thigh muscle bearing a tumor with 24 h following ACPL administration indicating area of active angiogenesis and $\alpha_v\beta_3$ expression in the tumor periphery (arrows). b: Axial images of a poorly visualized intramuscular tumor pre-contrast with subsequent enhancement post-ACPL administration. Reprinted with permission from [20].

Mild Hyperthermia Technique

A more generalized method of tumor targeting for chemotherapy delivery may be achieved by altering tumor physiology with external techniques such as local hyperthermia. Hyperthermia promotes increased perfusion and permeability of the tumor vasculature, thus improving drug delivery and subsequent accumulation in the perivasculature and tumor bed [22-25]. Other factors influenced by hyperthermia include tumor oxygenation, inhibition of DNA repair, and, at high enough temperatures, direct cytotoxicity [3,15,25-30].

As mentioned previously, one of the most influential factors and easily modifiable characters of tumor physiology is tumor perfusion, which affects drug and oxygen delivery

[15]. Preclinical models have shown that mild hyperthermia between 40-42°C administered to local areas caused increased perfusion, oxygenation, and permeability of tumor microvasculature [15,25,28]. In fact, between 40-42°C, accumulation of 100 nm liposomes was found to double with every degree increase (Figure 5)[15,25]. Mild hyperthermia is contrasted to thermal ablation as seen with RFA when temperatures reach >55°C, which creates a direct thermal cytotoxic effect [15]. This was supported by the observation that at higher temperatures above the 42°C, cytotoxic effects of vascular damage and tissue hypoxia resulting in hemorrhage and intravascular stasis were seen [28 25.]

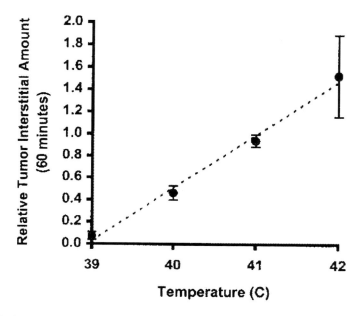

Figure 5. Correlation of relative tumor interstitial amount of fluorescent light intensities representing liposomal accumulation 60 minutes after applied temperature, as a function of temperature. The correlation coefficient was 0.99 (y = 0.48x + 18.82). Values are mean and SE (n = 6 for each temperature). Adapted and reprinted with permission from [25].

Hyperthermia has also been shown to enhance liposome extravasation for up to four hours after heat administration [22,23]. In addition to improved perfusion, the positive effects of hyperthermia on liposomal/drug accumulation was thought to be due to an increased endothelial pore size in order to allow greater permeation into the extravascular space [3,16,22]. This was not only shown by initial studies by Kong et al. but the effect of hyperthermia on endothelial pore size with extravascular permeation of elastin-like polypeptides was also shown in a similar study by Dreher et al [22,31]. In general, tumors physiologically tend to have large endothelial gaps and decreased vascular integrity due to the predilection of being comprised of immature vasculature [22]. In two preclinical studies by Matteucci et al. and Kleiter et al. in spontaneous feline sarcomas and transplanted rat fibrosarcomas, respectively, post-heat treatment showed increased liposomal accumulation [32,33]. This noted increase in permeability with mild hyperthermia was found to be unique to tumor vasculature, further allowing cultivation of targeted drug carriers to the tumor bed. Normal vasculature, in comparison, tend to be more structurally mature and without noticeable prolonged increases in permeability.

It should also be noted that hyperthermia has been utilized to enhance treatment in radiotherapy through improved oxygenation. Radiation therapy clinical trials have shown that hyperthermia may prolong progression-free survival due to the mechanism described above, but these studies will not be discussed in this article and can be found in other studies and reviews [30,34-39].

DRUG DELIVERY VEHICLES

The optimal drug delivery vehicle is capable of encapsulating, retaining, and releasing the contents at the desired location. Nanoscopic drug delivery carriers provide a potential solution to toxic side effects that are inherent to current systemic chemotherapeutic drug regimens [40 13]. The use of liposomes as a drug-carrying vehicle allows for manipulation of the encapsulated environment and lipid membrane to optimize the internalization of the drug and targeting/delivery, respectively. Due to the delivery vehicle's ability to confine the drug to the interior while traversing the bloodstream, the undesirable systemic side effects can be significantly decreased. To allow for enhanced delivery of the drug to the tumor bed, manipulation of the factors discussed above in "Optimizing Drug Delivery," including size, utilization of targeting epitopes, or even direct injection via a catheter may be used [15]. Once at the physical site, drug deposition and sustained retention within the tumor, requires the vehicles to respond to the local environment and trigger release of its contents, thus allowing for increased targeted delivered drug to the tumor at higher concentrations than previously possible with systemic chemotherapeutics. With these goals in mind, the development of several potential nanoparticle drug delivery vehicles has been investigated including polymersomes and liposomes [14,41]. Liposomes have been more extensively developed and will be the main model system investigated for the remainder of this paper.

Liposomes

Since the advent of liposomes as a drug carrier system in the 1960s, this nanoscale drug delivery vehicle has been gaining popularity. [1,3,22,42-45]. Comprised of spherical phospholipid layers surrounding an aqueous core, liposomes can be constructed to encapsulate and retain drugs that are placed inside the liposome's interior [4,22,44,45]. Ranging in diameter from 50-400 nm, liposomes naturally accumulate extravascularly into the tumor bed tissue [24]. Manipulation of the size, content, and phospholipid outer layer for controlled encapsulation, perfusion, and increasing extravasation are the qualities that potentially make liposomes an ideal drug delivery vehicle.

Although liposomes exhibit strong potential, several challenges as a targeted therapeutic vehicle exist. Two main challenges for liposomes as a delivery vehicle are the optimization of liposomal stability in the bloodstream and rapid, triggered release rates of liposomal contents at the targeted tumor site. With the development of polyethylene glycol (PEG) added to the liposomal formulation, improved liposomal stability in the bloodstream was achieved. Pegylated liposomes extended plasma half-life and reduced uptake by the reticuloendothelial system [45-49]. The second challenge to liposomes as an ideal drug delivery vehicle was overcoming slow liposomal content release such that the liposome could potentially traverse the tumor before its drug was released. Thus, an equally significant discovery was the ability to alter the phospholipid capsule at temperature or pH transition points, such that a triggered release of liposomal contents occurs when the external environment changes. For pH sensitive liposomes, triggered release is based on the concept that body pH remains constant with very little variation, except as noted in the tumor or metastatic regions where pH tends to be lower [50-53]. While thermal sensitive liposomes (TSL) use localized temperature variation to initiate content release from the liposomes due to a phase transition in the lipid membrane that occurs at temperatures above a designated transition temperature. Because tumor and body temperature are often similar, exogenous temperature application must be utilized in order to achieve the temperature variations required for liposomal content release. Extensive studies have been conducted examining exogenous mild hyperthermia application via an implanted catheter controlling triggered release of liposomal contents with great success [22,23,54]. Currently, TSLs are able to release its contents within tens of seconds of achieving a hyperthermic environment as will be discussed below [23-25,55-58]. With the development of TSL, liposomes have the potential to meet all three criteria - encapsulation, retention, and triggered drug release – to become the ideal drug delivery vehicle.

Temperature Sensitive Liposomes (TSL)

As mentioned above in the section "Optimizing Drug Delivery – Mild Hyperthermia Technique," liposomal accumulation in tumors can be augmented with mild hyperthermia by altering tumor physiology [3,15,59]. It should also be noted that the addition of heat not only alters the tumor physiology to promote permeability and delivery vehicle extravasation into the tissue, but it also destabilizes liposome membranes at the liposome's phase transition point to allow for release of the drug from the liposomes into the tumor bed. Initial TSL models showed destabilization that took unacceptably long times to release drug into the tumor site.

With the addition of lysolipid to the bilayer of the liposome, the development of true TSL with membrane destabilization happened within 20 seconds after the thermal transition point (39-41°C) was reached [56,58]. This allowed for rapid, controlled release of liposome contents at the heated site [1,57]. Under normothermic conditions, the liposome membrane is comprised of an evenly distributed heterogenous lipid mixture that desegregates under mild hyperthermia into multiple homogenous lipids rafts. These homogenous lipid rafts do not mix and form pseudo grain boundaries that have significantly increased permeability to aqueous solutions, allowing the drug to permeate through, down its concentration gradient [15].

These two developments of lysolipid incorporation into the liposome's phospholipid membrane creating a sensitive transition point and the mild hyperthermia technique allowed for fast, effective membrane destabilization and content release creating substantially improved liposomal targeted drug delivery to tumor sites [1]. The effectiveness of these TSLs have been shown to increase intratumoral drug concentrations almost up to 30-fold as seen in a study by Kong et al. in comparison to that of free drug treatments resulting in significantly delayed tumor growth [3,23,56,60,61]. Consideration of the properties of the drug delivery vehicle is just one half of the equation for optimizing targeted drug therapy delivery, while the other considerations depend on the type of imaging modality utilized to identify the location of drug release.

ROLE OF IMAGING IN MONITORING TUMOR RESPONSE

Currently, imaging is used to monitor drug therapy based on anatomical changes in the volume of the tumor, or activity in the uptake of a radiotracer. The ideal role of non-invasive imaging in targeted tumor therapy is to allow real-time monitoring of drug delivery; and to create a correlation between the drug delivered and subsequent treatment results. Monitoring may be accomplished through a variety of techniques depending on the type of imaging modality used, whether it may be ultrasound (US), PET/SPECT, CT, or magnetic resonance imaging (MRI). Ultimately, the images would be correlated with the drug concentration in order to map out a distribution profile. From the drug distribution profile, undertreated regions would ideally be identified and would be assessed for subsequent cancer therapy until the optimal drug dose delivery pattern is achieved for every individual patient. Conversely, if a beneficial drug distribution was observed, then the duration of planned treatment could be modified to limit drug exposure [3]. With the increasing role of imaging in oncologic assessment, non-invasive methods of monitoring treatment response are becoming more readily available [1,17,30,62,63]. Development of optimal imaging equipment to monitor targeted drug therapies have been limited by equipment resolution and detection sensitivity [15,64]. Presently, methods of tumor imaging include directly tagged molecules of interest, as in SPECT and PET, or the use of surrogate molecules of interest such as the contrast dye seen with MRI and CT [1,15].

Directly tagged molecules used in PET and SPECT provide functional drug concentration data with radiolabeled pharmaceuticals but are limited by poor spatial resolution and require a cyclotron for radioisotope production [1,32]. Additionally, with radioisotopes, the detection of agent release from drug carrier vehicles is limited, as the imaging properties of radioisotopes are unaffected by the presence of drug carrier vehicles [13]. Due to the poor spatial resolution with PET and SPECT, the use of CT and MRI with its improved spatial resolution is currently under research for monitoring targeted drug delivery systems [1,32,55,65,66]. CT provides excellent spatial resolution but requires the use of ionizing radiation for temporal imaging with high-density contrast agents [1,66,67]. The most advantageous imaging method at this time is MRI due to its excellent spatial and temporal resolution without the use of ionizing radiation [1]. An added benefit to MRI is the ability to detect a wide variety of contrast agents that can cause a signal change depending on encapsulated versus free solution of contrast once it enters the tumor bed. The two main limitations with MRI are its high cost and low signal to noise ratio (SNR) that can be encountered with contrast-labeled drugs [1,68,69]. With the wide variety of imaging modalities available, visualization of drug distribution has significant potential for future development.

IMAGING OF LIPOSOMES

With the advent of liposomes, the gamut of imaging modalities has been tested to identify the most viable imaging option. Ideally, the goal for successful, non-invasive imaging of liposomes include the following characteristics: high SNR at therapeutic drug concentrations, signal that can be correlated to drug concentrations, and high spatial and temporal resolution in order to detect real-time delivery and the boundaries of drug delivery [13]. Detection of free liposomes has been visualized using modalities such as MRI, PET, and SPECT. However, the drawback to PET and SPECT is that they utilize radioisotopes that are encapsulated in addition to the drug or are tagged onto the liposomes in order to trace drug delivery. Meanwhile, monitoring of contrast-encapsulated liposomes has been tested with ultrasound, CT, and MRI [3,63,70]. Although multiple modalities for liposomal imaging options are currently in development, the main focus of this review will be on that of MRI imaging of liposomes.

PET/SPECT Imaging

PET has excellent sensitivity and a linear quantification between signal and drug concentration with radiolabeled compounds, which can easily be established. However, poor spatial resolution limits the ability to accurately detect the distribution boundaries after administration of the liposomes in the setting of radioisotopes [33]. Testing with technetium-99m (^{99m}Tc), showed that hyperthermia therapy increased liposomal accumulation in target tissues two to thirteen times more than without increased temperatures [32,33]. An adequate correlation was also discovered with liposomes containing ^{99m}Tc in comparison to separate liposomes containing doxorubicin in tumor tissues under normothermic and hyperthermic conditions. Further details on these findings can be found in studies by Kleiter et al., 2006 and Matteucci et al., 2000. However, the limited resolution on PET/SPECT studies hinders the ability to delineate accurate peripheral tumor bed borders in order to identify and target missed areas during subsequent treatment [3]. An additional drawback to the utilization of PET and SPECT is that it does in fact use radioisotopes, which tend to be short-lived particles and requires nuclear medicine scanning, which increases systemic exposure to radioactive substances. Studies involving scintigraphic imaging for detection and quantification of liposomal delivery have been under investigation and are a topic that continues to currently undergo development [71 67].

IMAGEABLE LIPOSOMES WITH MRI

In the early 2000, imageable liposomes were developed using manganese (Mn) as a paramagnetic contrast agent with the intent of use for drug delivery monitoring. Groups have studied liposomes for drug delivery including the cancer therapies discussed here, anesthetic, analgesic, anti-parasitic, and vaccine agents as reviewed a couple times in the past [3,22,45]. By exploiting the manipulability of liposomal carrying contents and membrane features, research on improved targeting of liposomes have been conducted, resulting in the development of membrane-ligand recognition and triggered liposomal release as reviewed by Torchilin, 2005 [45].

The ability of liposomes to encapsulate drugs designed for content release has opened the door not only for targeted drug delivery, but also for imaging applications. A dual drug delivery and imaging vehicle liposomal formulation of doxorubicin as the chemotherapeutic and manganese as contrast agent (DOX-Mn) were developed and tested for imaging and targeted tumor delivery in preclinical models[1]. Doxorubicin is a cytotoxic anthracycline antibiotic isolated from bacterial cultures of *Streptomyces peucetius* var. *caesius*. The drug works by binding and intercalating with nucleic acids primarily within the DNA double helix, as well as the cell membranes and plasma proteins secondarily [2,13]. Mn, like the contrast agent gadolinium, is a paramagnetic transition metal that acts like a T1-weighted MRI contrast agent in vivo [1,13].

The theory of MR and the relationship between T1 and relaxivity is further explained by Tashjian et al [3]. Briefly, these MRI contrast agents shorten T1, the time constant for the amount of time it takes for a magnetic moment to realign with the magnetic field, by increasing the energy transfer from interaction of the water molecules with the contrast agent molecule. This allows the system to return to its equilibrium state faster, thus generating more detectable signal. This effect on T1 occurs in a concentration dependent manner, increasing the signal obtained from the tissue where the contrast agent has collected. This signal effect can be quantified by relating the signal difference between pre- and post-contrast administration to the T1 pre- and post-contrast value. The inverse change in T1 (Δ 1/T1) is linearly related to the change in concentration. The proportionality constant termed relaxivity is a physical dependent property of the contrast agent being used. Higher values of relaxivity yield an overall greater reduction in T1 for a given concentration, which in turn leads to a greater signal change for a given concentration of contrast agent.

In the liposome encapsulated drug/contrast agent, the lipid bilayer acts as a barrier between the contrast agent and the free water. Consequently, limiting signal-enhancing interactions. Although contrast in the image is seen, the contrast signal is limited by the water that is able to exchange across the membrane. When the liposomes are heated, however, there is rapid destabilization in the liposomal membrane. This allows rapid bidirectional exchange of water and contrast/drug agent in and out of the liposome causing an increase in the relaxivity and a significant increase in the measured signal [1,55]. Although this partitioning effect on signal is an advantageous and unique property of MR contrast agents within liposomes, it does have its limitation. If one does not have the information on the physical environment (in our case temperature) a measured signal that is strong could either be interpreted as a small number of liposomes that released their contents or a large number of intact liposomes. Therefore, quantification of the contrast agent requires knowledge of the temperature distribution [1].

Briefly, the method for calculating the DOX concentration from the signal intensity images will be described here. An initial T1 image is generated prior to contrast administration. Then, following the administration of the contrast agent, signal intensity images are acquired at a desired temporal resolution. If one assumes that all the signal change that occurs is due to T1 shortening (the time constant in the exponential signal equation), then the other measured values from the initial T1 image can be used to convert the signal change into a measured T1. Performing that analysis on a pixel-by-pixel basis would result in a dynamic T1 image. Subtracting the images from each other would yield a change in T1. Then knowing the temperature distribution in the tumor environment, the temperature dependent relaxivity of the liposome can be used to calculate the change in the concentration of the contrast agent that has occurred. Also assuming that the ratio of the contrast agent and the drug remains constant (i.e. the drug and the contrast agent remain spatially co-localized) then one can infer the concentration of the delivered drug (Figure 6) [1,15].

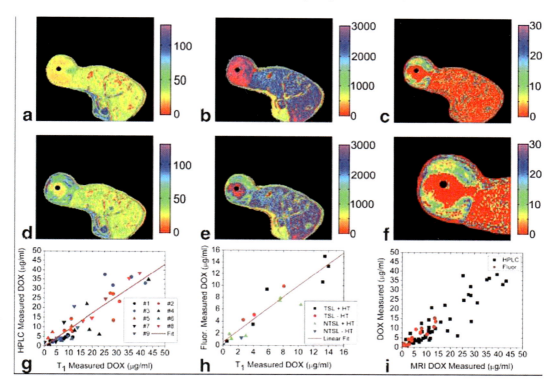

Figure 6. The procedure for calculating T1-based liposomal DOX concentration is shown in the first two rows. a: An initial (t _ 0 min) raw signal (0–125 a.u. color bar) intensity map shows an axial view of the rat bearing a flank fibrosarcoma (top left) with a central heating catheter. b: The initial calculated T1 intensity map (0 to 3000 ms color bar) from a series of multiple-flip-angle images. d: The raw signal intensity (0–125 a.u. color bar) map at 45 min after injection and content release of temperature sensitive lipsomes (TSL). e: The calculated T1 map (0 to 3000 ms color bar) 45 min after injection. Note that the regions that enhanced in d have reduced T1 intensity, indicating contrast/drug presence through T1 shortening. c: The calculated DOX concentration (ng/mg) on a pixel-by-pixel basis from images b and e. f: An enlarged image of c showing the heterogeneity in drug delivery that can be imaged and quantified by this MRI technique. Two independent studies in a rat FSA model indicate a great agreement between invasive DOX concentrations and T1-based DOX concentrations. g: The results for the HPLC validated DOX concentration measurements from each animal. Note that the measurements span the concentration range for most of the tested animals. T1-based DOX concentration measurements above 50 ng/ml were excluded from the regression analyses (red line) due to excessive systematic error. h: The results for the fluorescence validated DOX concentration measurements, for each liposome/treatment type. i: An overlay of both experiments is displayed, showing the precision and accuracy of MRI for measuring DOX at lower concentrations. Adapted and reprinted with permission from [1].

This analysis however, does have several assumptions that may affect quantification accuracy. The first assumption is that the fitted variables (proton density, T2, and noise) in the equation relating T1 and signal remain constant. This assumption breaks down as contrast agent concentration increases and T2 effects start to have an influence. A second assumption, which has been alluded to, is that the Mn:DOX ratio remains spatially constant after liposomal contents are released [1]. Given that DOX is a larger molecule than Mn, transport discrepancies between the two molecules in tumor tissue could disrupt the DOX:Mn ratio [1]. As a larger molecule DOX diffusion could be decreased and retention could be increased through the tumor tissue in comparison to Mn [1]. On the other hand, as a smaller agent Mn may have a faster washout period, also altering the initial DOX:Mn ratio [1].

Despite these potential limitations in determining DOX concentrations through the calculation algorithm, these errors do not significantly affect the utility of this MRI technique for measuring drug distribution [1]. This concentration calculated technique was independently validated in a rat fibrosarcoma model via two methods – direct tissue sampling with high-performance liquid chromatography (HPLC) and semi-quantitative histologic fluorescence [1]. A linear 1:1 relationship between DOX measured from the MRI and that with direct fluorescence was found, with a slope and intercept not statistically different from one and zero, respectively (Figure 6, g-i) [1]. These results indicated the DOX concentration could be accurately calculated from MRI.

MRI Role in Monitoring Drug Delivery Outcome in Practice

The advancement of noninvasive imaging techniques with Mn contrast-loaded liposomes in conjunction with mild hyperthermia treatment has a strong potential to drastically alter chemotherapeutic protocols. TSL with mild hyperthermia can increase DOX tumor concentration up to 30 times over that of free drug [23]. Currently, imaging is able to differentiate between ablated and residual tumor with imaging modalities such as CT and MRI after treatment [72]. With an imageable liposome, real-time evaluation of adequate targeted drug delivery and intratumoral distribution via MRI and possibly other imaging modalities opens the door for appropriate adjustment of chemodosimetry in order to predict and optimize individual patients' response to treatments [1, 3].

Although TSL with mild hyperthermia has immensely increased the capability of targeted drug delivery, the hyperthermia methods may lead to heterogeneous, non-uniform deposition of drug in the tumor bed [1]. In order to evaluate optimal relationships between liposome distribution and the utility of drug delivery imaging, therapeutic model studies were conducted varying the timing of liposomal infusion and hyperthermia administration [4]. This was studied using rat fibrosarcomas treated with intravenous Dox-Mn TSL administered before, during, and one half before and one half during hyperthermic conditions were achieved. Water heated to ~50°C passing through an exogenous catheter placed into the center of the tumor creating a radial temperature bed ranging from 45-46°C adjacent to the catheter to 38.5-39.5°C at the tumor border was used to achieve hyperthermic conditions (Figure 7)[15]. The effect of when hyperthermic conditions were applied in relation to the injection of liposomes was shown to affect the extended delayed tumor growth [4]. The most efficacious treatment combination was found with reaching steady state mild hyperthermia temperatures prior to infusion of TSL [4,15]. The result was more rapid doxorubicin accumulation and higher concentration of drug within the tumor in a peripheral distribution pattern. This suggested that TSL content release occurred once liposomes entered the heated tumor. This peripheral distrobution is optimal because the periphery is the region where the effects of hyperthermic cytotoxicity tapers off with direct ablation techniques. Thus, an optimal combination of cytoxic heat effect to the central tumor and delivery of therapeutic drug concentrations to the tumor periphery can be achieved with release of TSLs after steady state hyperthermia is achieved [4,15]. In comparison to the two other patterns of heat administration and liposome injection relationships, delivery of the liposome injection after steady-state hyperthermia was achieved produced the longest delay of tumor re-growth [13]. Although not as effective in short-term treatment, the other two patterns of heat and liposome administration did create unique drug distribution profiles. The administration of TSL prior to applying hyperthermic conditions created a central distribution of the liposomes due to accumulation of TSL in the center of the tumor before content release due to hyperthermic conditions, while the TSL administration half before and half after achieving hyperthermic steady state resulted in a diffuse uniform appearance of drug delivery (Figure 8) [4]. These varied patterns of drug distribution with differing hyperthermic/liposome techniques opens the possibility to accommodate for delivery of drug in variant anatomic tumor patterns.

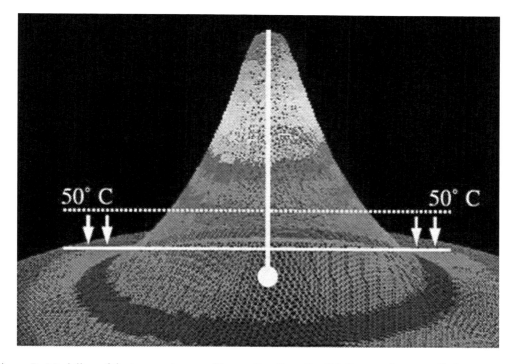

Figure 7. Modeling of the temperature profile as a function of radial distance from a radiofrequency ablation probe. The dashed line indicated the coagulation caused by elevated temperature alone. The solid line indicates isotherm where coagulation occurs with the presence of liposomal Doxorubicin. Adapted and reprinted with permission from [15].

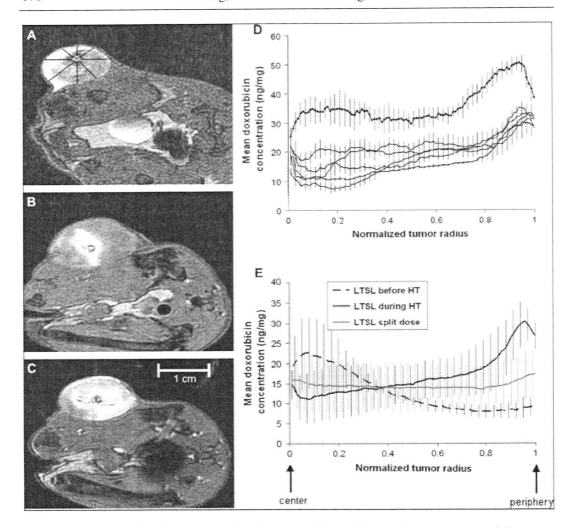

Figure 8. Tumor drug distribution after administration of doxorubicin- and manganese-containing lysolipid-based temperature-sensitive liposomes (TSL) and hyperthermia (HT) by three different schedules. (A – C) Axial pelvic magnetic resonance images show rats bearing flank fibrosarcomas (top left). Radial lines in (A) show the orientations of doxorubicin concentration profiles in (D) and (E). (A) TSLs administered during steady-state hyperthermia resulted in peripheral enhancement (liposome content release; white) at the edge of the tumor; (B) TSLs administered before hyperthermia resulted in central enhancement; and (C) TSLs administered in two equal doses, half before hyperthermia and the remainder after steady-state hyperthermia was reached, resulted in uniform enhancement. (D) T1-based mean tumor doxorubicin concentration (nanograms per milligram of tissue) after treatment with TSLs during hyperthermia, shown as a function of the normalized tumor radius for each rat. The bold profile is for the tumor shown in (A). Mean values are for 80 line profiles from each rat. (E) Mean doxorubicin concentration (nanograms per milligram of tissue) profiles for each of the three therapeutic groups as a function of the normalized tumor radius (n = 6 – 7 rats per group). Vertical lines in (D) and (E) correspond to 95% confidence intervals. Reprinted with permission from [4].

Liposome loading techniques and complex formation with $MnSO_4$ as a drug delivery system is a versatile concept that may be applied to many other chemotherapeutic combinations [1]. The use of Mn as a quantitative marker and a contrast agent has the potential to be utilized with many targeted therapy drug delivery systems, such as microspheres, peptide polymers, monoclonal antibodies, and cellular-based therapies.

Clinical Liposome Drug Trials

Several liposomal doxorubicin formulations are approved, such as DaunoSome and Doxil (Ortho Biotech), while others are currently undergoing clinical trials, such as Thermodox (Celsion) [73]. Doxil liposome is an approved carrier for human cancer therapy, including Kaposi sarcoma, advanced ovarian cancer, multiple myeloma [33,43 74 60 15]. Clinical trials are underway for use of Doxil in advanced breast cancer [2,3,43]. The benefit seen from these clinical and preclinical Doxil trials was a reduction in some, but not all, side effects. Most notably the toxic side effects that once limited the dosing range for doxorubicin, particularly the cardiac toxicity in therapeutic doseages was practically eliminated [75]. Thermodox, another liposomal chemotherapeutic drug, is currently undergoing phase III clinical trials for primary liver cancers, while undergoing phase I/II clinical trials for recurrent chest wall breast cancer. Other drugs currently under testing for use include Ambisome (Astellas Pharm), a liposome incorporating amphotericin B, and liposomal daunorubicin. Liposomal formulations have come a long way to become stable, realistic drug delivery vehicles, but evaluation of long-term effects of these treatments for human cancers have just begun.

FUTURE DIRECTIONS

Targeted cancer therapies are a vast area of research with strong development potential. The new techniques described above, quantitative contrast-enhanced liposomes that act as a dual drug delivery vehicle and mild hyperthermia, are widely applicable methods that could revolutionize chemodosimetry and individual response to treatment. The most promising combined application of cancer targeted therapies exists with RFA, which could be utilized as the heat source to achieve the hyperthermic conditions required for TSL release at the tumor bed. The similar temperature profile with central heating and peripheral temperature drop-off seen in prior studies described above, especially by Ponce et al., 2007, can be seen in RFA (Figure 7) [4,15].

Some liposomal drug formulations have been approved for clinical use, while several clinical trials are in progress. The addition of targeted chemodosimetry to possible applications for cancer treatments can contribute to improving local tumor control either independently or in conjunction with radiation therapy. In chemosensitive tumors, local treatment may help to shrink tumor burden to allow for surgical resection or allow for much higher concentrations of drug administration in order to overcome drug resistant tumors, thus breaking the limitation of the toxic systemic side effects seen with current free drug therapies.

Although liposome imaging studies in vivo, such as rat fibrosarcoma models as well as phase II clinical trials, are underway, the side effects of liposomes, Mn, and their byproducts require further study. Optimization of methods to improve liposomal imaging, such as the use of less toxic contrast agents, such as gadolinium has been conducted by Peller et al., and novel alternative pathways of manipulating tumor pharmacokinetics for targeted drug delivery are just two of many potential topics that require more exploration [76]. Although targeted cancer therapy is a new field with great untapped potential, these developments are just the beginning in the field of targeted chemotherapeutics.

REFERENCES

[1] Viglianti BL, Ponce AM, Michelich CR, et al. Chemodosimetry of in vivo tumor liposomal drug concentration using MRI. *Magn Reson Med* 2006;56(5):1011-1018.

[2] Holland J. F. & Frei E, editor. *Cancer Medicine*. 6 ed. Volume 1-2. Hamilton, Ontario: BC Decker Inc; 2003. 2700 p.

[3] Tashjian JA, Dewhirst MW, Needham D, Viglianti BL. Rationale for and measurement of liposomal drug delivery with hyperthermia using non-invasive imaging techniques. *Int J Hyperthermia* 2008;24(1):79-90.

[4] Ponce AM, Viglianti BL, Yu D, et al. Magnetic resonance imaging of temperature-sensitive liposome release: drug dose painting and antitumor effects. *J Natl Cancer Inst* 2007;99(1):53-63.

[5] Jain RK. Transport of molecules across tumor vasculature. *Cancer Metastasis Review* 1987;6:559-593.

[6] Jain RK. Transport of molecules in the tumor interstitium: a review. *Cancer Res* 1987;47(12):3039-3051.

[7] Baxter LT, Jain RK. Transport of fluid and macromolecules in tumors. I. Role of interstitial pressure and convection. *Microvasc Res* 1989;37(1):77-104.

[8] Baxter LT, Jain RK. Transport of fluid and macromolecules in tumors. II. Role of heterogeneous perfusion and lymphatics. *Microvasc Res* 1990;40(2):246-263.

[9] Jain RK. Physiological barriers to delivery of monoclonal antibodies and other macromolecules in tumors. *Cancer Res* 1990;50(3 Suppl):814s-819s.

[10] Jain RK. Haemodynamic and transport barriers to the treatment of solid tumours. *Int J Radiat Biol* 1991;60(1-2):85-100.

[11] Baxter LT, Jain RK. Transport of fluid and macromolecules in tumors. III. Role of binding and metabolism. *Microvasc Res* 1991;41(1):5-23.

[12] Baxter LT, Jain RK. Transport of fluid and macromolecules in tumors. IV. A microscopic model of the perivascular distribution. *Microvasc Res* 1991;41(2):252-272.

[13] Viglianti BL, Abraham SA, Michelich CR, et al. In vivo monitoring of tissue pharmacokinetics of liposome/drug using MRI: illustration of targeted delivery. *Magn Reson Med* 2004;51(6):1153-1162.

[14] Dreher MR, Liu W, Michelich CR, Dewhirst MW, Yuan F, Chilkoti A. Tumor vascular permeability, accumulation, and penetration of macromolecular drug carriers. *J Natl Cancer Inst* 2006;98(5):335-344.

[15] Viglianti BL. Target molecular therapies: methods to enhance and monitor tumor drug delivery. *Abdom Imaging* 2008.

[16] Yuan F, Dellian M, Fukumura D, et al. Vascular permeability in a human tumor xenograft: molecular size dependence and cutoff size. *Cancer Res* 1995;55(17):3752-3756.

[17] Yang DJ, Kim EE, Inoue T. Targeted molecular imaging in oncology. *Ann Nucl Med* 2006;20(1):1-11.
[18] Ahmed M, Goldberg SN. Combination radiofrequency thermal ablation and adjuvant IV liposomal doxorubicin increases tissue coagulation and intratumoural drug accumulation. *Int J Hyperthermia* 2004;20(7):781-802.
[19] Stauffer PR, Goldberg SN. Introduction: thermal ablation therapy. *Int J Hyperthermia* 2004;20(7):671-677.
[20] Sipkins DA, Cheresh DA, Kazemi MR, Nevin LM, Bednarski MD, Li KC. Detection of tumor angiogenesis in vivo by alphaVbeta3-targeted magnetic resonance imaging. *Nat Med* 1998;4(5):623-626.
[21] Brooks PC, Clark RA, Cheresh DA. Requirement of vascular integrin alpha v beta 3 for angiogenesis. *Science* 1994;264(5158):569-571.
[22] Kong G, Dewhirst MW. Hyperthermia and liposomes. *Int J Hyperthermia* 1999;15(5):345-370.
[23] Kong G, Anyarambhatla G, Petros WP, et al. Efficacy of liposomes and hyperthermia in a human tumor xenograft model: importance of triggered drug release. *Cancer Res* 2000;60(24):6950-6957.
[24] Kong G, Braun RD, Dewhirst MW. Hyperthermia enables tumor-specific nanoparticle delivery: effect of particle size. *Cancer Res* 2000;60(16):4440-4445.
[25] Kong G, Braun RD, Dewhirst MW. Characterization of the effect of hyperthermia on nanoparticle extravasation from tumor vasculature. *Cancer Res* 2001;61(7):3027-3032.
[26] Song CW. Effect of local hyperthermia on blood flow and microenvironment: a review. *Cancer Res* 1984;44(10 Suppl):4721s-4730s.
[27] Dewhirst MW, Viglianti BL, Lora-Michiels M, Hanson M, Hoopes PJ. Basic principles of thermal dosimetry and thermal thresholds for tissue damage from hyperthermia. *Int J Hyperthermia* 2003;19(3):267-294.
[28] Vujaskovic Z, Song CW. Physiological mechanisms underlying heat-induced radiosensitization. *Int J Hyperthermia* 2004;20(2):163-174.
[29] Song CW, Park HJ, Lee CK, Griffin R. Implications of increased tumor blood flow and oxygenation caused by mild temperature hyperthermia in tumor treatment. *Int J Hyperthermia* 2005;21(8):761-767.
[30] Viglianti BL, Lora-Michiels M, Poulson JM, et al. Dynamic contrast-enhanced magnetic resonance imaging as a predictor of clinical outcome in canine spontaneous soft tissue sarcomas treated with thermoradiotherapy. *Clin Cancer Res* 2009;15(15):4993-5001.
[31] Dreher MR, Liu W, Michelich CR, Dewhirst MW, Chilkoti A. Thermal cycling enhances the accumulation of a temperature-sensitive biopolymer in solid tumors. *Cancer Res* 2007;67(9):4418-4424.
[32] Matteucci ML, Anyarambhatla G, Rosner G, et al. Hyperthermia increases accumulation of technetium-99m-labeled liposomes in feline sarcomas. *Clin Cancer Res* 2000;6(9):3748-3755.
[33] Kleiter MM, Yu D, Mohammadian LA, et al. A tracer dose of technetium-99m-labeled liposomes can estimate the effect of hyperthermia on intratumoral doxil extravasation. *Clin Cancer Res* 2006;12(22):6800-6807.
[34] Datta NR, Bose AK, Kapoor HK, Gupta S. Head and neck cancers: results of thermoradiotherapy versus radiotherapy. *Int J Hyperthermia* 1990;6(3):479-486.

[35] Valdagni R, Amichetti M. Report of long-term follow-up in a randomized trial comparing radiation therapy and radiation therapy plus hyperthermia to metastatic lymph nodes in stage IV head and neck patients. *Int J Radiat Oncol Biol Phys* 1994;28(1):163-169.

[36] Overgaard J, Gonzalez Gonzalez D, Hulshof MC, et al. Randomised trial of hyperthermia as adjuvant to radiotherapy for recurrent or metastatic malignant melanoma. European Society for Hyperthermic Oncology. *Lancet* 1995;345(8949):540-543.

[37] van der Zee J, Gonzalez Gonzalez D, van Rhoon GC, van Dijk JD, van Putten WL, Hart AA. Comparison of radiotherapy alone with radiotherapy plus hyperthermia in locally advanced pelvic tumours: a prospective, randomised, multicentre trial. Dutch Deep Hyperthermia Group. *Lancet* 2000;355(9210):1119-1125.

[38] Thrall DE, LaRue SM, Yu D, et al. Thermal dose is related to duration of local control in canine sarcomas treated with thermoradiotherapy. *Clin Cancer Res* 2005;11(14):5206-5214.

[39] Jones EL, Oleson JR, Prosnitz LR, et al. Randomized trial of hyperthermia and radiation for superficial tumors. *J Clin Oncol* 2005;23(13):3079-3085.

[40] Allen TM, Cullis PR. Drug delivery systems: entering the mainstream. *Science* 2004;303(5665):1818-1822.

[41] Chilkoti A, Christensen T, MacKay JA. Stimulus responsive elastin biopolymers: Applications in medicine and biotechnology. *Curr Opin Chem Biol* 2006;10(6):652-657.

[42] Bangham AD, Standish MM, Watkins JC. Diffusion of univalent ions across the lamellae of swollen phospholipids. *Journal of Molecular Biology* 1965;13(1):238-252.

[43] Massing U. Cancer therapy with liposomal formulations of anticancer drugs. *International Journal of Clinical Pharmacology and Therapeutics* 1997;35:87-90.

[44] Massing U, Fuxius S. Liposomal formulations of anticancer drugs: selectivity and effectiveness. *Drug Resist Updat* 2000;3(3):171-177.

[45] 4Torchilin VP. Recent advances with liposomes as pharmaceutical carriers. *Nat Rev Drug Discov* 2005;4(2):145-160.

[46] Klibanov AL, Maruyama K, Torchilin VP, Huang L. Amphipathic polyethyleneglycols effectively prolong the circulation time of liposomes. *FEBS Lett* 1990;268(1):235-237.

[47] Needham D, Hristova K, McIntosh TJ, Dewhirst MW, Wu N, Lasic DD. Polymer-grafted Liposomes: Physical Basis for the "Stealth" Property. *Journal of Liposome Research* 1992;2(3):411-430.

[48] Gabizon AA. Pegylated liposomal doxorubicin: metamorphosis of an old drug into a new form of chemotherapy. *Cancer Invest* 2001;19(4):424-436.

[49] Gabizon AA. Stealth liposomes and tumor targeting: one step further in the quest for the magic bullet. *Clin Cancer Res* 2001;7(2):223-225.

[50] Karanth H, Murthy RS. pH-sensitive liposomes--principle and application in cancer therapy. *J Pharm Pharmacol* 2007;59(4):469-483.

[51] Lokling KE, Fossheim SL, Skurtveit R, Bjornerud A, Klaveness J. pH-sensitive paramagnetic liposomes as MRI contrast agents: in vitro feasibility studies. *Magn Reson Imaging* 2001;19(5):731-738.

[52] Lokling KE, Skurtveit R, Bjornerud A, Fossheim SL. Novel pH-sensitive paramagnetic liposomes with improved MR properties. *Magn Reson Med* 2004;51(4):688-696.

[53] Lokling KE, Skurtveit R, Fossheim SL, Smistad G, Henriksen I, Klaveness J. pH-sensitive paramagnetic liposomes for MRI: assessment of stability in blood. *Magn Reson Imaging* 2003;21(5):531-540.

[54] Lindner LH, Reinl HM, Schlemmer M, Stahl R, Peller M. Paramagnetic thermosensitive liposomes for MR-thermometry. *Int J Hyperthermia* 2005;21(6):575-588.

[55] Fossheim SL, Il'yasov KA, Hennig J, Bjornerud A. Thermosensitive paramagnetic liposomes for temperature control during MR imaging-guided hyperthermia: in vitro feasibility studies. *Acad Radiol* 2000;7(12):1107-1115.

[56] Needham D, Anyarambhatla G, Kong G, Dewhirst MW. A new temperature-sensitive liposome for use with mild hyperthermia: characterization and testing in a human tumor xenograft model. *Cancer Res* 2000;60(5):1197-1201.

[57] Needham D, Dewhirst MW. The development and testing of a new temperature-sensitive drug delivery system for the treatment of solid tumors. *Adv Drug Deliv Rev* 2001;53(3):285-305.

[58] Mills JK, Needham D. Lysolipid incorporation in dipalmitoylphosphatidylcholine bilayer membranes enhances the ion permeability and drug release rates at the membrane phase transition. *Biochim Biophys Acta* 2005;1716(2):77-96.

[59] Yatvin MB, Cree TC, Tegmo-Larsson IM, Gipp JJ. Liposomes as drug carriers in cancer therapy: hyperthermia and pH sensitivity as modalities for targeting. *Strahlentherapie* 1984;160(12):732-740.

[60] Hauck ML, LaRue SM, Petros WP, et al. Phase I trial of doxorubicin-containing low temperature sensitive liposomes in spontaneous canine tumors. *Clin Cancer Res* 2006;12(13):4004-4010.

[61] Ponce AM, Vujaskovic Z, Yuan F, Needham D, Dewhirst MW. Hyperthermia mediated liposomal drug delivery. *Int J Hyperthermia* 2006;22(3):205-213.

[62] Barboriak DP, Macfall JR, Viglianti BL, Dewhirst Dvm MW. Comparison of three physiologically-based pharmacokinetic models for the prediction of contrast agent distribution measured by dynamic MR imaging. *J Magn Reson Imaging* 2008;27(6):1388-1398.

[63] Myhr G. Multimodal ultrasound mediated drug release model in local cancer therapy. *Med Hypotheses* 2007;69(6):1325-1333.

[64] Webb A. Introduction to biomedical imaging. Hoboken, N.J.: Wiley-*Interscience*; 2003. xiii, 252 p. p.

[65] Fossheim SL, Fahlvik AK, Klaveness J, Muller RN. Paramagnetic liposomes as MRI contrast agents: influence of liposomal physicochemical properties on the in vitro relaxivity. *Magn Reson Imaging* 1999;17(1):83-89.

[66] Mukundan S, Jr., Ghaghada KB, Badea CT, et al. A liposomal nanoscale contrast agent for preclinical CT in mice. *AJR Am J Roentgenol* 2006;186(2):300-307.

[67] Bhatnagar A, Hustinx R, Alavi A. Nuclear imaging methods for non-invasive drug monitoring. *Adv Drug Deliv Rev* 2000;41(1):41-54.

[68] Bacic G, Niesman MR, Bennett HF, Magin RL, Swartz HM. Modulation of water proton relaxation rates by liposomes containing paramagnetic materials. *Magn Reson Med* 1988;6(4):445-458.

[69] Unger E, Shen DK, Wu GL, Fritz T. Liposomes as MR contrast agents: pros and cons. *Magn Reson Med* 1991;22(2):304-308; discussion 313.

[70] Dromi S, Frenkel V, Luk A, et al. Pulsed-high intensity focused ultrasound and low temperature-sensitive liposomes for enhanced targeted drug delivery and antitumor effect. *Clin Cancer Res* 2007;13(9):2722-2727.

[71] Goins BA, Phillips WT. The use of scintigraphic imaging as a tool in the development of liposome formulations. *Prog Lipid Res* 2001;40(1-2):95-123.

[72] Goldberg SN, Gazelle GS, Mueller PR. Thermal ablation therapy for focal malignancy: a unified approach to underlying principles, techniques, and diagnostic imaging guidance. *AJR Am J Roentgenol* 2000;174(2):323-331.

[73] Wang X, Wang Y, Chen ZG, Shin DM. Advances of cancer therapy by nanotechnology. *Cancer Res Treat* 2009;41(1):1-11.

[74] Krown SE, Northfelt DW, Osoba D, Stewart JS. Use of liposomal anthracyclines in Kaposi's sarcoma. *Semin Oncol* 2004;31(6 Suppl 13):36-52.

[75] Alberts DS, Garcia DJ. Safety aspects of pegylated liposomal doxorubicin in patients with cancer. *Drugs* 1997;54 Suppl 4:30-35.

[76] Peller M, Schwerdt A, Hossann M, et al. MR characterization of mild hyperthermia-induced gadodiamide release from thermosensitive liposomes in solid tumors. *Invest Radiol* 2008;43(12):877-892.

In: Neuro-Oncology and Cancer Targeted Therapy
Editor: Lucía M. Gutiérrez pp.183-198
ISBN 978-1-61668-708-3
© 2010 Nova Science Publishers, Inc.

Chapter 7

EFFECTS OF HYPOXIA ON ANGIOGENESIS AND SURVIVAL OF GLIOBLASTOMA MULTIFORME

Alok Bhushan[*], *Sandeep Sheth, Aditi Jain and James C K Lai*

Department of Biomedical and Pharmaceutical Sciences
College of Pharmacy and Idaho Biomedical Research Institute
Idaho State University, Pocatello, ID 83209, USA

ABSTRACT

Glioblastoma multiforme (GBM) is one of the most vascular, aggressive and malignant forms of primary brain tumors. The presence of pseudopalisading necrosis and glomeruloid microvascular hyperplasia distinguishes GBM from other lower-grade astrocytomas. In GBM, a critical correlation exists between the presence of hypoxic regions and its angiogenic phenotype. Pseudopalisading necrosis is the result of vascular pathologies and both can generate regions of hypoxia around them. Hypoxia can also be caused by high metabolic activity of the tumor. The presence of glomeruloid bodies in the regions adjacent to the necrotic foci indicates an aggressive angiogenic phenotype. Hypoxia seems to be an important physiological stimulus that gives rise to the incidence of necrosis, formation of pseudopalisading cells and glomeruloid bodies: these are the critical events in the progression of GBM. Hypoxia sets off various signals that initiate angiogenesis by upregulating the expression of hypoxia inducible factor-1 (HIF-1) and secreting pro-angiogenic growth factors like vascular endothelial growth factor (VEGF) and interleukin-8 (IL-8). This review will focus upon the emerging concept regarding mechanisms responsible for the accelerated growth in GBM, emphasizing a link between hypoxia and angiogenesis. Since no significant advances have occurred in the past twenty five years in the treatment of GBM, it is imperative to understand the underlying

---

[*] Address for correspondence:
Alok Bhushan
Department of Biomedical and Pharmaceutical Sciences
College of Pharmacy
Idaho State University
Pocatello, ID 83209-8334
Ph No. 208-282-4408
Email: abhushan@pharmacy.isu.edu

molecular mechanisms taking place in the development of GBM and then come up with a treatment strategy that can at least increase the survival rate of the patients if not eradicate the disease.

Key words: Glioblastoma, Hypoxia, Angiogenesis.

INTRODUCTION

Glioblastoma multiforme (GBM) is one of the most aggressive and common tumors in brain. Despite multimodal therapy, the prognosis of the patients with glioblastoma remains poor and the mean survival time is less than 12 months after diagnosis. The main reason of such low survival rate is that total removal of the tumor by surgery is difficult as the tumor cells invade into surrounding normal brain tissue, leading to malignant transformation (Figure 1). The molecular mechanisms responsible for rendering this tumor highly malignant and rapidly progressive are not fully understood. From the existing literature it is clear that glioblastomas show two distinct histopathological features: microvascular hyperplasia including glomeruloid vascular proliferation and necrosis with pseudopalisading cells surrounding it.

Necrosis in GBM develops in areas where metabolic demand exceeds oxygen supply [1]. Various findings have demonstrated that the pseudopalisading cells surrounding the necrotic foci are severely hypoxic [2]. Conversely, before the necrosis has occurred, hypoxia is induced by the high metabolic activity of the tumor.

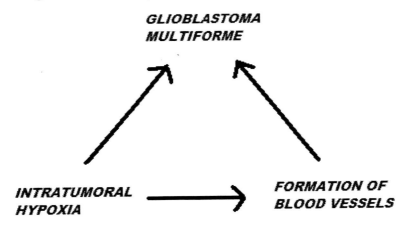

Figure 1. Hypothetical correlation between hypoxia and angiogenesis in the development of glioblastoma multiforme.

Hypoxia sets off a variety of signals that initiates angiogenesis [3]. In this process, the hypoxic cells up-regulate the expression of various angiogenic growth factors especially vascular endothelial growth factor (VEGF). This response is mediated by transcription factors of the hypoxia-inducible factor (HIF) family. HIF-1, when stabilized under hypoxic condition, is translocated into the nucleus and binds to hypoxia-responsive element (HRE) within the VEGF promoter thereby increasing its transcription. VEGF stimulates angiogenesis by initiating the proliferation of endothelial cells that restores the high oxygen demand of the hypoxic tumor cells. Some of the new treatment strategies for GBM include targeting VEGF/VEGF receptors (VEGFR) by monoclonal antibody or VEGFR traps, respectively [4].

CANCER OVERVIEW

Tumor is the name given to the swelling or lesion caused by the uncontrolled growth of abnormal cells. Neoplasm is the abnormal proliferation of genetically altered cells; however, currently this word is synonymously used with tumor. Neoplasm can be benign or malignant. Cancer, a malignant neoplasm, is a group of diseases characterized by uncontrolled growth and spread of abnormal cells. Uncontrolled cellular growth, invasion or infiltration into adjacent tissues and spreading to distant organs in the body (metastasis) are the three properties of a malignant neoplasm, which, if not treated, could be harmful and ultimately lethal. On the other hand, benign tumors impose less danger to the host.

Based upon the site of origin, cancer can be classified into primary or secondary. Primary tumors are cancers that are at the original site where it first arose, while secondary tumors are those that have metastasized from a primary location.

The 2009 report of American Cancer Society on cancer statistics reports that 562,340 Americans are expected to die of cancer and is the second most common cause of death after heart disease [5].

OVERVIEW OF GLIOMA

Tumors of central nervous system are classified based on their tissue of origin, such as neuroepithelial type and non-neuroepithelial type. Neuroepithelial type of tumors includes the astrocytic tumors which are the tumors developed from astrocytes. As astrocytes are a type of glial cells, astrocytic tumors can collectively be called as astrocytomas, glial tumors or gliomas.

From the microscopic appearance and behavior, gliomas are graded into low-grade or high-grade. Again, the malignancy grading of World Health Organization (WHO) classifies gliomas into four grades [6]. Grade I gliomas indicate a specific type of astrocytoma, i.e., pilocytic astrocytoma occurring in children. Supratentorial astrocytomas, which is classified into diffuse astrocytomas, is a grade II glioma and it usually occurs in adults. Grade I and Grade II gliomas are low-grade and grow slowly over many years [7]. The mean survival time of the patients following surgical resection of grade I and grade II gliomas is generally more than 5 years, though the time varies with individuals, with some cases remaining latent for several years and others progressing rapidly to grade III and grade IV tumors [6]. Anaplastic astrocytoma is a grade III tumor (high-grade) and the mean survival time of patients with this type of astrocytoma is 2-3 years [6]. Glioblastoma Multiforme (GBM) is classified as grade IV (high-grade) astrocytoma and is known to be the most aggressive, malignant, highly invasive primary brain tumor [7]. In the literature, GBM is commonly referred as glioblastoma.

STATISTICS OF GBM

Affecting patients mostly between 40 and 70 years of age [8, 9], GBM most commonly develops in the cerebral hemispheres, more often in the frontal lobes than the temporal lobes or basal ganglia and very rarely in the cerebellum or spinal cord [8, 10]. Children also get affected in fewer than 10% of the cases; however, their brainstem is affected more commonly than in adults [8]. As per the SEER (Surveillance, Epidemiology, and End Results Program) report by Central Brain Tumor Registry of the United States [11], the incidence rate of primary malignant brain and central nervous system tumors for 2004-2005 was 18.16 per 100,000 person-years. This rate is higher in females (19.16 per 100,000 person-years) than males (17.08 per 100,000 person-years). However, the incidence rate of glioma was found to be higher in males (7.09 per 100,000 person-years) than in females (4.96 per 100,000 person-years) [11]. GBM is the most frequently occurring brain tumor in humans and represent 12-15% of all intracranial tumors and 50-60% of astrocytic tumors [7, 11]. The average estimated 5-year survival rates for primary brain tumors is 28% overall, but the range is large and is dominated by patients with low-grade tumors. The 5-year survival rate exceeds 85% for low-grade tumors such as pilocytic astrocytoma and oligodendroglioma; however, it is less than 5% for patients with high-grade tumors like GBM [3].

The prognosis of patients with GBM largely depends upon whether effective treatment regimes are available. Despite multimodal aggressive treatment, comprising surgical resection, local radiotherapy and systemic chemotherapy, the median survival time after diagnosis is still around 10-12 months, with fewer than 20% surviving longer than one year and approximately 5% surviving longer than 5 years [10, 12].

CLASSIFICATION OF GBM

Noticing the growth pattern of glioblastoma, in 1940, a German neuropathologist named Hans-Joachim Scherer was the first person to clearly distinguish primary glioblastoma from secondary glioblastoma [13]. In the majority of the cases, primary glioblastoma is found in older patients. It can develop *de novo,* i.e., without any clinical or histopathological evidence of a pre-existing, less malignant precursor cells as a result of key genetic alterations [7,14,15]. This single-step malignant transformation can take place just within 3 months [7]. Secondary glioblastoma, on the other hand, generally develop in younger patients (<45 years) [7]. Secondary glioblastoma is also referred to as progressive glioblastoma: it develops through a series of genetic steps and malignant progression from diffuse astrocytoma (WHO grade II) or anaplastic astrocytoma (WHO grade III) over a period of time [7]. Based on the genetic typing, the primary and secondary glioblastomas have also been termed glioblastomas type 2 and 1, respectively [14, 16].

VASCULAR PHENOTYPE IN GBM

In a normal brain, all the cells receive nutrients and oxygen through passive diffusion from the nearest blood vessel. However, in a pathological condition like tumor formation, the passive diffusion of nutrients and oxygen is unable to fulfill the increasing metabolic demands of proliferating cells. In order to survive, the growing tumor cells recruit blood vessels from surrounding host blood vessels. The blood vessel density within and surrounding the tumor also increases with tumor progression.

Low-grade infiltrating astrocytomas (WHO grade II) have a vessel density not much different than that in normal brain. The density of tumor capillary blood vessels increases as the low-grade infiltrating astrocytomas become more cellular and atypical, to form anaplastic astrocytoma (WHO grade III) and is the highest in glioblastoma (WHO grade IV). The vascular architecture also changes from normal to dilated to highly irregular vessels as the tumor grade increases [7, 9]. The two distinguishing features of GBM are necrosis with pseudopalisading cells and microvascular hyperplasia though their exact order of occurrence is not known.

Necrosis

Multiple small, irregularly-shaped necrotic regions are found in anaplastic astrocytomas where high metabolic demands for oxygen of rapidly dividing cells exceed that supplied [1, 18]. Larger necroses can be formed because of vaso-occlusion and infarction following intravascular thrombosis, which sets in due to insufficient blood supply and is a very common finding in GBM [19]. By the time necrosis is found in astrocytomas, the tumor cells have achieved a highly malignant character [1]. Thus, tumor necrosis itself does not result directly in aggressive behavior.

Microvascular Hyperplasia

Microvascular hyperplasia is a structurally distinct form of angiogenesis. It does not refer to an increased number of blood vessels, but to the morphological structure of vascular bundles emerging from the parent vessels, lined by hyperplastic endothelial cells, surrounded by basal lamina and an incomplete layer of pericytes [17, 20, 21]. Microvascular hyperplasia can be due to hypoxia-induced growth of new blood vessels. These newly formed vessels arrange in tufts, resemble renal glomeruli and so are called as glomeruloid bodies [17]. It is interesting to note that glomeruloid bodies are also found in gastrointestinal carcinomas and lymphomas and are the markers of poor prognosis in melanoma, prostate cancer, breast cancer, endometrial cancer, and non-small cell lung cancer [22, 23]. The presence of glomeruloid bodies in most cases indicates an aggressive angiogenic phenotype in the regions close to those showing necrosis [17].

These histopathological features of GBM prompt the hypothesis that hypoxia could be the driving force behind the occurrence of necrotic regions and formation of pseudopalisading cells and glomeruloid bodies.

INDUCTION OF HYPOXIA IN GBM

Immunohistochemistry using pimonidazole, a hypoxia-marker, has shown that tumor cells located more than ten cell layers away from a vessel are hypoxic [24]. Several mechanisms have been suggested to explain the appearance of hypoxia in GBM. The necrotic zones caused by intravascular thrombosis can lead to hypoxia in the tissues surrounding these zones [1]. Alternatively, the high metabolic activity of the tumor cells could also lead to hypoxia even before necrosis has occurred [1]. Yet another possibility is that the tumor cells present at the greatest distance from arterial supplies become hypoxic after a critical point in tumor growth due to their increased metabolic demands [19].

Vascular Regression-induced Hypoxia in GBM

Experiments on animal models of gliomas have suggested that the initial stages of tumor angiogenesis actually involve regression of blood vessels [26, 27]. Before initiating angiogenesis, the hypoxic glioma cells initially acquire their blood supply by 'co-opting' the host's normal blood vessels, making them a 'non-angiogenic tumor' [28]. The co-opted host vasculature then undergoes regression resulting in massive tumor cell death in the center of the tumor [19, 29]. The regression of the initially co-opted vessels can be hypothesized as a host defense mechanism [28]. Angiopoietin-2 (Ang-2), in the absence of VEGF, seems to be a key regulator in the regression of initially co-opted tumor vessels [19, 29]. Only the endothelial cells of high-grade gliomas but not the low-grade gliomas or the normal brain overexpresses Ang-2 [30, 31]. Ang-2 acts in an autocrine manner on the tumoral vessels as a Tie-2 receptor antagonist.

In the absence of VEGF, Tie-2 receptor blockade by Ang-2 leads to vascular destabilization, endothelial cell apoptosis and vascular regression causing acute hypoxia, ultimately leading to tumor cell death in the center of the tumor [19, 29]. Co-option of existing vasculature in the brain by tumor cell has been proposed to induce vaso-occlusive events leading to acute hypoxia/necrosis [19]. The remaining tumor cells which were able to overcome this regression have been demonstrated to release some factors that inhibit the apoptosis of endothelial cells and initiate a robust angiogenic response [32] by increasing the expression of VEGF in a HIF-dependent manner on the tumor periphery [19].

The events involving vessel co-option suggests that most tumors originate as an avascular mass which co-opt with host vessels and then are rescued to form malignant and aggressive tumors that have the ability to metastasize [28]. Apart from GBM, vessel co-option has also been observed in other tumor types like murine Lewis lung carcinoma, murine ovarian cancer, human melanoma, and human Kaposi sarcoma [33-36].

HYPOXIA-INDUCED TUMOR CELL MIGRATION

As a compensatory mechanism to overcome the hypoxic situation, the tumor (glioma) cells migrate towards the nearby vessels moving outwards and away from the central hypoxic area. The wave of actively migrating tumor cells forms pseudopalisades and leave behind an enlarged central zone filled with fibrillar processes and non-migrating extremely hypoxic tumor cells undergoing necrosis [37].

The formation of pseudopalisading cells can be thought to be induced by hypoxia [19, 37]. This observation is supported by the evidence that hypoxic GBM cells migrate more rapidly than normoxic cells *in vitro*; and hypoxic cells *in vitro* as well as pseudopalisading cells in GBM tissue sections express extracellular matrix proteases, including MMP-2 and uPAR [2, 38, 39]. MMP-2 exhibits gelatinase activity; thus, it can digest gelatin in the extracellular matrix. uPAR, on binding with urokinase plasminogen activator (uPA), converts inactive plasminogen to active plasmin. The active plasmin brings about the lysis of various extracellular matrix components. Consequently, the expression of MMP-2 and uPAR in pseudopalisading cells in GBM is associated with tumor cell migration and invasion [40].

ANGIOGENESIS IN GBM

Tumor progression involves several steps including tumor-vascular interaction, formation of blood vessels and growth of tumor cells in a suitable microenvironment [41]. The development of the blood vessels by tumor cells is referred to as tumor angiogenesis and is due to tumor-vascular cell interaction. Endothelial cells form the inner lining of the blood vessels. Their proliferation, migration and tube formation result in angiogenesis [42]. Tumor angiogenesis starts with the stimulation of endothelial cells by pro-angiogenic growth factors secreted by the tumor cells that bind to their specific receptors on endothelial cells. The basement membrane and extracellular matrix, surrounding the endothelial cells, are degraded by extracellular proteases (MMPs and uPA) thereby allowing the activated endothelial cells to divide and invade into the surrounding matrix. The endothelial cells then migrate through the extracellular matrix towards the tumor in response to different pro-angiogenic growth factors and cytokines. Migrating endothelial cells then assemble themselves to form a central lumen, and an immature blood vessel is formed. The immature vessel matures by the formation of a new basement membrane around the new vessel. The angiogenic response of the endothelial cells is important for the tumor cells to survive under conditions of oxygen deprivation. Angiogenesis is necessary for invasion and metastasis.

All the biological steps involved in angiogenesis are well regulated, and depend upon the balance between opposing pro- and anti-angiogenic factors, called the 'Angiogenic Switch' [43, 44]. This switch is regulated between 'on' and 'off' and was first proposed by Judah Folkman that the 'Switch' from avascular ('off') to the vascular ('on') phenotype is the key event for the progression and metastasis of tumors [43]. The presence of microvascular hyperplasia in glioblastoma indicates that angiogenesis has occurred to support the neoplastic growth [17].

HYPOXIA-ANGIOGENESIS CORRELATION IN GBM

Angiogenesis is believed to be the physiological response to hypoxia. In GBM, the tumor cells undergo an array of biological responses to hypoxic conditions. Pseudopalisading cells are hypoxic and adapt to such an environment as is seen from its nuclear overexpression of

HIF-1α [2, 45]. HIF-1 activation results in the up-regulation of pro-angiogenic growth factors with the eventuality of furthering the process of angiogenesis [46]. Recent literature demonstrates that pseudopalisading cells secrete increased levels of pro-angiogenic growth factors such as VEGF [47-50] and IL-8 (Interleukin-8) [51]. Overall, in GBM, there is a clear indication that hypoxia induces HIF-1α expression, VEGF expression, and tumor angiogenesis [50, 52].

HYPOXIA-INDUCIBLE FACTOR-1: THE ANGIOGENIC MASTER SWITCH

HIF-1 is a transcription factor activated under low oxygen tension. HIF-1 is a DNA-binding heterodimer made up of an oxygen- and growth factor-regulated HIF-1α subunit and a constitutively-active HIF-1β subunit [53]. Under normoxia, prolyl-hydroxylases results in the degradation of HIF-1α subunit by the proteasome. As prolyl-hydroxylases uses oxygen as a co-substrate, its activity is decreased and eventually stabilizing HIF-1α. HIF-1α protein stabilization is the rate-limiting step in HIF-1 activation. Hypoxic conditions activate HIF-1, which in turn binds to HIF-1β and this complex is translocated into the nucleus of the hypoxic cells where it binds to the hypoxia-responsive elements (HREs). The HIF-1 activation leads to induction of transcription and expression of numerous hypoxia-responsive genes like VEGF. These genes are involved in tumor angiogenesis, invasion, cell survival and glucose metabolism [25].

REGULATIONS OF HIF-1

Intracellular Signals Regulating HIF-1

HIF-1 can also be activated by physiological or pathological activation of growth factor and cell adhesion pathways. Growth factor induced activation of tyrosine kinase receptors leads to stabilization and activation of HIF-1. Upon ligand (EGF, TNF-α, PDGF, etc.) binding, receptor tyrosine kinase dimerizes and becomes activated leading to a cascade of downstream signaling starting with the activation of phosphatidylinositol 3-kinase (PI3K). PI3K phosphorylates phosphatidylinositol (4,5)-biphosphate (PIP2) to form phosphatidylinositol (3,4,5)-triphosphate (PIP3) which in turn activates AKT. AKT is a serine/threonine kinase well known for its pro-survival and anti-apoptotic properties. Activation of AKT has been observed to increase HIF-1α protein translation by the AKT/FRAP/mTOR pathway [54, 55].

Activated receptor tyrosine kinase can also activate HIF-1α by signaling through Ras/MAPK (mitogen activated protein kinase) pathway [56]. Common genetic alterations in GBM have been suggested to increase the activities of AKT and Ras which can together increase the transcriptional activity of HIF-1 [57]. Additionally, the PI3K/AKT pathway is also activated by extracellular matrix adhesion mediated by integrins [58]. Integrin ligation activates integrin-linked kinase, which has been shown to increase HIF-1α expression as well as VEGF production by PI3K/AKT/FRAP/mTOR pathway resulting in tumor angiogenesis [59]. Increased activity of integrin-linked kinase has also been reported in gliomas [60].

Genetic Alterations Regulating HIF-1 in Gliomas

There is a correlation between glioblastoma tumor grade and HIF-1α overexpression [53]. Through different mechanisms, the expression of HIF-1α is also upregulated by mutations in tumor suppressor genes (e.g., *p53* and *PTEN*) and oncogenes (e.g., *EGFR*) [55, 61, 62]. The above genetic alterations modulate HIF-1 expression in a way that enhances hypoxia-induced new vessel growth.

One critical function of the tumor supressor p53 gene is a transcription factor in regulating mitogenesis and is also involved in the control of angiogenesis [63]. Following DNA damage [64] by stressors such as chronic/severe hypoxia, p53 protein accumulates and is activated, inducing apoptosis and arrest of the cell cycle. This mechanism helps to maintain the genetic integrity of the cells. Most low-grade infiltrative astrocytomas show mutations in p53 gene; but in primary glioblastomas, it is less frequent [7]. Mutated p53 has no ability to induce apoptosis or cell cycle arrest, resulting in chromosomal abnormalities [64]. In addition, expression of wild-type p53 has been suggested to decrease angiogenesis by down-regulating the expression of VEGF [69] and HIF-1 [61]: thus, mutated p53 may initiate neovascularization [63]. Wild-type p53 blocks the activation of HIF-1 in hypoxia by the interaction of HIF-1α with MDM2. This interaction induces the ubiquitination of HIF-1α and targets it for degradation. In summary, p53 mutations suppress hypoxia-mediated apoptosis, induce HIF-1α expression, and upregulates HIF-1 mediated transactivation of VEGF and other target genes.

The tumor-suppressor gene *PTEN* (phosphatase and tensin homolog; *MMAC1*) located on the 10q23.3 chromosome is mutated in 15 to 40% of glioblastomas and almost exclusively in primary glioblastomas [66]. *PTEN* códes for a phosphatase that converts PIP3 into PIP2 thereby, blocking the PI3K-AKT-mTOR pathway that initiates cell survival and cell cycle entry. Zundel et al. [62] proposed that loss of *PTEN* function during malignant progression contributes to tumor expansion and angiogenesis through the deregulation of AKT activity and HIF-1-regulated gene expression whereas increase in wild-type *PTEN* in glioblastoma cells suppresses HIF-1α expression.

EGFR is a cell-surface tyrosine kinase receptor that becomes activated through the binding of growth factors (e.g., EGF, TGF-α) on its extracellular domain. As discussed above, EGFR activation regulates several downstream signal transduction pathways, principally PI3K-AKT-mTOR pathway and Ras-MAPK signaling pathway resulting in increased cell proliferation and cell survival by blocking apoptosis. Mutation in *EGFR* gene occurs in high percentages (~ 40% - 60%) of primary glioblastomas but rarely (< 10%) in secondary glioblastomas [15]. The most frequent *EGFR* gene mutation is the truncation of trans-membrane protein which renders the receptor constitutively active and ligand-independent. The constitutively active form of EGFR, like the one found in glioblastomas, is known to increase HIF-1α expression and VEGF production by a PI3K-AKT-mTOR-dependent [67] and possibly Ras/MAPK-dependent pathway.

ANGIOGENESIS DRIVEN BY PRO-ANGIOGENIC GROWTH FACTORS IN GBM:

Angiogenesis is required for survival of any tumor growth like pseudopalisades formed on the periphery of necrotic areas. To support the growth of these palisades, microvascular hyperplasia is often found adjacent to them. Pseudopalisading cells are severely hypoxic and express high levels of different hypoxia-inducible pro-angiogenic growth factors including VEGF [47, 49], IL-8 [51] and hepatocyte growth factor (HGF) [68].

Hypoxia is a potent stimulator of VEGF, increasing its expression not only at the mRNA level but also at the protein level [25]. VEGF concentrations have been found to be 200-300-fold higher in cystic fluid of human GBMs than in the serum [69]. Such high levels of VEGF result from HIF-mediated activation of transcription of *VEGF* gene by binding to specific promoter sequences in hypoxic pseudopalisading cells and inhibition of this HIF-VEGF pathway have been demonstrated to suppress tumor growth [70]. Following the expression and secretion by the tumor cells, extracellular VEGF binds to its high-affinity tyrosine kinase receptors, VEGFR-1 (Flt-1) and VEGFR-2 (Flk-1/KDR) which are up-regulated in the endothelial cells of high-grade gliomas and not in the endothelial cells of normal brain. Binding of VEGF to their receptors initiates a signaling cascade that leads to endothelial cell proliferation and migration. The resulting new blood vessel that is formed provides oxygen and nutrients to the growing tumor.

In addition to hypoxia, HGF has also been found to induce up-regulation and secretion of VEGF in human glioma cells [71]. HGF is upregulated in human gliomas and its expression level correlates with tumor grade [68]. HGF also possesses pro-angiogenic effects *in vitro* and can cause endothelial cell proliferation, migration and tube formation [68] while its up-regulation in gliomas in a xenograft model leads to increased angiogenesis and tumor growth. Although hypoxia has been known to increase the expression of HGF and its receptor, the expression of HGF in pseudopalisading cells of glioblastomas has not been demonstrated [72].

IL-8 is another pro-angiogenic factor that is highly up-regulated within the hypoxic pseudopalisades of GBMs [51]. However, unlike VEGF, hypoxic regulation of IL-8 is not directly the result of HIF activation, because there is no hypoxia responsive element within its promoter. IL-8 works in an autocrine manner by binding to its receptors, CXCR1 and CXCR2, and shows invasive and metastatic effects in neoplastic cells in addition to inducing angiogenesis [73].

Remarkably, hypoxia also induces the up-regulation of other pro-anagiogenic factors like angiopoietin and its receptors, erythropoetins, endothelin-1, and transforming growth factor α and β [46], but down-regulates thrombospondin-1 [74], brain angiogenesis inhibitors (BAIs) [75]. However, a detailed discussion of all these factors and their potential role in gliomagenesis is beyond the scope of this review [46].

CONCLUSION

Glioblastoma multiforme (GBM) is one of the most vascularized human primary brain tumors and represents the most malignant stage of astrocytoma progression. The prognosis of the patients with GBM is poor and the reasons include: (i) complete surgical resection is almost impossible because the aggressive tumor cells infiltrate into the surrounding brain tissues, and (ii) the tumor cells are genetically resistant to adjuvant therapies like local radiotherapy and systemic chemotherapy [19]. The patients will eventually die of the disease within 12 months of diagnosis when the tumor cells invade nervous system structures critical for life.

The novelty of this review lies in identifying a correlation between the presence of hypoxia in GBM and its induction of angiogenesis to facilitate tumor progression and invasion to adjacent normal brain tissue. The two major characteristic features and diagnostic markers that distinguish GBM from other lower-grade astrocytomas are necrosis with pseudopalisades and microvascular hyperplasia forming glomeruloid bodies. Pseudopalisading necrosis is a typical GBM morphology that links vascular pathology, hypoxia, angiogenesis, and enhanced tumorigenicity. The generation of hypoxia in the regions surrounding vascular pathology like intravascular thrombosis or endothelial cell apoptosis (vascular regression) results in the migration of tumor cells forming pseudopalisades. Non-migrating cells which are left behind by pseudopalisades are extremely hypoxic and eventually undergo necrosis. Hypoxia is the key physiological stimulus that drives various events in the progression of GBM. Intratumoral hypoxia and genetic alterations provide dual mechanisms for the induction of HIF-1. HIF-1 is a 'master angiogenic switch', which when turned 'on', can change the tumor vasculature to the pro-angiogeic phenotype by inducing the transcription of its downstream target genes, including VEGF.

The angiogenic response induced by HIF-1 leads to the formation of tumor-specific blood vessels (microvascular hyperplasia) that takes place early during the process of tumor progression. Hypoxia may also facilitate the downregulation of anti-angiogenic factors. The summation of all these effects is enhanced tumorigenicity at the cellular level. Such an increase in malignancy no doubt leads to an increased metabolic demand, which may facilitate the occurrence of more regions of hypoxia and necrosis, completing the vicious cycle [1].

As angiogenesis greatly contributes to the aggressive behavior of glioblastoma, therapeutic approach for its treatment should therefore focus on inhibiting angiogenesis. Anti-angiogenic agents like VEGF/VEGFR inhibitors (bevacizumab), tyrosine kinase inhibitors (sorafenib, cetuximab, etc.), thalidomide, and the like are being tested in clinical trials against malignant gliomas [4]. However, the drawback of anti-angiogenic therapy is that it can affect the normal cell differentiation and physiology. Perhaps further research will resolve this dichotomy. Nevertheless, this review highlights the importance of the use of anti-angiogenic agents. The combination of anti-angiogenic therapy with chemotherapeutic agents and/or radio therapy could prove synergistic for the treatment of GBM and other solid tumors.

REFERENCES

[1] Louis, D.N. (1997). A molecular genetic model of astrocytoma histopathology. *Brain Pathol, 7*, 755-764.

[2] Brat, D.J., Castellano-Sanchez, A.A., Hunter, S.B., Pecot, M., Cohen, C., Hammond, E.H., Devi, S.N., Kaur, B. & Van Meir, E.G. (2004). Pseudopalisades in glioblastoma are

hypoxic, express extracellular matrix proteases, and are formed by an actively migrating cell population. *Cancer Res, 64*, 920-927.

[3] Evans, S.M., Judy, K.D., Dunphy, I., Jenkins, W.T., Hwang, W.T., Nelson, P.T., Lustig, R.A., Jenkins, K., Magarelli, D.P., Hahn, S.M., Collins, R.A., Grady, M.S. & Koch, C.J. (2004). Hypoxia is important in the biology and aggression of human glial brain tumors. *Clin Cancer Res, 10*, 8177-8184.

[4] Anderson, J.C., McFarland, B.C. & Gladson, C.L. (2008). New molecular targets in angiogenic vessels of glioblastoma tumours. *Expert Rev Mol Med, 10*, e23.

[5] American Cancer Society. Cancer facts and figures 2009. 2009. Available from: URL: www.cancer.org

[6] Louis, D.N., Ohgaki, H., Wiestler, O.D., Cavenee, W.K., Burger, P.C., Jouvet, A., Scheithauer, B.W. & Kleihues, P. (2007). The 2007 WHO classification of tumours of the central nervous system. *Acta Neuropathol, 11*, 97-109.

[7] Kleihues, P., & Cavenne, W.K. (2000). *World Health Organization classification of tumors: Pathology and genetics of tumors of the nervous system.* Lyon, France: IARC Press.

[8] Altman, D.A., Atkinson, D.S. Jr., Brat, D.J. (2007). Best cases from the AFIP: glioblastoma multiforme. *Radiographics, 27*, 883-888.

[9] Brat, D.J. & Mapstone, T.B. (2003). Malignant glioma physiology: cellular response to hypoxia and its role in tumor progression. *Ann Intern Med, 138*, 659-668.

[10] Smith, J.S. & Jenkins, R.B. (2000). Genetic alterations in adult diffuse glioma: occurrence, significance, and prognostic implications. *Front Biosci, 5*, D213-231.

[11] CBTRUS. CBTRUS Statistical Report: Primary brain tumors in the United States, 2004-2005. 2009. Available from: URL: www.cbtrus.org

[12] Krex, D., Klink, B., Hartmann, C., von Deimling, A., Pietsch, T., Simon, M., Sabel, M., Steinbach, J.P., Heese, O., Reifenberger, G., Weller, M. & Schackert, G. (2007). Long-term survival with glioblastoma multiforme. *Brain, 13*, 2596-2606.

[13] Scherer, H.J. (1940). Cerebral astrocytomas and their derivatives. *American Journal of Cancer, 40*, 159-198.

[14] Kleihues, P. & Ohgaki, H. (1999). Primary and secondary glioblastomas: from concept to clinical diagnosis. *Neuro Oncol, 1*, 44-51.

[15] Ohgaki, H. & Kleihues, P. (2007). Genetic pathways to primary and secondary glioblastoma. *Am J Pathol, 170*, 1445-1453,.

[16] von Deimling, A., von Ammon, K., Schoenfeld, D., Wiestler, O.D., Seizinger, B.R. & Louis, D.N. (1993). Subsets of glioblastoma multiforme defined by molecular genetic analysis. *Brain Pathol, 3*, 19-26.

[17] Brat, D.J. & Van Meir, E.G. (2001). Glomeruloid microvascular proliferation orchestrated by VPF/VEGF: a new world of angiogenesis research. *Am J Pathol, 158*, 789-796.

[18] Lantos, P.L., VandenBerg, S.R., & Kleihues, P. (1996). Tumors of the nervous system. In D.I. Graham, & P.L. Lantos (Eds.), *Greenfield's Neuropathology* (edition 6th.583-879). London:Arnold.

[19] Brat, D.J. & Van Meir, E.G. (2004). Vaso-occlusive and prothrombotic mechanisms associated with tumor hypoxia, necrosis, and accelerated growth in glioblastoma. *Lab Invest, 84*, 397-405.

[20] Rojiani, A.M. & Dorovini-Zis, K. (1996). Glomeruloid vascular structures in glioblastoma multiforme: an immunohistochemical and ultrastructural study. *J Neurosurg, 85,* 1078-1084.

[21] Wesseling, P., Schlingemann, R.O., Rietveld, F.J., Link, M., Burger, P.C. & Ruiter, D.J. (1995). Early and extensive contribution of pericytes/vascular smooth muscle cells to microvascular proliferation in glioblastoma multiforme: an immuno-light and immuno-electron microscopic study. *J Neuropathol Exp Neurol, 54,* 304-310.

[22] Straume, O., Chappuis, P.O., Salvesen, H.B., Halvorsen, O.J., Haukaas, S.A., Goffin, J.R., Begin, L.R., Foulkes, W.D. & Akslen, L.A. (2002). Prognostic importance of glomeruloid microvascular proliferation indicates an aggressive angiogenic phenotype in human cancers. *Cancer Res, 62,* 6808-6811.

[23] Tanaka, F., Oyanagi, H., Takenaka, K., Ishikawa, S., Yanagihara, K., Miyahara, R., Kawano, Y., Li, M., Otake, Y. & Wada, H. (2003). Glomeruloid microvascular proliferation is superior to intratumoral microvessel density as a prognostic marker in non-small cell lung cancer. *Cancer Res, 63,* 6791-6794.

[24] Evans, S.M., Hahn, S.M., Magarelli, D.P. & Koch, C.J. (2001). Hypoxic heterogeneity in human tumors: EF5 binding, vasculature, necrosis, and proliferation. *Am J Clin Oncol, 24,* 467-472.

[25] Kaur, B., Tan, C., Brat, D.J., Post, D.E. & Van Meir, E.G. (2004). Genetic and hypoxic regulation of angiogenesis in gliomas. *J Neurooncol, 70,* 229-243.

[26] Holash, J., Wiegand, S.J. & Yancopoulos, G.D. (1999). New model of tumor angiogenesis: dynamic balance between vessel regression and growth mediated by angiopoietins and VEGF. *Oncogene, 18,* 5356-5362.

[27] Zagzag, D., Amirnovin, R., Greco, M.A., Yee, H., Holash, J., Wiegand, S.J., Zabski, S., Yancopoulos, G.D. & Grumet, M. (2000). Vascular apoptosis and involution in gliomas precede neovascularization: a novel concept for glioma growth and angiogenesis. *Lab Invest, 80,* 837-849.

[28] Hillen, F. & Griffioen, A.W. (2007). Tumour vascularization: sprouting angiogenesis and beyond. *Cancer Metastasis Rev, 26,* 489-502.

[29] Brat, D.J., Castellano-Sanchez, A., Kaur, B. & Van Meir, E.G. (2002). Genetic and biologic progression in astrocytomas and their relation to angiogenic dysregulation. *Adv Anat Pathol, 9,* 24-36.

[30] Stratmann, A., Risau, W. & Plate, K.H. (1998). Cell type-specific expression of angiopoietin-1 and angiopoietin-2 suggests a role in glioblastoma angiogenesis. *Am J Pathol, 153,* 1459-1466.

[31] Zagzag, D., Hooper, A., Friedlander, D.R., Chan, W., Holash, J., Wiegand, S.J., Yancopoulos, G.D. & Grumet, M. (1999). In situ expression of angiopoietins in astrocytomas identifies angiopoietin-2 as an early marker of tumor angiogenesis. *Exp Neurol, 159,* 391-400.

[32] Ezhilarasan, R., Mohanam, I., Govindarajan, K. & Mohanam, S. (2007). Glioma cells suppress hypoxia-induced endothelial cell apoptosis and promote the angiogenic process. *Int J Oncol, 30,* 701-707.

[33] Dome, B., Paku, S., Somlai, B. & Timar, J. (2002). Vascularization of cutaneous melanoma involves vessel co-option and has clinical significance. *J Pathol, 197,* 355-362.

[34] Holash, J., Maisonpierre, P.C., Compton, D., Boland, P., Alexander, C.R., Zagzag, D., Yancopoulos, G.D. & Wiegand, S.J. (1999). Vessel cooption, regression, and growth in tumors mediated by angiopoietins and VEGF. *Science, 284,* 1994-1998.

[35] Kim, E.S., Serur, A., Huang, J., Manley, C.A., McCrudden, K.W., Frischer, J.S., Soffer, S.Z., Ring, L., New, T., Zabski, S., Rudge, J.S., Holash, J., Yancopoulos, G.D., Kandel, J.J. & Yamashiro, D.J. (2002). Potent VEGF blockade causes regression of coopted vessels in a model of neuroblastoma. *Proc Natl Acad Sci U S A, 99,* 11399-11404.

[36] Zhang, L., Yang, N., Park, J.W., Katsaros, D., Fracchioli, S., Cao, G., O'Brien-Jenkins, A., Randall, T.C., Rubin, S.C. & Coukos, G. (2003). Tumor-derived vascular endothelial growth factor up-regulates angiopoietin-2 in host endothelium and destabilizes host vasculature, supporting angiogenesis in ovarian cancer. *Cancer Res, 63,* 3403-3412.

[37] Rong, Y., Durden, D.L., Van Meir, E.G. & Brat, D.J. (2006). 'Pseudopalisading' necrosis in glioblastoma: a familiar morphologic feature that links vascular pathology, hypoxia, and angiogenesis. *J Neuropathol Exp Neurol, 65,* 529-539.

[38] Pennacchietti, S., Michieli, P., Galluzzo, M., Mazzone, M., Giordano, S. & Comoglio, P.M. (2003). Hypoxia promotes invasive growth by transcriptional activation of the met protooncogene. *Cancer Cell, 3,* 347-361.

[39] Yamamoto, M., Mohanam, S., Sawaya, R., Fuller, G.N., Seiki, M., Sato, H., Gokaslan, Z.L., Liotta, L.A., Nicolson, G.L. & Rao, J.S. (1996). Differential expression of membrane-type matrix metalloproteinase and its correlation with gelatinase A activation in human malignant brain tumors in vivo and in vitro. *Cancer Res, 56,* 384-392.

[40] Puli, S., Lai, J.C. & Bhushan, A. (2006). Inhibition of matrix degrading enzymes and invasion in human glioblastoma (U87MG) cells by isoflavones. *J Neurooncol, 79,* 135-142.

[41] Naumov, G.N., Folkman, J., Straume, O. & Akslen, L.A. (2008). Tumor-vascular interactions and tumor dormancy. *APMIS, 116,* 569-585.

[42] Adair, T.H. (2005). Growth regulation of the vascular system: an emerging role for adenosine. *Am J Physiol Regul Integr Comp Physiol, 289,* R283-R296.

[43] Folkman, J. (1971). Tumor angiogenesis: therapeutic implications. *N Engl J Med, 285,* 1182-1186.

[44] Nyberg, P., Xie, L. & Kalluri, R. (2005). Endogenous inhibitors of angiogenesis. *Cancer Res, 65,* 3967-3979.

[45] Zagzag, D., Zhong, H., Scalzitti, J.M., Laughner, E., Simons, J.W. & Semenza, G.L. (2000). Expression of hypoxia-inducible factor 1alpha in brain tumors: association with angiogenesis, invasion, and progression. *Cancer, 88,* 2606-2618.

[46] Kaur, B., Khwaja, F.W., Severson, E.A., Matheny, S.L., Brat, D.J. & Van Meir, E.G. (2005). Hypoxia and the hypoxia-inducible-factor pathway in glioma growth and angiogenesis. *Neuro Oncol, 7,* 134-153.

[47] Plate, K.H. (1999). Mechanisms of angiogenesis in the brain. *J Neuropathol Exp Neurol, 58,* 313-320.

[48] Plate, K.H., Breier, G., Weich, H.A., Mennel, H.D. & Risau, W. (1994). Vascular endothelial growth factor and glioma angiogenesis: coordinate induction of VEGF receptors, distribution of VEGF protein and possible in vivo regulatory mechanisms. *Int J Cancer, 59,* 520-529.

[49] Plate, K.H., Breier, G., Weich, H.A. & Risau, W. (1992). Vascular endothelial growth factor is a potential tumour angiogenesis factor in human gliomas in vivo. *Nature, 359,* 845-848.

[50] Shweiki, D., Itin, A., Soffer, D. & Keshet, E. (1992). Vascular endothelial growth factor induced by hypoxia may mediate hypoxia-initiated angiogenesis. *Nature, 359,* 843-845.

[51] Brat, D.J., Bellail, A.C. & Van Meir, E.G. (2005). The role of interleukin-8 and its receptors in gliomagenesis and tumoral angiogenesis. *Neuro Oncol, 7,* 122-133.

[52] Semenza, G.L. (2000). HIF-1: using two hands to flip the angiogenic switch. *Cancer Metastasis Rev, 19,* 59-65.

[53] Semenza, G.L. (2000). HIF-1: mediator of physiological and pathophysiological responses to hypoxia. *J Appl Physiol, 88,* 1474-1480.

[54] Laughner, E., Taghavi, P., Chiles, K., Mahon, P.C. & Semenza, G.L. (2001). HER2 (neu) signaling increases the rate of hypoxia-inducible factor 1alpha (HIF-1alpha) synthesis: novel mechanism for HIF-1-mediated vascular endothelial growth factor expression. *Mol Cell Biol, 21,* 3995-4004.

[55] Zhong, H., Chiles, K., Feldser, D., Laughner, E., Hanrahan, C., Georgescu, M.M., Simons, J.W. & Semenza, G.L. (2000). Modulation of hypoxia-inducible factor 1alpha expression by the epidermal growth factor/phosphatidylinositol 3-kinase/PTEN/AKT/FRAP pathway in human prostate cancer cells: implications for tumor angiogenesis and therapeutics. *Cancer Res, 60,* 1541-1545.

[56] Wang, F.S., Wang, C.J., Chen, Y.J., Chang, P.R., Huang, Y.T., Sun, Y.C., Huang, H.C., Yang, Y.J. & Yang, K.D. (2004). Ras induction of superoxide activates ERK-dependent angiogenic transcription factor HIF-1alpha and VEGF-A expression in shock wave-stimulated osteoblasts. *J Biol Chem, 279,* 10331-10337.

[57] Holland, E.C., Celestino, J., Dai, C., Schaefer, L., Sawaya, R.E. & Fuller, G.N. (2000). Combined activation of Ras and Akt in neural progenitors induces glioblastoma formation in mice. *Nat Genet, 25,* 55-57.

[58] Frederick, L., Wang, X.Y., Eley, G. & James, C.D. (2000). Diversity and frequency of epidermal growth factor receptor mutations in human glioblastomas. *Cancer Res, 60,* 1383-1387.

[59] Tan, C., Cruet-Hennequart, S., Troussard, A., Fazli, L., Costello, P., Sutton, K., Wheeler, J., Gleave, M., Sanghera, J. & Dedhar, S. (2004). Regulation of tumor angiogenesis by integrin-linked kinase (ILK). *Cancer Cell, 5,* 79-90.

[60] Obara, S., Nakata, M., Takeshima, H., Katagiri, H., Asano, T., Oka, Y., Maruyama, I. & Kuratsu, J. (2004). Integrin-linked kinase (ILK) regulation of the cell viability in PTEN mutant glioblastoma and in vitro inhibition by the specific COX-2 inhibitor NS-398. *Cancer Lett, 208,* 115-122.

[61] Ravi, R., Mookerjee, B., Bhujwalla, Z.M., Sutter, C.H., Artemov, D., Zeng, Q., Dillehay, L.E., Madan, A., Semenza, G.L. & Bedi, A. (2000). Regulation of tumor angiogenesis by p53-induced degradation of hypoxia-inducible factor 1alpha. *Genes Dev, 14,* 34-44.

[62] Zundel, W., Schindler, C., Haas-Kogan, D., Koong, A., Kaper, F., Chen, E., Gottschalk, A.R., Ryan, H.E., Johnson, R.S., Jefferson, A.B., Stokoe, D. & Giaccia, A.J. (2000). Loss of PTEN facilitates HIF-1-mediated gene expression. *Genes Dev, 14,* 391-396.

[63] Dameron, K.M., Volpert, O.V., Tainsky, M.A. & Bouck, N. (1994). Control of angiogenesis in fibroblasts by p53 regulation of thrombospondin-1. *Science, 265,* 1582-1584.

[64] Kastan, M.B., Onyekwere, O., Sidransky, D., Vogelstein, B. & Craig, R.W. (1991). Participation of p53 protein in the cellular response to DNA damage. *Cancer Res, 51,* 6304-6311.

[65] Bouvet, M., Ellis, L.M., Nishizaki, M., Fujiwara, T., Liu, W., Bucana, C.D., Fang, B., Lee. J.J. & Roth, J.A. (1998). Adenovirus-mediated wild-type p53 gene transfer downregulates vascular endothelial growth factor expression and inhibits angiogenesis in human colon cancer. *Cancer Res, 58,* 2288-2292.

[66] Tohma, Y., Gratas, C., Biernat, W., Peraud, A., Fukuda, M., Yonekawa, Y., Kleihues, P. & Ohgaki, H. (1998). PTEN (MMAC1) mutations are frequent in primary glioblastomas (de novo) but not in secondary glioblastomas. *J Neuropathol Exp Neurol, 57,* 684-689.

[67] Clarke, K., Smith, K., Gullick, W.J. & Harris, A.L. (2001). Mutant epidermal growth factor receptor enhances induction of vascular endothelial growth factor by hypoxia and insulin-like growth factor-1 via a PI3 kinase dependent pathway. *Br J Cancer, 84,* 1322-1329.

[68] Abounader, R. & Laterra, J. (2005). Scatter factor/hepatocyte growth factor in brain tumor growth and angiogenesis. *Neuro Oncol, 7,* 436-451.

[69] Takano, S., Yoshii, Y., Kondo, S., Suzuki, H., Maruno, T., Shirai, S. & Nose, T. (1996). Concentration of vascular endothelial growth factor in the serum and tumor tissue of brain tumor patients. *Cancer Res, 56,* 2185-2190.

[70] Kung, A.L., Wang, S., Klco, J.M., Kaelin, W.G. & Livingston, D.M. (2000). Suppression of tumor growth through disruption of hypoxia-inducible transcription. *Nat Med, 6,* 1335-1340.

[71] Moriyama, T., Kataoka, H., Hamasuna, R., Yokogami, K., Uehara, H., Kawano, H., Goya, T., Tsubouchi, H., Koono, M. & Wakisaka, S. (1998). Up-regulation of vascular endothelial growth factor induced by hepatocyte growth factor/scatter factor stimulation in human glioma cells. *Biochem Biophys Res Commun, 249,* 73-77.

[72] Dong, S., Nutt, C.L., Betensky, R.A., Stemmer-Rachamimov, A.O., Denko, N.C., Ligon, K.L., Rowitch, D.H. & Louis, D.N. (2005). Histology-based expression profiling yields novel prognostic markers in human glioblastoma. *J Neuropathol Exp Neurol, 64,* 948-955.

[73] Hjortoe, G.M., Petersen, L.C., Albrektsen, T., Sorensen, B.B., Norby, P.L., Mandal, S.K., Pendurthi, U.R., Rao, L.V. (2004). Tissue factor-factor VIIa-specific up-regulation of IL-8 expression in MDA-MB-231 cells is mediated by PAR-2 and results in increased cell migration. *Blood, 103,* 3029-3037.

[74] Tenan, M., Fulci, G., Albertoni, M., Diserens, A.C., Hamou, M.F., El Atifi-Borel, M., Feige, J.J., Pepper, M.S., Van Meir, E.G. (2000). Thrombospondin-1 is downregulated by anoxia and suppresses tumorigenicity of human glioblastoma cells. *J Exp Med, 191,* 1789-1798.

[75] Kee, H.J., Koh, J.T., Kim, M.Y., Ahn, K.Y., Kim, J.K., Bae, C.S., Park, S.S., Kim, K.K. (2002). Expression of brain-specific angiogenesis inhibitor 2 (BAI2) in normal and ischemic brain: involvement of BAI2 in the ischemia-induced brain angiogenesis. *J Cereb Blood Flow Metab, 22,* 1054-1067.

In: Neuro-Oncology and Cancer Targeted Therapy
Editor: Lucía M. Gutiérrez pp.199-212
ISBN 978-1-61668-708-3
© 2010 Nova Science Publishers, Inc.

Chapter 8

TEMOZOLOMIDE IN HIGH-GRADE GLIOMAS: RATIONALE, SCHEDULES AND SYNERGISM WITH RADIATION

Stefano Dall'Oglio, Anna D'Amico, Fabio Pioli and Sergio Maluta
Department of Radiation Oncology, University Hospital,
Verona, Italy

ABSTRACT

High-grade gliomas (HGG)—glioblastoma multiforme (GBM) and anaplastic astrocytoma (AA)—are still characterized by a dismal prognosis despite recent advances in treatment options (new radiotherapy techniques including IMRT and radiosurgery, new alkylating agents such as Temozolomide [TMZ], molecular targeted drugs). Gold-standard therapy has involved maximum possible resection, followed by adjuvant irradiation plus TMZ followed by maintenance TMZ. TMZ has also proven its efficacy on tumors of oligodendroglial origin. The conventional "5 out of 28 days" schedule of TMZ achieved an overall survival rate at 2 years of 26.5%; in patients with methylation of methylguanine methyltrasnsferase (MGMT) promoter, better results can be achieved but MGMT methylation status determination is feasible only in a few centres. Dose-intensity TMZ schedules have the capability of depleting MGMT in tumor cells, thus promising a better outcome also in non-methylated patients. Alternative schedules, such as the "weekly alternating" or the "21 out of 28 days" ones, have been tried in relapsed patients and recently also in newly diagnosed ones. Sporadic cases of severe bone marrow aplasia with high doses of TMZ have been reported, which required bone marrow transplantation. This chapter tries to find a possible rationale for intensified regimens of TMZ administration and reviews its possible benefits and risks, focusing on results of clinical trials and reported toxicity cases.

INTRODUCTION: RATIONALE FOR TEMOZOLOMIDE IN HIGH-GRADE GLIOMAS

The infiltrating nature of high-grade glioma makes complete resection virtually impossible, even when possible resection can be associated with severe neurological damage. Thus, standard treatment generally consists of cytoreductive surgery followed by radiotherapy. Over a period of almost 30 years, several randomised trials have explored the use of adjuvant chemotherapy, with research mostly focusing on nitrosoureas, which are used because they are lipid soluble and cross the blood-brain barrier [1,2]; most of these trials have shown inconclusive results.

In 1980, Robert Stone, a research student at Aston University, synthesized the first examples of mitozolomide, a new ring-system imidazo[5, 1-d]-1,2,3,5-tetrazine. The development of mitozolomide was abandoned because of the unpredictable and long-lasting haematological toxic effects seen in early clinical trials. TMZ, the N-methyl congener of mitozolomide (Figure 1), has a demonstrably different toxicological profile; whereas mitozolomide cross-linked DNA, TMZ is a monofunctional agent which has good tissue distribution and was shown to be schedule-dependent in terms of its antitumour activity. Additionally, TMZ is a neat and robust molecule, stable at acid pH allowing it to be absorbed intact after oral administration, and has excellent bio-distribution, including penetration into the central nervous system.

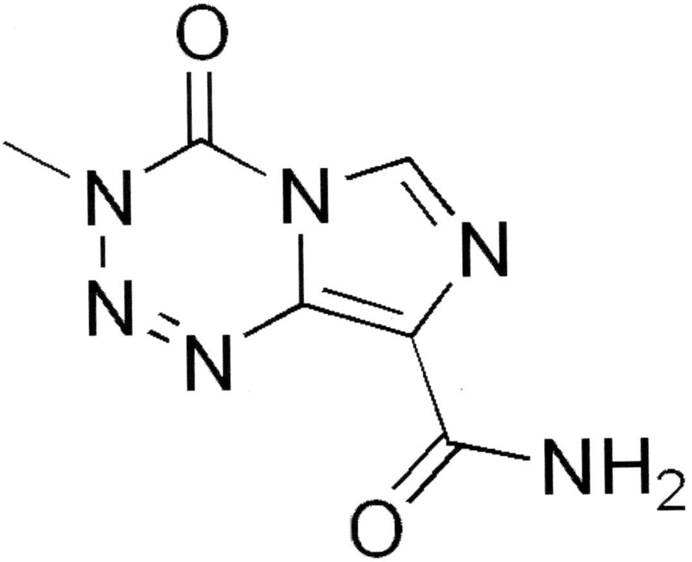

Figure 1. TMZ structure.

When TMZ is hydrolysed, the first product is the methyl triazene MTIC which ultimately transfers its methyl group to a nucleophile. The pH stability profile of TMZ has a number of consequences for TMZ as a drug; most importantly, the acid stability means that it survives the strong acid of the stomach so it can be administered orally in capsules.

The antitumour activity of TMZ is largely attributed to the methylation of DNA which is dependent upon formation of a reactive methyldiazonium cation. The cytotoxicity of TMZ is affected by three DNA-repair activities, in particular:

1) O^6-alkylguanine-DNA alkyltransferase. Much evidence suggests that the cytotoxicity of TMZ can be correlated with the formation of O^6- methylguanine, despite the fact that this lesion accounts for only a small percentage of the total DNA adducts formed. Adducts produced at the O^6-position of guanine are, however, considered particularly mutagenic and cytotoxic.
2) DNA-mismatch repair. O^6-methylguanine produced in DNA by TMZ is thought to be cytotoxic as a consequence of its processing by a DNA mismatch repair pathway which normally corrects GT mismatch replication errors.
3) Base excision repair and poly(ADP-ribose) polymerase. Methyl adducts produced at N^7-guanine and N^3-adenine by TMZ could also hinder DNA-replication, as enzymatic or spontaneous depurination will ultimately result in DNA strand breakage.

TMZ after oral administration is characterized by a rapid absorption phase (the peak plasma concentration of TMZ being achieved within 30 min of administration), and mono-exponential elimination (with an elimination half-life of 1.29 h). The predominant route of TMZ elimination is by renal excretion and occurs largely as intact drug, although an unidentified acidic urinary metabolite is also produced.

The first Phase I trial of TMZ was conducted in the UK and the results were published in 1992 [3]. The starting dose of TMZ was 50 mg/m^2, initially given intravenously as a 1-h infusion. The pharmacology of TMZ was examined following both intravenous and oral administration. Good oral bio-availability was confirmed at a dose of 200 mg/m^2.

All subsequent clinical studies have been with TMZ given orally. The doses of TMZ were escalated from 50 mg/m^2 up to 1200 mg/m^2, when leukopenia and thrombocytopenia became dose limiting on the single-dose schedule. Because of the schedule dependency in the pre-clinical screen, TMZ was given five times daily at doses of 750, 1000 and 1200 mg/m^2 in 42 patients. Again, myelosuppression was dose limiting at 1200 mg/m^2. A well-tolerated schedule for clinical use was identified giving TMZ 150 mg/m^2 orally for five consecutive days (total dose 750 mg/m^2 for the first course), and if no myelosuppression was detected on day 22 of the 4-week cycle, subsequent courses were given at 200 mg/m^2 for 5 days (total dose 1 g/m^2 on a 4-week cycle).

On the basis of preclinical data suggesting an increased activity with repeated exposure to TMZ, the schedule of daily treatment for 5 days was developed [4]. A daily dose of 200 mg/m^2 (150 mg/m^2 for the first cycle in patients who have received chemotherapy previously) was established as the maximally tolerated dose and recommended for phase II testing. The dose-limiting toxic effect with the intermittent schedule has been thrombocytopenia. At the recommended dose of 200 mg/m^2 daily, grade 4 thrombocytopenia is observed in less than 10% of patients, and grade 3/4 neutropenia in less than 5%. Nausea can easily be prevented by standard antiemetics or paediatric doses of 5-HT3 antagonists. Some patients complain of fatigue in the week after therapy.

Other schedules of TMZ administration have been explored. In a phase I trial, the feasibility of continuous daily administration of TMZ over 6–7 weeks was assessed. Doses were increased gradually from 50 mg/m^2 to 100 mg/m^2 daily [5]. Myelosuppression was identified as the dose-limiting toxic effect; other side-effects with continuous administration are minor. Antiemetic prophylaxis is not required in most cases. The recommended dose for further studies using continuous administration is 75 mg/m^2 given daily for 6–7 weeks. This schedule allows the administration of 2.1 g/m^2 for each 4 weeks, which is twice the dose that is administered when TMZ is given in cycles of daily doses for 5 days. Whether continuous low-dose administration and higher dose intensity lead to improved efficacy remains unclear.

Other schedules of continuous daily administration were investigated. With the administration of TMZ for 7 days every 2 weeks (7 days on, 7 days off), myelosuppression and thrombocytopenia were again dose limiting at 175 mg/m^2, and a daily dose of 150 mg/m^2 is recommended for further studies. A schedule of daily TMZ for 21 days in each 28 days was explored, and a dose of 100 mg/m^2 recommended for phase II studies. In all trials, myelosuppression with neutropenia and thrombocytopenia are the dose-limiting side-effect. Continuous administration of TMZ is associated with a high frequency of lymphocytopenia [6].

The present chapter is trying to answer the question if intensified TMZ schedules can achieve better results than conventional ones and how is their impact on bone marrow toxicity. The authors review the most important trials with alternative TMZ regimens.

THE CURRENT USE OF TEMOZOLOMIDE IN HIGH-GRADE GLIOMAS

The standard of care in operated HGG is concurrent TMZ – radiotherapy (75 mg/m^2) plus adjuvant TMZ (150–200 mg/m^2 with the 5/28 – day schedule). Nevertheless, alternative ones are being tried. To fully understand the motivations that stand behind the choice of one schedule or another, it is important to briefly recall the role of MGMT, the enzyme that "repair" the DNA once it has been methylated by TMZ, and the mechanisms that are beyond the synergism between TMZ and radiation.

MGMT: MECHANISMS OF ACTION

The DNA repair protein MGMT is ubiquitously expressed in normal tissues, although levels vary tremendously among organs and individuals. Its evolutionary conservation suggests a fundamental role in the maintenance of genome integrity [7,8]. The MGMT gene is located on chromosome 10q26 and encodes a DNA repair protein that removes alkyl groups from the O6 position of guanine, a target of alkylating agents such as TMZ. Restoration of the DNA consumes the MGMT that must be resynthesized in the cell. In tumors, high expression of MGMT has been associated with resistance to treatment with alkylating agents [9]. Methylation of the O6 position of guanine induced by TMZ yields one of the most biologically important adducts triggering a cytotoxic response that if left unrepaired could eventually lead to cell death [10]. Inactivation of the MGMT gene by promoter methylation diminishes DNA repair activity and has been associated with longer overall survival in patients with GBM treated using alkylating agents.

The epigenetic silencing of the MGMT gene has an important role in MGMT expression; in a study upon specimens of brain tumors from 47 consecutive patients, the MGMT promoter was methylated in gliomas from 19 ones (40%) [11]. Several studies acknowledged the methylation status of MGMT promoter as a prognostic factor for patients with GBM [12,13]. From these studies it turns out that treatment strategies to overcome must be explored to overcome the MGMT – mediated chemoresistance. One of these strategies consists in using dose – intensified TMZ schedules to deplete MGMT activity in tumor tissue [14]. Prolonged TMZ administration can substantially deplete MGMT; in an Italian study on 103 patients, apart from the MGMT – promoter methylation status, those patients who received less than six TMZ cycles had an overall survival (OS) of 13.7 months, while those who received six cycles had an OS of 34.8 months [15].

According to other authors, MGMT - methylation status determination is crucial before starting TMZ chemotherapy: the determination of MGMT promoter methylation status by methylation-specific PCR may allow the selection of patients most likely to benefit from TMZ treatment; patients whose tumors are not methylated at the MGMT promoter seem to achieve little or no benefit from the addition of TMZ to radiotherapy. For these patients, alternative treatments with a different mechanism of action or methods of inhibiting MGMT should be developed [16].

THE STANDARD USE OF TMZ

The recent trial by the European Organisation for Research and Treatment of Cancer (EORTC) and National Cancer Institute of Canada (NCIC) Clinical Trials Group (EORTC 26981/22981-NCIC CE3) was the first study to demonstrate unequivocally that the addition of TMZ to radiotherapy early in the course of GBM provides a statistically significant and clinically meaningful survival benefit [17]. Nevertheless, in that study the two-year survival rate was 26.5 percent in the group with radiotherapy plus TMZ, as compared with 10.4 percent in the group with radiotherapy alone. Patients were randomly assigned to receive radiotherapy alone or radiotherapy plus continuous daily TMZ (75 mg/m^2, 7 days per week from the first to the last day of radiotherapy), followed by six cycles of adjuvant TMZ (150 to 200 mg/m^2 for 5 days during each 28 - day cycle). No grade 3 or 4 hematologic toxic effects were observed in the radiotherapy group. During concomitant TMZ therapy, grade 3 or 4 neutropenia was documented in 4% of patients, and grade 3 or 4 thrombocytopenia occurred in 3% of them. Overall, 7% of patients had any type of grade 3 or 4 hematologic toxic effect. During adjuvant TMZ therapy, 14% of patients had any grade 3 or 4 hematologic toxic effect, 4% had grade 3 or 4 neutropenia, and 11% had grade 3 or 4 thrombocytopenia. The most common nonhematologic adverse event during radiotherapy was moderate-to-severe fatigue in 26% of patients in the radiotherapy group and 33% in the radiotherapy-plus-TMZ group. Pneumonia was reported in five patients in the radiotherapy group and three in the radiotherapy-plus-TMZ group.

A recent update of that study [18], with 5 – year follow – up results, showed that the survival advantage of combined treatment lasted for up to 5 years of follow-up: 5 - years OS was 9.8% for the patients in the TMZ – radiation arm and 1.9% for the patients in the radiation alone arm. Most patients successfully treated with combined therapy eventually had tumour recurrence and died. Survival does not plateau, and combined treatment is unlikely to be curative for many patients. Most patients treated with radiotherapy alone in the present study have received salvage chemotherapy at recurrence or progression, and about half the patients initially treated with TMZ received further chemotherapy at progression; salvage therapy was prescribed to more patients initially treated with radiotherapy alone. Survival nevertheless favours combined treatment, which supports the conclusion that the addition of chemotherapy early in the disease course and concomitantly with radiotherapy is the best strategy to incorporate new drugs.

Because of these high mortality rates, some investigators tried to explore new strategies of TMZ administration, in order to overcome the chemoresistance due to TMZ; that is the matter of the next chapter.

TEMOZOLOMIDE AND RADIOTHERAPY

New Radiotherapy Techniques in the Treatment Strategy of HGG

To improve the outcome of radiation therapy in HGG, various irradiation modalities have been tested, including increased dose, fractionation schedules, and addition of chemotherapy. Randomized trials failed to demonstrate any benefit from hyperfractionated or accelerated schedules and also various irradiation techniques studied to increase the tumoral dose, such as intraoperative electron radiotherapy, brachytherapy and stereotactic irradiation. The RTOG 83-02 randomize study including 800 patients affected by anaplastic glioma and glioblastoma showed no differences in outcome increasing dose of hyperfractionated radiotherapy from 64.8 Gy up 81.6 Gy or by using different doses of accelerated hyperfractionated radiotherapy in the range of 48 – 54.4 Gy. Radiosensitizing agents such as hydroxyurea, misonidazole, carboplatin and etoposide, didn't produce any significant improvement in survival when combined with radiotherapy. Also antiangiogenic drugs such as interferon-alpha did not confer any benefit.

Being no evidence-based demonstration of an improvement obtained by increasing dose of radiation in HGG the current standard dose is until now considered 60 Gy in 6 weeks. In spite of the consideration that hypofractionated and stereotactic radiotherapy failed to demonstrate a better survival rates, the irradiation new techniques and the new imaging now available allow the delivery of higher doses to selected volumes with acceptable toxicity rate. Recently a boost technique was used in several prospective randomized studies (RTOG 9305, RTOG 0023) and in retrospectives studies. None of these studies showed improved survival rates over those obtained with conventional irradiation [19].

To overcome the poor results with radiotherapy alone in the post – operative setting of HGG, the TMZ – radiation interaction has been tested.

TMZ Concomitant with Radiation: Is There a Rationale for That?

For many decades radiotherapy and chemotherapy have been considered to produce devastating damage to cells and many antitumor drugs are known to induce directly or indirectly DNA damage without their selective action was been completely understand. Why cancer cells are more sensitive to alkylating agents than normal replicating cells is still unknown. In response to DNA damage, the p53 tumor suppressor factor promotes cell-cycle arrest or apoptosis. The first one can be used to repair the damage, the second one to eliminate cells when the repair cannot be performed. The DNA repair systems allow cells to compete with sources of DNA damage, whereas the absence of p53 function is considered the most common molecular abnormality in tumor cells playing an important role in developing cancer. Apoptosis is the key to explain how anticancer therapy works and cells resistant to apoptosis may be resistant to chemotherapy.

Apoptosis is the prevalent model to understand how ionizing radiations and alkylating agents have some success in anticancer therapy, but other mechanisms are also important in the tumor cell death. Different cell death pathways may be activated and at least eight different non-apoptotic types can be defined.

Mitotic catastrophe (cell death occurring during or after faulty mitosis), senescence (cells do not divide), autophagy (programmed cell death in which the cell digests itself) and necrosis are the most important antiproliferative response and cell death pathways observed upon antitumor therapy.

Regarding this topic, necrosis is the most relevant pathway to be described, because in some cases it could be confused with a disease progression.

Necrosis in the past has been considered as an uncontrolled and pathological cell death type as a passive process without any cellular control. Recent reports indicate that this modality of death is under a partial control of cell and it has been suggested that the alkylating DNA damage agents induces a regulated form of necrosis. Also apoptosis may be accompanied by necrosis. Necrosis requires activation of a DNA repair protein (poly-ADP-ribose polymerase). The capacity of alkylating agents to selectively kill cancer cells also in case of p53 deficiency, could be explained with the poly-ADP-ribose polymerase-mediated necrosis. It should be interesting to determine if the tumor DNA alkylating agents resistant have acquired a loss of poly-ADP-ribose polymerase activity.

It has been suggested that TMZ administered concurrently with radiation seems to have significantly greater antitumor effect compared with sequential administration [20]. The benefit is most pronounced in cells deficient in functional MGMT protein, and this benefit seems to occur from enhancement of the cytotoxic effects both of TMZ and radiation. The mechanisms of action seem to involve an increased degree of radiation-induced apoptosis and enhanced double – stranded (ds) DNA damage, which have been reported to be critical factors underlying radiation-induced cell death. The observed increase in dsDNA damage may be secondary to either decreased repair capacity or increased degree of breaks on combined TMZ plus radiation. The pattern of cell death in tumor cells treated with radiation alone is characterized primarily by this early phase of cell death. It is possible that with the additional degree of dsDNA damage observed in radiation + TMZ – treated MGMT - negative GBM cells, TMZ acts as a catalyst in promoting this latter phase of cell death.

Table 1. TMZ Administration schedules

Schedule	Dose(mg/m2)	Dose Intensity (mg/m2/week)	Tumor Categories	Ref.
Daily for 5 days, repeat every 28 days	150-200	250	Relapsed AA or AOA	Yung 1999 [21]
Daily for 42-49 days, every 70 days	75-85	315	Refractory HGG	Brock 1998 [6]
Daily for 7 days, repeat every 14 days	150	525	Refractory or relapsed HGG	Tolcher 2003 [22], Wick 2004 [24]
Daily for 3 days, every 14 days	300	450	Relapsed HGG	Vera 2004 [23]

Table 2. Hematological adverse events (grade 3-4)

N. Patients	Leukopienia (%)	Neutropenia (%)	Lymphocytopenia (%)	Thrmphocytopenia (%)	Infection (%)	Ref.
Standard administrtion schedule (5 days every 28 days)						
138	9	NR	13	2 (pulm.)		Brada 2001 [25]
162	2	NR	6	NR		Yung 1999 [21]
112	1	NR	7	NR		Yung 2000 [26]
49	NR	54	7	0		Stupp 2002 [27]
223	5	NR	11	NR		Stupp 2005 [17]
Low-dose continuous administration schedules						
7	0	0	0	0		Brock 1998 [6]
62	NR	6	7	5		Stupp 2002 [27]
284	2	4	3	NR		Stupp 2005 [17]
Dose-dende administration schedules						
39	NR	16	13	1		Wick 2005 [28]
51	NR	7.8	3.9	0		Tosoni 2006 [29]

COMPARISON OF THE STANDARD TEMOZOLOMIDE SCHEDULE WITH THE ALTERNATIVE ONES

Different TMZ administration schedules and treatment durations are used in practice, mostly in relapsed HGG, but also in newly diagnosed ones (Table 1) [6,21–24]. The toxicities of these schedules are reported in various articles (Table 2) [6,17,21–25].

The investigational continuous dose-dense schedules, such as 7 days on/7 days off or 3 of 4 weeks, allow one to double the dose intensity; however, to date no definite increase in antitumor activity has been demonstrated. One particularity of the continuous administration schedule is the induction of profound, albeit reversible, lymphopenia together with diminished CD4 counts similar to those seen in patients with acquired immunodeficiency syndrome. This continuous administration together with the frequent use of corticosteroid agents adds to an immunodeficient state, predisposing the patient to opportunistic infections. Monitoring of CD4 counts and antibiotic prophylaxis has been proposed in such case.

In the study by Yung [21], TMZ was administered with the 5/28 – day schedule in 162 patients with AA or anaplastic oligo – astrocytoma (AOA), for a maximum of 2 years or until unacceptable toxicity or tumor progression occurred. Myelosuppression was noncumulative and typically resolved with a one-dose level reduction; consequently, therapy could be administered continuously, and although the median number of administered cycles was five, 23% of patients received 12 cycles and one patient received as many as 22 cycles. The majority of reported side effects were mild to moderate in severity. Nausea and vomiting, the most frequently reported adverse events, were also mild to moderate and could be readily controlled with the administration of standard antiemetics. The noncumulative toxicity and favorable adverse events profile of TMZ make this agent a logical choice against recurrent malignant astrocytomas and suggest that it could be used effectively at relapse.

Brock [6] conducted a phase I trial of TMZ in 24 patients (mostly HGG) with recurrent tumors refractory to treatment, using an extended continuous oral schedule (TMZ 75 - 85 mg/m^2 daily for 42 – 49 days) and a second 6 - or 7 - week cycle was given if the patient showed a clinical or radiological response with no adverse toxicity. The maximum tolerated dose (MTD) resulted of 85 mg/m^2/day over 6 weeks. The overall response rate was 33% (41% in patients with recurrent gliomas and an additional 25% in patients maintaining stable disease).

A schedule with TMZ administration of 3 days every 14 days with dose escalation was tried by Vera in 70 patients with refractory gliomas (prior surgery and/or radiotherapy) [23]. Patients were assigned to one of four groups to receive TMZ at daily doses of 200 (seven patients), 250 (13 patients), 300 (38 patients) and 350 mg/m^2/day (12 patients). Fifty per cent of treated patients completed at least three cycles and the other half more than four cycles at the planned dose. Grade 3 neutropenia was observed 7.9% of patients ($n = 70$); grade 3 thrombocytopenia occurred 13.1% of them. Complete responses were observed in three patients: one anaplastic oligodendroglioma, one oligoastrocytoma and one oligodendroglioma. Ten partial responses were observed. Objective responses were observed in six chemotherapy-naïve patients and in four patients previously exposed to nitrosoureas.

A weekly –alternating schedule was tried by Wong in 25 patients with recurrent or progressive high-grade gliomas [30]. TMZ was administred at a dose of 150 mg/m^2 daily. There were no grade 4 toxicities, no episodes of neutropenic sepsis nor treatment-related deaths. Thrombocytopenia was the most common haematological toxicity. One patient achieved a CR and four patients (16%) achieved a PR.

Our institution performed a phase II study in newly diagnosed HGG with concomitant TMZ and radiotherapy followed by a weekly alternating TMZ schedule with dose escalation [31]. Thirty-four patients were enrolled (32 GBM and 2 AA). Each patient after surgery received standard radiotherapy plus concomitant TMZ 75 mg/m^2 for a maximum of 49 days. After a 4-week break, patients were then to receive 12 cycles of 1-week-on/1-week-off TMZ, with 75 mg/m^2 for the first cycle, 100 mg/m^2 for the second, 125 mg/m^2 for the third, and 150 mg/m^2 from the fourth to the 12th. No grade-3 hematological toxicity was observed. Only one patient had a grade-4 thrombocytopenia plus grade 1 neutropenia and grade 1 anemia, and interrupted TMZ. One patient had a *Pneumocystis carinii* pneumonitis. The OS rate was 59% for all patients, but it must be considered that 50% of patients had a partial resection.

Anaplastic (Grade-III) Gliomas

Anaplastic gliomas, classified as WHO grade - III tumors, are more prognostic favorable tumors as compared to WHO grade - IV astrocytomas, known as GBM. Histologically, they consist of pure AA, pure oligodendrogliomas and oligoastrocytomas, which show a better outcome as compared to AA. The standard therapeutic approach is a neurosurgical resection followed by postoperative radiation. Median survival times reported in these tumors range from 18 up 50 months. In spite of this different outcome, in the majority of reports grade - III tumors and GBM are taken together and results are not analyzed separately, often producing a sort of misunderstanding in the evaluation of therapy effectiveness. Only few publications reported the outcome of radiotherapy in patients with anaplastic gliomas [32].

Until today radiotherapy is considered the most effective treatment in anaplastic gliomas, even if many prospective randomized phase III trials were initiated in order to better clarify the role of chemotherapy, especially in patients affected by oligodendroglial tumors (RTOG 9402, EORTC 26951, NOA-04).

TEMOZOLOMIDE-RELATED TOXICITY

The adverse events associated with TMZ are mild to moderate and generally predictable; the most serious are non-cumulative and reversible myelosuppression and, in particular, thrombocytopenia, which occurs in less than 5% of patients.

Aplastic anemia is a rare hemopoitic stem cell disorder that results in pancytopenia and hypocellular bone marrow. Aplastic anemia is classified as congenital, acquired or idiopathic depending on etiology and non-severe, severe or very severe on the basis of degree of blood pancytopenia. TMZ being an alkylating agent is, however, more likely to be capable of inducing treatment related myelodysplasia. The question remains whether a patient has an underlying cause or a genetic predisposition to aplastic anemia which was unmasked with TMZ. Cotrimoxazole administered for concurrent TMZ – RT may contribute to toxicity.

In a recent case-report of TMZ–induced bone marrow aplasia, although treatment options such as bone marrow transplantation were considered, the patient died due to septicaemia [33].

With the classical 5/28 – day schedule, myelosuppression and, in particular, thrombocytopenia occur in 5 to 10% of patients, with a nadir between Days 21 and 28 of each treatment cycle. If severe myelosuppression is observed, the dose for subsequent cycles should be reduced by 25%. In a phase II study conducted by Brada [25], there was no evidence of cumulative hematological toxicity. Only 9% of therapy cycles required a dose reduction due to thrombocytopenia. Nausea and, to a lesser extent, vomiting may occur after TMZ intake, although such symptoms can be prevented by standard antiemetic prophylaxis. Other mild adverse effects associated with TMZ therapy include headache (41%), fatigue (34%), and constipation (33%).

Continuous administration of TMZ for up to 49 days was evaluated in a Phase I trial [6]. Again, myelosuppression and, in particular, thrombocytopenia were found to be dose limiting. Profound lymphopenia was observed in the majority of patients but was considered clinically nonsignificant.

Continuous daily TMZ administration during radiotherapy was evaluated in a randomized phase III trial [17]. Overall, tolerance was considered excellent; in particular, mild to moderate fatigue was reported in 9% of the patients receiving TMZ and radiotherapy compared with 6% in those receiving radiotherapy alone. Antiemetic prophylaxis was required in a minority of patients only during continuous low-dose TMZ therapy. However, opportunistic infections have been observed due to profound lymphopenia and were possibly exacerbated by concurrent corticosteroid administration. *Pneumocystis carinii* pneumonia prophylaxis with either pentamidine inhalations or

Trimethroprim - sulfamethoxazole has been recommended during concomitant TMZ and radiotherapy or when CD4 lymphocyte counts decrease below 200/μL.

CONCLUSION

In newly diagnosed GBM, continuous low-dose TMZ and concomitant radiotherapy are the approved standard of care. The current administration schedule is 150–200 mg/m² for 5 days every 28 days. More intense dosing regimens aimed at exhausting the DNA repair enzyme MGMT are still under investigation. Molecular studies suggest that specific tumor characteristics, such as a silenced MGMT gene, may allow tailoring of treatments for individual patients.

The development of TMZ has greatly fuelled research in brain tumors. Never before have so many agents and strategies been tested for activity against HGG. New agents will be tested as first-line therapy in addition to standard TMZ-radiation therapy or at recurrence. Ongoing or planned trials in GBM evaluate the addition of anti-angiogenic treatments (cilengitide, PTK/ZK, bevacizumab). We need to take this increased interest and awareness to incorporate biological end points in our trials.

All new trials using TMZ or other alkylating agents will need to stratify patients according to the MGMT-promoter methylation status of the tumor. Patients in whom MGMT is active can be treated with dose-intensity TMZ schedules; nevertheless, in the near future they will be offered alternative, more promising or still investigational therapies.

REFERENCES

[1] Stenning, SP; Freedman, LS; Bleehen NM. An overview of published results from randomised studies of nitrosoureas in primary high grade malignant glioma. *Br J Cancer,* 1987; 56, 89–90.

[2] Fine, HA; Dear, KBG; Loeffler, JS; Black, PM; Canellos, GP. Metaanalysis of radiation therapy with and without adjuvant chemotherapy for malignant gliomas in adults. *Cancer,* 1993; 71, 2585–2597.

[3] Newlands, ES; Blackledge, GR; Slack, JA; Rustin, GJ; Smith, DB; Stuart, NS; Quarterman, CP; Hoffman, R; Stevens, MF; Brampton, MH. Phase I trial of temozolomide (CCRG 81045: M&B 39831: NSC 362856). *Br J Cancer,* 1992; 65, 287-291.

[4] Stevens, MFG; Hickman, JA; Langdon, SP; Chubb, D; Vickers, L; Stone, R; Baig, G; Goddard, C; Gibson, NW; Slack, JA; Newton, C; Lunt, E; Fizames, C; Lavelle, F. Antitumor Activity and Pharmacokinetics in Mice of 8-Carbamoyl-3-methylimidazo[5,l-on-l,2,3,5-tetrazin-4(37/)-one (CCRG 81045; M & B 39831), a Novel Drug with Potential as an Alternative to Dacarbazine. *Cancer Res.* 1987; 47, 5846-5852.

[5] Figueroa, J; Tolcher, A; Denis, L. Protracted cyclic administration of temozolomide is feasible; a phase I, pharmacokinetic and pharmacodynamic study. *Proc Am Soc Clin Oncol.* 2000; 19, 222a (abstr 868).

[6] Brock, CS; Newlands, ES; Wedge, SR; Bower, M; Evans, H; Colquhoun, I; Roddie, M; Glaser, M; Brampton, MH; Rustin, GJ. Phase I trial of temozolomide using an extended continuous oral schedule. *Cancer Res.* 1998; 58, 4363-4367.

[7] Gerson, SL. Clinical relevance of MGMT in the treatment of cancer. *J Clin Oncol.* 2002; 20, 2388–2399.

[8] Gerson, SL. MGMT: its role in cancer aetiology and cancer therapeutics. *Nat Rev Cancer,* 2004; 4, 296–307.

[9] Belanich, M; Pastor, M; Randall, T; Guerra, D; Kibitel, J; Alas, L; Li, B; Citron, M; Wasserman, P; White, A; Eyre, H; Jaeckle, K; Schulman, S; Rector, D; Prados, M; Coons, S; Shapiro, W; Yarosh D. Retrospective study of the correlation between the DNA repair protein alkyltransferase and survival of brain tumor patients treated with carmustine. *Cancer Res.* 1006; 56, 783–788.

[10] Kaina, B; Christmann, M. DNA repair in resistance to alkylating anticancer drugs. *Int J Clin Pharmacol Ther.* 2002; 40, 354–367.

[11] Esteller, M; Garcia-Foncillas, J; Andion, E; Goodman, SN; Hidalgo, OF; Vanaclocha, V; Baylin, SB; Herman, JG. Inactivation of the DNA-repair gene MGMT and the clinical response of gliomas to alkylating agents. *N Engl J Med.* 2000; 343, 1350-1354.

[12] Martinez, R; Schackert, G; Yaya-Tur, R; Rojas-Marcos, I; Herman, JG; Esteller, M. Frequent hypermethylation of the DNA repair gene MGMT in long-term survivors of glioblastoma multiforme. *J Neurooncol.* 2007; 83, 91–93.

[13] Zawlik, I; Vaccarella, S; Kita, D; Mittelbronn, M; Franceschi, S; Ohgaki, H. Promoter methylation and polymorphisms of the MGMT gene in glioblastomas: a population-based study. *Neuroepidemiology,* 2009; 32, 21–29.

[14] Wick, W; Platten, M; Weller, M. New (alternative) temozolomide regimens for the treatment of glioma. *Neuro Oncol.* 2009; 11, 69-79.

[15] Brandes, AA; Franceschi, E; Tosoni, A; Blatt, V; Pession, A; Tallini, G; Bertorelle, R; Bartolini, S; Calbucci, F; Andreoli, A; Frezza, G; Leonardi, M; Spagnolli, F; Ermani, M. MGMT promoter methylation status can predict the incidence and outcome of pseudoprogression after concomitant radiochemotherapy in newly diagnosed glioblastoma patients. *J Clin Oncol.* 2008; 26, 2192-2197.

[16] Hegi, ME; Diserens, AC; Gorlia, T; Hamou, MF; de Tribolet, N; Weller, M; Kros, JM; Hainfellner, JA; Mason, W; Mariani, L; Bromberg, JE; Hau, P; Mirimanoff, RO; Cairncross, JG; Janzer, RC; Stupp, R. MGMT gene silencing and benefit from temozolomide in glioblastoma. *N Engl J Med.* 2005; 352, 997–1003.

[17] Stupp, R; Mason, WP; van den Bent, MJ; Weller, M; Fisher, B; Taphoorn, MJ; Belanger, K; Brandes, AA; Marosi, C; Bogdahn, U; Curschmann, J; Janzer, RC; Ludwin, SK; Gorlia, T; Allgeier, A; Lacombe, D; Cairncross, JG; Eisenhauer, E; Mirimanoff, RO; European Organisation for Research and Treatment of Cancer Brain Tumor and Radiotherapy Groups; National Cancer Institute of Canada Clinical Trials Group. Radiotherapy plus concomitant and adjuvant temozolomide for glioblastoma. *N Engl J Med.* 2005; 352, 987-996.

[18] Stupp, R; Hegi, ME; Mason, WP; van den Bent, MJ; Taphoorn, MJ; Janzer, RC; Ludwin, SK; Allgeier, A; Fisher, B; Belanger, K; Hau, P; Brandes, AA; Gijtenbeek, J; Marosi, C; Vecht, CJ; Mokhtari, K; Wesseling, P; Villa, S; Eisenhauer, E; Gorlia, T; Weller, M; Lacombe, D; Cairncross, JG; Mirimanoff, RO; European Organisation for Research and Treatment of Cancer Brain Tumour and Radiation Oncology Groups; National Cancer Institute of Canada Clinical Trials Group. Effects of radiotherapy with concomitant and adjuvant temozolomide versus radiotherapy alone on survival in glioblastoma in a randomised phase III study: 5-year analysis of the EORTC-NCIC trial. *Lancet Oncol.* 2009; 10, 459-466.

[19] Pirtoli, L; Rubino, G; Marsili, S; Oliveri, G; Vannini, M; Tini, P; Miracco, C; Santoni, R. Three-dimensional conformal radiotherapy, temozolomide chemotherapy, and high-dose fractionated stereotactic boost in a protocol-driven, postoperative treatment schedule for high-grade gliomas. *Tumori,* 2009; 95, 329-337.

[20] Chakravarti, A; Erkkinen, MG; Nestler, U; Stupp, R; Mehta, M; Aldape, K; Gilbert, MR; Black, PM; Loeffler, JS. Temozolomide-mediated radiation enhancement in glioblastoma: a report on underlying mechanisms. *Clin Cancer Res.* 2006; 12, 4738-4746.

[21] Yung, WK; Prados, MD; Yaya-Tur, R; Rosenfeld, SS; Brada, M; Friedman, HS; Albright, R; Olson, J; Chang, SM; O'Neill, AM; Friedman, AH; Bruner, J; Yue, N; Dugan, M; Zaknoen, S; Levin, VA. Multicenter phase II trial of temozolomide in patients with anaplastic astrocytoma or anaplastic oligoastrocytoma at first relapse. Temodal Brain Tumor Group. *J Clin Oncol.* 1999; 17, 2762-2771.

[22] Tolcher, AW; Gerson, SL; Denis, L; Geyer, C; Hammond, LA; Patnaik, A; Goetz, AD; Schwartz, G; Edwards, T; Reyderman, L; Statkevich, P; Cutler, DL; Rowinsky, EK. Marked inactivation of O6-alkylguanine-DNA alkyltransferase activity with protracted temozolomide schedules. *Br J Cancer,* 2003; 88, 1004-1011.

[23] Vera, K; Djafari, L; Faivre, S; Guillamo, JS; Djazouli, K; Osorio, M; Parker, F; Cioloca, C; Abdulkarim, B; Armand, JP; Raymond, E. Dose-dense regimen of temozolomide given every other week in patients with primary central nervous system tumors. *Ann Oncol.* 2004; 15, 161-171.

[24] Wick, W; Steinbach, JP; Küker, WM; Dichgans, J; Bamberg, M; Weller, M. One week on/one week off: a novel active regimen of temozolomide for recurrent glioblastoma. *Neurology* 2004; 62, 2113–2115.

[25] Brada, M; Hoang-Xuan, K; Rampling, R; Dietrich, PY; Dirix, LY; Macdonald, D; Heimans, JJ; Zonnenberg, BA; Bravo-Marques, JM; Henriksson, R; Stupp, R; Yue, N; Bruner, J; Dugan, M; Rao, S; Zaknoen, S. Multicenter phase II trial of temozolomide in patients with glioblastoma multiforme at first relapse. *Ann Oncol.* 2001; 12, 259-266.

[26] Yung, WK; Albright, RE; Olson, J; Fredericks, R; Fink, K; Prados, MD; Brada, M; Spence, A; Hohl, RJ; Shapiro, W; Glantz, M; Greenberg, H; Selker, RG; Vick, NA; Rampling, R; Friedman, H; Phillips, P; Bruner, J; Yue, N; Osoba, D; Zaknoen, S; Levin, VA. A phase II study of temozolomide vs. procarbazine in patients with glioblastoma multiforme at first relapse. *Br J Cancer,* 2000; 83, 588-593.

[27] Stupp, R; Dietrich, PY; Ostermann Kraljevic, S; Pica, A; Maillard, I; Maeder, P; Meuli, R; Janzer, R; Pizzolato, G; Miralbell, R; Porchet, F; Regli, L; de Tribolet, N; Mirimanoff, RO; Leyvraz, S. Promising survival for patients with newly diagnosed glioblastoma multiforme treated with concomitant radiation plus temozolomide followed by adjuvant temozolomide. *J Clin Oncol.* 2002; 20, 1375-1382.

[28] Wick, W; Weller, M. How lymphotoxic is dose-intensified temozolomide? The glioblastoma experience. *J Clin Oncol.* 2005; 23, 4235-4236.

[29] Tosoni, A; Cavallo, G; Ermani, M; Scopece, L; Franceschi, E; Ghimenton, C; Gardiman, M; Pasetto, L; Blatt, V; Brandes, AA. Is protracted low-dose temozolomide feasible in glioma patients? *Neurology* 2006; 66, 427-429.

[30] Wong, S; Rosenthal, MA; Dowling, A; Jennens, R; Woods, AM; Ashley, D; Cher, L. Phase II study of two-weekly temozolomide in patients with high-grade gliomas. *J Clin Neurosci.* 2006; 13, 18-22.

[31] Dall'Oglio, S; D'Amico, A; Pioli, F; Gabbani, M; Pasini, F; Passarin, MG; Tabacchi, A; Turazzi, S; Maluta, S. Dose-intensity temozolomide after concurrent chemoradiotherapy in operated high-grade gliomas. *J Neurooncol.* 2008; 90, 315-319.

[32] Nagy, M; Schulz-Ertner, D; Bischof, M; Welzel, T; Hof, H; Debus, J; Combs, SE. Long-term outcome of postoperative irradiation in patients with newly diagnosed WHO grade III anaplastic gliomas. *Tumori,* 2009; 95, 317-324.

[33] Jalali, R; Singh, P; Menon, H; Gujral, S. Unexpected case of aplastic anemia in a patient with glioblastoma multiforme treated with Temozolomide. *J Neurooncol.* 2007; 85, 105-107.

In: Neuro-Oncology and Cancer Targeted Therapy
Editor: Lucía M. Gutiérrez pp.213-226
ISBN 978-1-61668-708-3
© 2010 Nova Science Publishers, Inc.

Chapter 9

INTRA-ARTERIAL TARGETED DELIVERY OF LIPOPHILIC PHOTOSENSITIZER FOR PHOTODYNAMIC THERAPY OF PROSTATE CANCER

Ronald B. Moore MD[*], Zhengwen Xiao, Richard J. Owen and John Tulip

Departments of Oncology, Surgery, Radiology and Diagnostic Imaging, Electric and Computer Engineering, University of Alberta, Edmonton, Alberta, Canada. T6G 2B7

ABSTRACT

Introduction: Prostate cancer (PCa) is the most common malignancy in western men. The stage and grade of the disease at diagnosis directly determine survival. Recently widespread PCa screening has greatly improved the ability to detect small and early stage cancer. Consequently many men with low-risk cancers have undergone radical therapies, suffering side effects from treatments without significant survival benefits. Minimally invasive therapies are being developed that may offer options for men with low-risk disease who want to balance the benefits and risks of treatment. Interstitial photodynamic therapy (PDT) is one such option. PDT uses a photosensitizing drug (photosensitizer) that is activated in the prostate by laser light of a specific wavelength, delivered by optical fibers. In the presence of oxygen, tissue necrosis occurs at the site of interaction between the photosensitizer and light. Current limitations of interstitial PDT for treatment of prostate cancer include low drug selectivity after intravenous (i.v.) administration and incomplete ablation of glandular tissue. To overcome these limitations, we have been exploring intra-arterial (i.a.) delivery of photosensitizer into the prostate. We have tested this strategy in rat and canine models, as well as in humans. In this chapter we report our observations and propose future targeted therapies to the prostate.

Methods: Biodistribution studies of ^{99m}Technetium labeled Macro-Aggregated Albumin (^{99m}Tc MAA) were carried out using whole body scintigraphy and ex-vivo

---
[*] Email: ron.moore@albertahealthservices.ca

tissue imaging. Hypocrellin B derivative SL052 (a lipophilic photosensitizer), formulated in liposomes or dissolved in dimethyl sulphoxide (DMSO), was injected i.a. via the prostate arteries and compared to i.v. administration. Optical fibers were inserted into the prostate and 630nm laser light delivered through fibers in a cyclic fashion. Drug concentration (fluorescence) and light transmission in prostate tissue were monitored during the course of PDT. Side effect profile and completeness of prostate gland ablation were the major parameters compared between treatment groups.

Results and conclusion: Intra-arterial injection of ^{99m}Tc MAA or SL052 dissolved in DMSO selectively targeted the prostate and attained an extremely high therapeutic ratio (18:1). With PDT there was complete ablation of the prostate glandular tissue with a significant reduction of prostate volume when compared pre-PDT ($p < 0.0001$). PDT with i.a. injection of lipophilic SL052-DMSO has the potential to provide an effective treatment for both prostate cancer and benign prostate enlargement. Intra-arterial delivery of drugs has the potential to be extended to targeted gene and molecular therapies for diseased solid organs.

Keywords: Intra-arterial drug delivery; minimally invasive therapy; targeted photochemotherapy; prostate; switched light delivery.

ABBREVIATIONS

DMSO	dimethyl sulphoxide
i.a.	intra-artery
PDT	photodynamic therapy
SL052	cyclohexane-1,2-diamino hypocrellin B derivative
SL052-DMSO	SL052 dissolved in DMSO
SL052-lipo	SL052 formulated in liposomes

INTRODUCTION

Benign prostatic hyperplasia (BPH) is a progressive disease and a common problem in aging men [1], resulting in lower urinary tract symptoms such as frequency and acute urinary retention. With significant advances in the diagnosis and treatment of BPH in recent years, medical therapies and minimally invasive techniques are the primary treatments [2]. Prostate cancer (PCa) is the most common cancer in American men [3], and the staging and grade (Gleason score) of the disease at diagnosis directly determine the survival. Many men (94%) live for 10 years after diagnosis without suffering morbidity and mortality attributable to the PCa. These men are believed to harbor low-risk cancers (Gleason score ≤ 6, stage < T2a, small tumor) [4], and these observations have been used to justify active surveillance (or watchful waiting) in men with low-risk PCa and short life expectancies [4, 5]. The widespread use of prostate-specific antigen (PSA) screening has greatly improved the ability to detect low-risk prostate cancer and has resulted in an increased diagnosis of PCa in younger, healthier men. The challenge is which treatment option should be selected for those younger men with localized PCa. Klotz reported that 34% of men initially selecting active surveillance ultimately pursue radical therapies because of disease progression or the psychological burden of potentially compromising their survival [7]. This suggests that active surveillance is not a long-term, viable alternative in younger cases.

Current available curative therapies for localized PCa are radical prostatectomy and radiotherapy. Adverse effects of radical prostatectomy include immediate postoperative complications and long-term urinary and sexual complications. External beam or interstitial radiation therapy in men with localized prostate cancer may also lead to urinary, gastrointestinal, and sexual complications [8]. Significant late effects include radiation necrosis and induction of bladder and colorectal cancers. Younger men diagnosed with low-risk PCa desire minimally invasive therapies that aim to offer similar treatment effects to current radical therapies, while reducing the associated adverse effects, especially sexual dysfunction. Several minimally invasive techniques are being developed, and interstitial photodynamic therapy (IPDT) is one such option. IPDT uses a photosensitizing drug (photosensitizer) that is activated in the prostate by specific wavelength laser light, delivered by optical fibers. In the presence of oxygen, tissue necrosis and apoptosis occur at the site of interaction between the photosensitizer and light. Recently, preclinical and clinical trials have supported interstitial PDT as a promising alternative therapy for PCa, because the prostate can be selectively irradiated by multiple fibers, with fiber placement techniques established in brachytherapy [9, 10, 11, 12]. Unlike radiotherapy, PDT is non-carcinogenic and may be applied repeatedly without accumulated toxicity.

For PDT of prostate cancer, the whole gland should be treated, as multiple tumor foci are commonly present. However, this requires highly selective drug (photosensitizer) and light delivery strategies to ensure treatment of the entire prostate volume, while sparing adjacent normal tissues to avoid complications to the rectum, bladder and neurovascular bundles controlling erection. First and foremost, the photosensitizer should specifically target the prostate and ideally only the prostate cancer. To date, photosensitizers are routinely injected intravenously (i.v.) However following i.v. injection, the majority of the photosensitizer is taken up by the reticuloendothelial system, resulting in low bioavailability to the target tissues. Therefore, in order to achieve adequate tissue drug concentration in the prostate excessive drug dosing is needed and this leads to high drug accumulation in normal tissues, especially in the skin resulting in photocutaneous toxicity. Based on our previous studies in the dog, photosensitizers can be delivered in a highly selective fashion to the prostate via intra-arterial (i.a.) injection to the prostate arteries. This new drug delivery strategy improved the targeting selectivity by reducing drug accumulation in tissues surrounding the prostate (i.e. rectum & bladder) and it also increased drug availability by avoiding first pass loss of the photosensitizer in the systemic circulation. Second, light delivery or dosimetry is another challenge for complete treatment of the prostate. Considering the size and contour of the prostate, multiple fibers are inserted into the prostate to deliver light. Real-time monitoring of dynamic changes in tissue oxygen and optic characteristics during PDT allows the end-points of therapy to be determined. In addition, oxygen sparing light delivery strategies, such as computer-driven switched light delivery system (Tulip J. et al., U.S. patent 60/646/656), have shown superior PDT effect to standard continuous illumination in rat prostate tumor models [14]. In this chapter we summarize our research observations and propose future targeted therapies to the prostate.

PHOTOSENSITIZERS

For over 15 years, our group has selected hypocrellins from perylenequinonoid pigments (PQP), as a practical platform upon which to develop improved photosensitizers [15, 16, 17]. Hypocrellin derivatives can be readily synthesized from the parent compound, hypocrellin B (HB), a natural product of the fungus, *Hypocrella bambusae sacc.*, a phytopathogen of bamboo [18]. HB derivatives are pure monomeric forms and may be derivatized to optimize properties of red light absorption, tissue biodistribution and toxicity. SL052 and SL017 are derivatives of hypocrellin B and were synthesized by QuestPharmaTech Inc., (Edmonton, AB, Canada). SL052 has a much higher absorption peak between 600 and 700 nm than hypocrellin B, which allows use of longer wavelength light for excitation. This wavelength range allows for maximal tissue penetration, with sufficient energy to excite the photosensitizer. The liposomal formulation of SL052 (SL052-lipo, ~200 nm in diameter) and SL052 dissolved in dimethyl sulphoxide (SL052-DMSO) were also generated by QuestPharmaTech Inc. Other photosensitizers, such as benzoporphyrin derivative (BPD), QLT0074 (QLT Inc., Vancouver, Cananda) and Aluminum phthalocyanine chloride (AlPC, New Jersey, USA) were also used in our preclinical studies based on their reported properties and for comparison to HB.

COMPUTER-DRIVEN FRACTIONATED LIGHT DELIVERY SYSTEM.

PDT efficacy depends on tissue photosensitizer concentration, light dose, and tissue oxygenation. During PDT, a rapid photochemical reaction occurs, yielding reactive oxygen species derived from tissue oxygen, which leads to depletion of oxygen [19, 20]. There is no PDT effect in the absence of oxygen and oxygen-preserving strategies have thus been developed, which include lowering fluence rate and fractionating light illumination (light/dark cycles) to allow tissue re-oxygenation during PDT. A significant limitation of using low fluence rate and manually fractionating illumination is the prolonged treatment time required. Clinical application of PDT generally seeks to minimize treatment time. This problem may be partially addressed during interstitial PDT of the prostate when multiple optical fibers are used and light delivery is controlled by a computer-controlled switch (Figure 1). With this technique, fractionated illumination can be achieved, without interruption of light delivery. Furthermore, the fibers can also be used to detect tissue fluorescence feedback, which makes real-time monitoring of photosensitizer concentration and PDT end-point possible. To speed up the treatment time, two or more lasers can be used simultaneously. This switched light delivery system was tested in rat models of prostate tumors and compared with continuous light delivery. Two Dunning rat prostate tumors with the opposite extremes of cell differentiation and blood perfusion (oxygenation) were treated with interstitial PDT. Tumor response (growth control) and tissue perfusion were monitored. Tumor response to PDT with fractionated light delivery was PDT dose dependent in both tumor models. Rats bearing anaplastic (poorly-differentiated) tumor treated by fractionated light had a median survival of 51 days with 25% tumor cures compared with that of 26 days with no tumor cure by continuous illumination ($P = 0.015$). Rats bearing well-differentiated tumor treated by fractionated light had a median survival of 82 days compared with 65 days by continuous illumination ($P = 0.001$). Thus PDT with fractionated light delivery improves efficacy in solid tumor treatment and will likely shorten treatment times depending on the light delivery set-up.

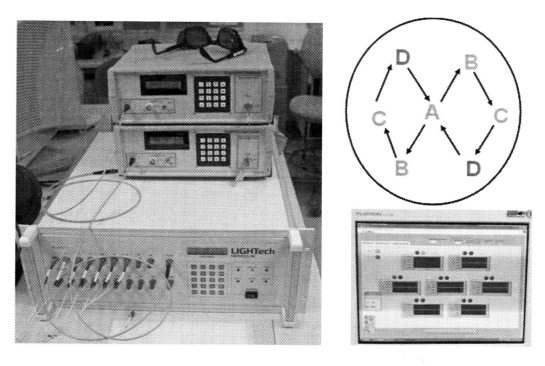

Figure 1. Computer-driven switched light delivery system for interstitial photodynamic therapy of the prostate. The picture on the left shows that two diode laser machines send the light to light switch, the switch then deliver the light to the fibers in the prostate in cycles (right upper panel). As shown in this diagram, an illumination cycle starts from fiber A (100 seconds), switching to fiber B, then C, then D, and back to A. The light delivery cycles are controlled by modified LabVIEW® programs (right lower panel).

TARGETED INTRA-ARTERIAL ADMINISTRATION OF LIPOPHILIC PHOTOSENSITIZERS

Photosensitizers are routinely administered by intravenous injection. Since photosensitizers *per se* are not significantly tumor selective, the majority of the drug is distributed to the skin, liver, spleen and kidneys due to macrophage uptake in the reticuloendothelial system, with only a small amount of the drug accumulating in the prostate [21]. To increase drug concentration in target tissue, excess amount of photosensitizer is needed, resulting in high drug accumulation in normal tissues, which leads to skin phototoxicity and collateral tissue damage by PDT. To selectively deliver photosensitizer to the prostate and reduce the waiting time of light illumination after drug administration, photosensitizers were injected via the prostate arteries into the prostate. This targeted delivery of drug was studied first in a canine model with BPH The canine model is the only preclinical model that develops prostate disease (BPH and PCa) like humans and has comparable vessels for vascular access.

There were two parts to our initial study. The first part aimed to determine drug distribution, and the second to determine the toxicity and effectiveness of this targeted therapy. All procedures and experimental animal use were first approved by the University Health Sciences Animal Policy and Welfare Committee according to the guidelines set by the Canadian Council on Animal Care.

To gain access to the prostate arteries, angiographic procedures were performed using standard equipment and fluoroscopic guidance. Anesthetized animals were positioned supine on a radiolucent surgical table and the lower abdomen and groin skin prepared with Betadine. The right common femoral artery was percutaneously cannulated using a standard Seldinger technique. A 5 Fr vascular sheath was placed. A 2.3 Fr microcatheter and 0.018-inch platinum guidewire were then used to cannulate the ipsilateral prostatovesical artery, which is a visceral branch of the internal iliac artery (Figure 2). After the prostate artery was cannulated with the 2.3 Fr microcatheter one milliliter (1.0 ml) of photosensitizer (liposomal QLT0074, or liposomal SL052, or SL052-DMSO) was injected. Subsequently the contralateral internal iliac artery and prostate artery were cannulated using a similar technique and another 1.0 ml photosensitizer was infused. After drug administration, the catheter and sheath were removed and the right femoral artery compressed to achieve hemostasis. In animals treated with PDT, light illumination of the prostate followed immediately.

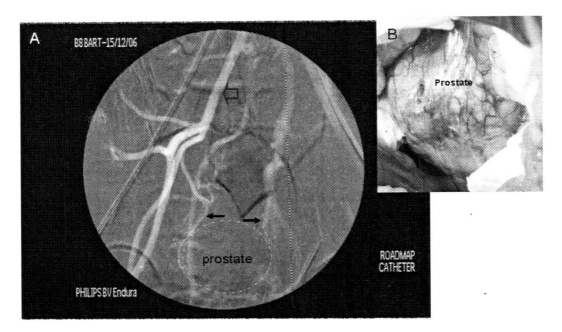

Figure 2. Targeted intra-arterial injection of photosensitizer to the canine prostate. A. Angiography shows that the two prostate arteries (solid arrows) which are branches from the internal iliac arteries (open arrow showing the right side) provide blood supply to the prostate (circled area). B. The prostate turns blue in color following intra-arterial injection of 9 mg SL052-DMSO.

In the initial drug distribution study, AlPC dissolved in DMSO and 99m-Technetium labeled macro-aggregated albumin (^{99m}Tc-MAA, 100MBq/ml, Edmonton Radiopharmaceutical Center) were used. Since ^{99m}Tc-MAA temporarily embolizes in the microvasculature, it was believed to be a good surrogate marker for studying lipophilic photosensitizers drug distribution when administered dissolved in DMSO. In addition, ^{99m}Tc-MAA can be detected either in whole-body scans by single photon emission computed tomographic imaging (SPECT) or in *ex vivo* organs/tissues by gamma camera imaging. Animals for drug distribution studies were sacrificed 30 min after drug injection into the second prostate artery and subjected to whole-body and pelvic SPECT imaging of the organs. Following whole-body SPECT imaging, the bladder, prostate, membranous urethra, penis, and rectum were surgically removed *en bloc* and subjected to *ex vivo* planar imaging. The intensity of ^{99m}Tc-MAA in pelvic organs/tissues was measured with Medisplay View software. For comparative analysis, portions (by weight) of the organs were also analyzed by well-counting in scintillation vials. In addition, animals receiving intra-arterial (i.a.) injection of photosensitizer were sacrificed and tissue samples were taken from bladder, right and left prostate lobes, membranous urethra, penis, and rectum wall for determination of photosensitizer concentration and localization. To achieve this one portion of tissue samples was processed for photosensitizer extraction analysis and the other matching set was cryo-sectioned for confocal microscopic imaging. Dogs receiving unilateral artery injection of ^{99m}Tc-MAA showed that only half of the prostate accumulated the radio-isotope, and whereas the whole prostate was highlighted by radiotracer following bilateral injection. This initial study indicated that prostate arterial delivery was highly selective in targeting the prostate. Except for the bladder neck, tissues adjacent to the prostate showed very low activity even after bilateral injection of ^{99m}Tc-MAA. On average, the prostate accumulated 10 times more radioactivity per gram of tissue compared to that of surrounding tissue as detected by well counting. In particular, both the bladder and rectum showed very low intensity relative to the high drug intensity detected in the prostate. Chemical extraction analysis revealed that photosensitizer concentration in the prostate was 18 times higher than that in the bladder and rectum ($P = 0.04$). Confocal microscopy confirmed these findings and showed that the photosensitizer selectively accumulated in the glandular tissue. Normally with i.v. administration the therapeutic ratio was less than 5:1 relative to surrounding normal tissue.

INTERSTITIAL PDT OF THE PROSTATE

With the encouraging drug distribution data, the first PDT experiments were started in 10 male dogs with BPH receiving i.a. injection of liposomal QLT0074 bilaterally (4 mg drug per prostate) Immediately after intra-arterial infusion of photosensitizer a lower mid-abdomen incision was made to expose the prostate anterior surface. Laser light (690 nm) was delivered through 7 optic fiber with 1.5 cm cylindrical light diffusing tips placed in after-loading needle sheaths. The fibers were inserted in a hexagonal pattern into the prostate in an anteroposterior direction, spaced ~10 mm apart and 5 mm away from the capsule edge. Two diode lasers (Optical Fiber Systems) were used and light delivery was controlled by a computer-driven switch with multiple light outputs (LIGHTech Fiberoptics, San Leandro, CA). The 7 fibers were sequentially illuminated 2 at a time for 100 seconds of each cycle. The total accumulative light dose delivered to the prostate was 900 J. After PDT the surgical incision was sutured closed. Animals were observed carefully for signs of complications including sepsis, bleeding, urinary retention, and bowel and erectile function in metabolic cages. Prophylactic antibiotics and analgesic were given for a week. Catheterization was performed when residual urine was evident.

This study demonstrated that the animals tolerated the PDT procedures well without evidence of skin phototoxicity. The most common complication encountered was urinary retention, presumably due to prostate swelling, which was readily managed by catheterization. To examine the early PDT effects, dogs were terminated <6 days post-PDT. At necropsy the prostate showed complete hemorrhagic and coagulative necrotic changes. To examine late effects other animals were sacrificed 3 to 11 months after PDT. In these animals the prostate volumes were reduced by 56% to 71% compared to the pre-PDT volumes ($P = 0.014$). Urodynamic investigations did not detect noticeable deleterious effects on bladder or urethral sphincter function. No damage to the rectum wall was observed. However, on close microscopic scrutiny there was a variable amount of surviving glandular tissue in the prostate, which might be a concern in the treatment of prostate cancer.

To further overcome the observed limitations of incomplete ablation of the gland and low drug selectivity after i.a. and i.v. administration of liposomal photosensitizer, we further refined the targeted PDT procedures and conducted further tests in 20 mature husky dogs with BPH [22]. SL052, a lipophilic photosensitizer, was formulated in liposomes or dissolved in DMSO, which was injected intra-arterially via the prostate arteries (2 to 18 mg drug per prostate). For comparison, liposomal SL052 was i.v. injected into 2 dogs (160 mg drug per dog). Light (635 nm) from 2 diode laser sources was delivered by the computer-controlled switch system as detailed above. Light illumination was started 3 hours after i.v. and 1 hour after i.a. drug delivery. Light doses of 200 to 600 J/cm^3 of prostate volume were applied. Drug concentration (fluorescence) and light transmission in the prostate tissue were monitored during the course of PDT. Control animals received i.a. SL052-DMSO without light or light only (no drug). Thirteen dogs were treated by PDT with i.a. injection of SL052-DMSO and attained either complete ablation of the prostatic glandular tissue (Figure 3) or significant reduction of the prostate volume (mean pre-PDT volume = 18 cm^3, mean post-PDT volume = 3 cm^3, $P < 0.0001$). Urinary retention was still the most common complication. Also, in those dogs receiving high PDT doses, over-treatment of the prostate was observed, which caused obstructive damage to the bladder and impaired renal function. However, there were no adverse effects on erectile or sphincter control. In comparison, PDT with i.v. injection of SL052 in liposome caused only early tissue damage, while its long term effect to the prostate was very limited (Figure 4). The liposomal formulated drug being soluble in serum was observed to be quickly cleared from the prostate with resulting whole body distribution. Where as the non-liposomal formulation, which immediately aggregated in serum, had a profound first pass effect following i.a., with the majority accumulating uniformly in the prostate. This was so dramatic that we had to reduce both the drug and light dose. We also explored simple embolization of the prostate, but this did not have as profound effect as PDT.

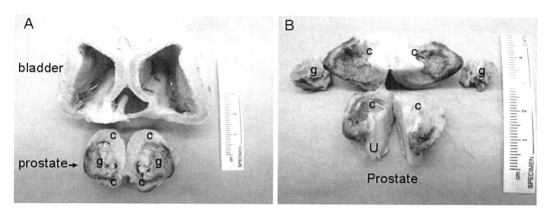

Figure 3. Interstitial PDT of the canine prostate with intra-arterial injection of 9 mg SL052-DMSO. A. Images show the bladder (sagital view) with a normal appearance and the prostate (cross section) demonstrating necrotic prostate glandular tissue (g) and the less damaged capsule (c), 3 months post-PDT. B. A picture of the same prostate (sagital and cross section views) shows that the necrotic glandular tissue (g) is easily separated from the capsule (c), this could cause urinary retention if it sloughs from the capsule and not removed in time. Clinically it can readily be removed with cystoscopy. The pre- and post-PDT volumes of this prostate were 38 cm^3 and capsule only (~4 cm^3), respectively. U denotes the membrane urethra.

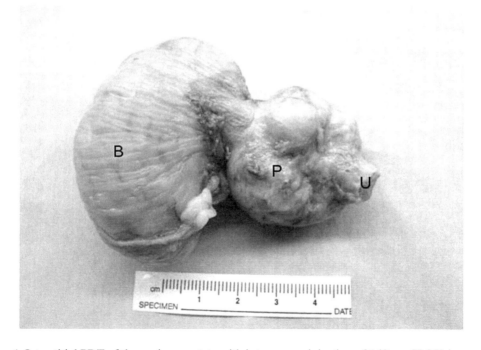

Figure 4. Interstitial PDT of the canine prostate with intravenous injection of 160 mg SL052 in liposomes. The bladder (B), prostate (P) and urethra (U) show little response to PDT at 4 months. The pre- and post-PDT volumes of the prostate were 12.8 cm^3 and 13 cm^3, respectively.

TRANSLATION TO HUMANS

Based on the selective targeting and complete PDT effect observed in the dog model, we proposed studies in humans for selective intra-arterial drug administration. An initial literature search revealed no prior reported studies on which to base this clinical study. Ethics approval was obtained from the University of Alberta Human Ethics Research Organization (HERO) for i.a. of ^{99m}Tc-MAA initially and to be followed by SL052. These studies are currently underway; however the findings to date are consistent with those observed in the preclinical dog model. With unilateral administration there is delivery to only one half of the prostate (Figure 5).

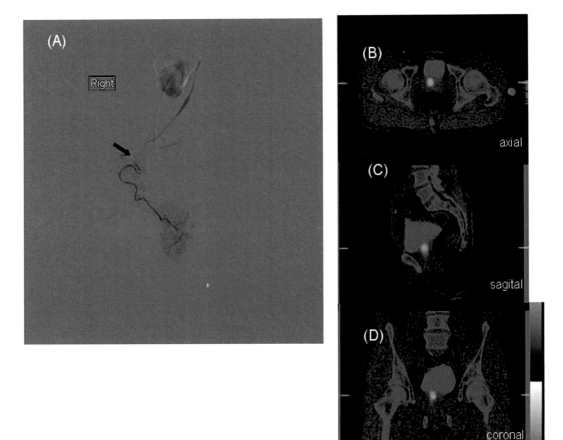

Figure 5. Selective intra-arterial drug delivery to human prostate. A. The right prostatovesical artery was cannulated with a 2.5Fr Miraflex micro-angiocatheter (arrow). Following confirmation of placement 30MBq ^{99m}Tc MAA was injected and SPECT Imaging performed. Images demonstrate only the right side of the prostate showing radioactivity (B-D).

OTHER APPLICATIONS OF TARGETED INTRA-ARTERIAL DRUG DELIVERY

Trans-arterial therapy has been used in the treatment of inoperable hepatocellular carcinoma. Chemotherapeutic agents combined with lipiodol (Ezem Canada) or radiation-emitting microspheres were injected via a transarterial route, because hepatic malignancies are primarily supplied by the hepatic artery [23, 24], as opposed to the portal system. Transarterially administered gene therapy is still in the early stages of investigation [25, 26]. Development of neutralizing antibodies after i.v. administration of recombinant adenovirus has been reported, and this antibody response has been postulated to limit transgene expression after subsequent cycles of treatment. A cellular toxic lymphocyte response to recombinant adenovirus has also been reported to limit the duration of transgene expression *in vivo* and cause an inflammatory response to transduced cells. Following arterial administration of recombinant adenoviral-p53, high local concentrations of recombinant p53 gene may enable transgene expression even in the presence of serum antibodies and cytotoxic lymphocytes. In addition, the local inflammatory lymphocyte response to positively transduced tumor cells may result in antitumor effects. Transarterial embolization (TAE) has been used in the treatment of musculoskeletal tumors [27], refractory hematuria of prostatic origin (benign and malignant) [27], renal hemorrhage (malignant and benign[29], [29], high-flow priapism (persistent penile erection) [30], and symptomatic uterine fibroids [32, 33]. From a cancer perspective, simple selective embolization of the cancer has only been used in a palliative setting is not likely to be curative without the addition of hypoxic bioreductive agents.

CONCLUSION

Targeted intra-arterial infusion can not only selectively deliver drugs to the prostate (or target tissue), but also can deliver lipophilic photosensitizers in various formulations, such as in liposomes (as for i.v. injection) or in DMSO. SL052-DMSO delivered by i.a. injection appears to have a longer transit time in the prostate (related to temporary lipophilic aggregation) than SL052 in liposome following i.a. injection and a large first-pass-effect thus requiring much lower drug dose (80 times less than i.v. delivery). The large therapeutic ratio relative to surrounding tissue makes the selective targeting of PDT with light a much easier and complete process with higher isodose curves out to the periphery of the target tissue. In addition the low total body drug dose reduces the chance of drug accumulation in normal tissues and therefore the risk of skin phototoxicity. Following i.a. injection of photosensitizer, light illumination can be started immediately with the PDT effect targeting both the glandular and vascular elements of the prostate. Based on our research and observations to date we believe that IPDT with intra-arterial injection of photosensitizer may become one of the treatment options for those patients with low-risk localized PCa or BPH. Further phase I/II clinical trials are currently in progress.

ACKNOWLEDGMENT

The authors thank the staff in Health Sciences Laboratory Animal Services (HSLAS) and Surgical-Medical Research Institute (SMRI) of University of Alberta for technical support and animal care. We acknowledge the financial support from National Cancer Institute of Canada (NCIC), Alberta Cancer Board (ACB), Alberta Heritage Foundation for Medical Research (AHFMR), Henry Gusse Foundation and QuestPharmaTech, Inc.

REFERENCES

[1] Emberton M, Cornel EB, Bassi PF, Fourcade RO, Gomez JM, Castro R. Benign prostate hyperplasia as a progressive disease: a guide to the risk factors and options for medical management. *Int J Clin Pract*. 2008;62:1076-86.

[2] Tanguay S, Awde M, Brock G, et al. Diagnosis and management of benign prostatic hyperplasia in primary care. *Can Urol Assoc J*. 2009;3(Suppl 2):S92-S100.

[3] Jemal A, Siegel R, Ward E, et al. Cancer statistics, 2008. *CA Cancer J Clin*. 2008;58:71–96.

[4] Carter HB, Walsh PC, Landis P, Epstein JI. Expectant management of stage T1c prostate cancer with curative intent: preliminary results. *J Urol*.2002;167:1231-1234.

[5] Carter HB, Kettermann A, Warlick C, et al. Expectant management of prostate cancer with urative intent: an update of the Johns Hopkins experience. *J Urol*.2007;178:2359-2364.

[6] Lu-Yao GL, Albertsen PC, Moore DF, et al. Outcomes of localized prostate cancer following conservative management. *JAMA*,2009;302(11):1202-1209.

[7] Klotz L. Active surveillance for prostate cancer: for whom? *J Clin Oncol*.2005;23:8165-8169.

[8] Michaelson MD, Cotter SE, Gargollo PC, Zietman AL, Dahl DM, Smith MR. Management of complications of prostate cancer treatment. CA Cancer J Clin 2008;58:196–213

[9] Xiao Z, Dickey D, Owen RJ, Tulip J, Moore RB. Interstitial photodynamic therapy of the anine prostate using intra-arterial administration of photosensitizer and computerized pulsed light delivery. *J Urol*.2007;178:308-13.

[10] Nathan TR, Whitelaw BE, Chang SC, et al. Photodynamic therapy for prostate cancer recurrence after radiotherapy: a phase I study. *J Urol*.2002;168:1427-32.

[11] Trachtenberg J, Weersink RA, Davidson SRH, et al. Vascular-targeted photodynamic therapy padoporfin, WST09) for recurrent prostate cancer after failure of external beam radiotherapy: a study of escalating light doses. *BJU int*.2008;102:556-62.

[12] Moore CM, Pendse D, Emberton M, Medscape. Photodynamic therapy for prostate cancer—a review of current status and future promise. *Nat Clin Pract Urol*.2009; 6:18-30.

[13] Moore RB, Xiao Z, Owen RJ, et al. Photodynamic therapy of the canine prostate: intra-arterial drug delivery. *Cardiovasc Intervent Radiol*.2008;31:164–76.

[14] Xiao Z, Halls S, Dickey D, Tulip J, Moore RB. Fractionated versus standard continuous light delivery in interstitial photodynamic therapy of Dunning prostate carcinomas. *Clin Cancer Res*.2007;13:7496-7505.

[15] Diwu Z, Lown JW. Photosensitization by anticancer agents 12. Perylene quinonoid pigments, a novel type of singlet oxygen sensitizer. *J Photochem Photobiol A Chem*.1992;64:273-287.

[16] Miller GG, Brown K, Ballangrud AM, et al. Preclinical assessment of hypocrellin B and hypocrellin B derivatives as sensitizers for photodynamic therapy of cancer: progress update. *Photochem Photobiol*.1997;65:714-722.

[17] Paul BT, Babu MS, Santhoshkumar TR, et al. Biophysical evaluation of two red-shifted hypocrellin B derivatives as novel PDT agents. *J Photochem Photobiol B Biology*, 009;94:38-44.

[18] Diwu Z. The study on the photochemotherapeutic mechanism of hypocrellin. PhD Dissertation, Institute of Photographic Chemistry, Academia Sinica, Beijing. 1988.

[19] Tromberg BJ, Orenstein A, Kimel S, et al. In vivo tumor oxygen tension measurements for the evaluation of the efficiency of photodynamic therapy. *Photochem Photobiol*.1990;52:375-85.

[20] Henderson BW, Busch TM, Vaughan LA, et al. Photofrin photodynamic therapy can significantly deplete or preserve oxygenation in human basal cell carcinamoas during treatment, depending on fluence rate. *Cancer Res*.2000;60:525-529.

[21] Pantelides ML, Moore JV, Forbes E, et al. The uptake of porphyrin and zinc-metalloporphyrin by the primate prostate. *Photochem Photobiol*.1993;57:838-841.

[22] Xiao Z, Owen RJ, Liu W, et al. Administration of lipophilic photosensitizer via the prostate arteries for photodynamic therapy of the canine prostate. *Photodiagn Photodyn Ther*.(submitted 2009, PDPDT-09-37).

[23] Lo CM, Ngan H, Tso WK, et al. Randomized controlled trial of transarterial lipiodol chemoembolization for unresectable hepatocellular carcinoma. *Hepatology*, 2002;35:1164-1171

[24] Kalva SP, Thalbet A, Wicky S. Recent advances in transarterial therapy of primary and secondary liver malignancies. *Radiographics*,2008;28:101-117.

[25] Anderson SC, Johnson DE, Harris MP, et al. P53 gene therapy in a rat model of hepatocellular carcinoma: intra-arterial delivery of a recombinant adenovirus. *Clin Cancer Res*. 1998;4:1649-1659.

[26] Okimoto T, Yahata H, Itou H, et al. Safety and growth suppressive effect of intra-hepatic arterial injection of AdCMV-p53 combined with CDDP to rat liver metastatic tumors. *J Exp Clin Cancer Res*. 2003; 22:399-406.

[27] Owen RJ. Embolization of musculoskeletal tumors. *Radiol Clin N Am*. 2008; 46:535-543.

[28] Rastinehad AR, Caplin DM, Ost MC, et al. Selective arterial prostatic embolization (SAPE) for refractory hematuria of prostatic origin. *Urology*, 2008; 71:181-184.

[29] Munro NP, Woodhams S, Nawrocki JD, Fletcher MS, Thomas PJ. The role of transarterial embolization in the treatment of renal cell carcinoma. *BJU International*; Aug2003, Vol. 92 Issue 3, p240-244.

[30] Jain V, Ganpule A, Vyas J, et al. Management of non-neoplastic renal hemorrhage by transarterial embolization. *Urology*, 2009; 74:522-527.

[31] Ciampalini S, Savoca G, Buttazzi L, et al. High-flow priapism: treatment and long-term follow-up. *Urology*, 2002; 59:110-113.

[32] Pinto I, Chimeno P, Romo A, et al. Uterine fibroids: uterine artery embolization versus abdominal hysterectomy for treatment – a prospective, randomized, and controlled clinical trial. *Radiology*, 2003; 226:425-431.

[33] Spies JB, Cooper JM, Worthington-Kirsch R, et al. Out-come of uterine embolization and hysterectomy for leiomyomas: results of a multicenter study. *Am J Obstet Gynecol.* 2004; 191:22-31.

Chapter 10

CERVICAL SPINE DEFORMITY ASSOCIATED WITH LAMINOPLASTY FOR RESECTION OF SPINAL CORD TUMORS IN CHILDREN

Peter Kan, M.D. and Meic H. Schmidt,[*]
Department of Neurosurgery, University of Utah School of Medicine,
Salt Lake City, Utah

ABSTRACT

Cervical deformity is a well-known complication of cervical laminectomy, especially for tumor resection in children. Despite the lack of evidence of its efficacy, cervical laminoplasty is often advocated in place of laminectomy in children to prevent such postoperative deformities. Our objective was to compare laminoplasty and laminectomy techniques in terms of postoperative spinal alignment and incidence of kyphotic deformity. The authors describe a case of a 28-year-old woman who developed a severe cervical kyphotic deformity after cervical laminoplasty for tumor resection performed 14 years earlier. The patient was treated with a posterior decompression and instrumentation, followed by multilevel anterior cervical discectomies and fusions. On the basis of our review of the literature, there appears to be no benefit to laminoplasty over laminectomy in terms of postoperative spinal alignment and incidence of kyphotic deformity.

Key words: Cervical deformities; laminoplasty; spinal cord tumors.

---

[*] Corresponding author: Meic H. Schmidt, M.D.
Department of Neurosurgery
University of Utah School of Medicine
175 N. Medical Drive East
Salt Lake City, UT 84132
Phone: 801-581-6908
Fax: 801-581-4138
Email: neuropub@hsc.utah.edu

INTRODUCTION

Sagittal cervical deformities such as kyphosis and 'swan-neck deformities' are not uncommon in patients, especially in children who have undergone a cervical laminectomy for resection of spinal cord tumors (1-3). Laminoplasty is often advocated in place of a laminectomy to prevent such deformities (4), despite a lack of clinical evidence of its advantages over laminectomy. We report a case of a severe cervical kyphosis requiring surgical correction that developed after a cervical laminoplasty for resection of an intradural neurofibroma. We review the literature on postlaminoplasty cervical spine deformities, focusing on their incidence, risk factors, and management as they relate to resection of cervical spinal cord tumors in children.

ILLUSTRATIVE CASE

History and Examination

A 28-year-old woman, who had a C3 to C6 cervical laminoplasty for resection of a C5 intradural extramedullary neurofibroma at the age of 14 years, presented with neck pain, paresthesia and loss of dexterity in her left hand, and numbness in both feet. She does not carry a diagnosis of neurofibromatosis.

On examination, her left upper arm revealed severe spasticity. Her strength was normal but she was markedly myelopathic, with 4+ hyperreflexia throughout, sustained clonus in both feet, and positive Babinski and Hoffman signs bilaterally.

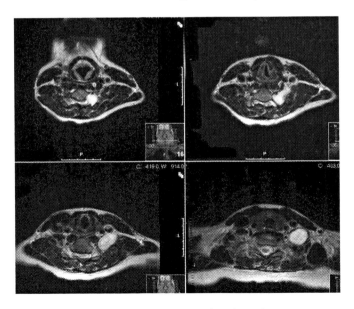

Figure 1. Axial T2-weighted magnetic resonance images showing a large recurrent tumor at C5 extending into the left brachial plexus.

Imaging

Magnetic resonance imaging of her cervical spine revealed a large recurrent tumor at the C5 level extending into her left brachial plexus (Figure 1). In addition, although she had a normal cervical alignment pre- and postlaminoplasty documented on plain radiographs, the patient had developed a 45-degree cervical kyphotic deformity centered at C4 to C7, with severe spinal canal stenosis and abnormal T2 cord signal changes (Figure 2). On plain radiographs, the deformity was mildly flexible but did not significantly reduce in extension (Figure 3). Computerized tomography images showed evidence of nonunion of the laminoplasty and the residual laminae were "free floating" (Figure 4).

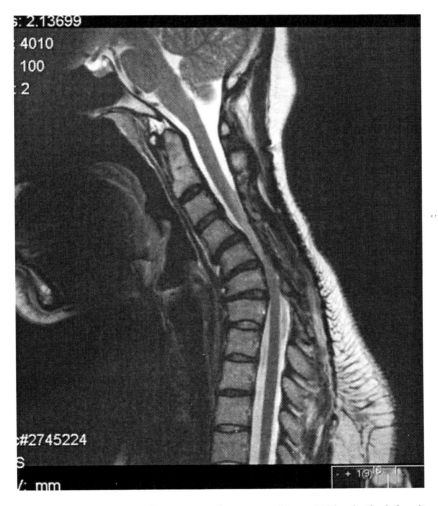

Figure 2. Sagittal T2-weighted magnetic resonance image revealing a 45° kyphotic deformity centered at C4-7, with severe spinal canal stenosis and abnormal cord signal changes.

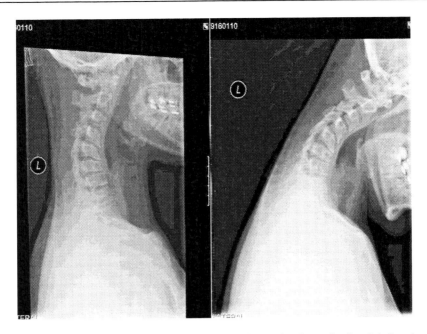

Figure 3. Extension (A) and flexion (B) views on plain radiographs showed a fixed deformity without significant reduction on extension.

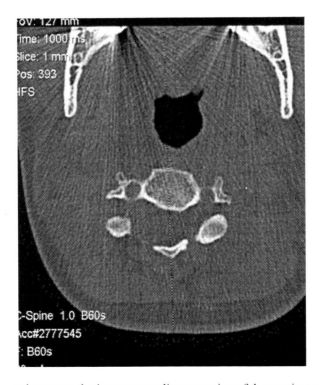

Figure 4. Axial computed tomography images revealing nonunion of the previous cervical laminoplasty with free-floating laminae.

Operation

Given that the patient had progressive myelopathy from a severe cervical kyphosis and recurrent tumor, a 3-stage operation was planned. Stage one of the surgery consisted of removal of the laminoplasty bone, resection of the medial part of the tumor that was compressing the spinal cord along with the C5 dorsal root, lateral mass instrumentation from C3 to C7, and a posterior release (Figure 5). After the posterior release, decompression, and instrumentation, the patient underwent an anterior cervical diskectomy and fusion from C4 to C7 for further correction of the kyphotic deformity. Lastly, after the final correction was accomplished, the patient was turned back into the prone position for final placement of rods and tightening of the instrumentation. Intraoperative monitoring with somatosensory evoked potentials and motor evoked potentials was used during all stages of the operation.

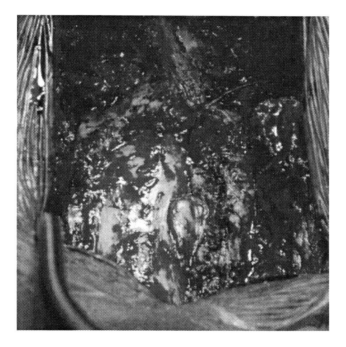

Figure 5. Intraoperative photograph showing the removal of previous laminoplasty and the medial portion of the tumor abutting the spinal cord.

Postoperative Course

The patient did well and was discharged on postoperative day 4 in a rigid cervical collar. Her neurologic status remained stable after surgery. Postoperative radiographs (Figure 6) revealed a good correction of her kyphotic deformity. The patient was pain free at a follow-up visit 3 years after surgery, with minimal loss of correction and without recurrent tumor.

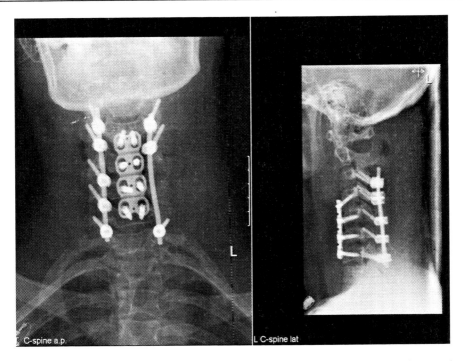

Figure 6. Postoperative anteroposterior (A) and lateral (B) radiographs showing a good correction of the kyphotic deformity.

DISCUSSION

In adults, cervical laminectomy is a common procedure for treating multilevel cervical stenosis in association with spondylosis, disc herniations, or ossification of the posterior longitudinal ligaments. In children, resection of spinal cord tumors is one of the more common reasons to perform a cervical laminectomy. Cervical laminoplasty was developed in Japan in the 1970s as an alternative to laminectomy because of concerns about spinal deformity and instability associated with cervical laminectomy.

In the normal lordotic cervical spine, the weight-bearing axis lies posterior to the vertebral bodies (VBs). To oppose cervical kyphosis, the anterior elements of the spine provide resistance to compression while the posterior elements provide tension to maintain the normal lordotic alignment. The loss of posterior ligamentous and bony elements after cervical laminectomy can shift the weight-bearing axis forward, resulting in a loss of lordosis or a change to a straight or even a kyphotic alignment. This, in turn, increases the compressive load on the anterior elements and places the remaining posterior elements under further tension, resulting in a progression of the kyphotic deformity (Figure 7) (5-7). At an advanced stage, the kyphotic deformity is often accompanied by a compensatory lordosis distal in the spine; these are commonly known as 'swan-neck' deformities.

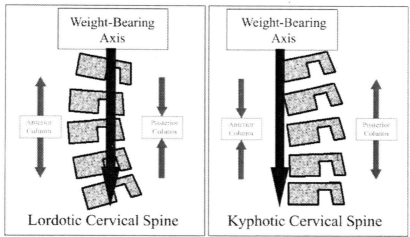

Figure reproduced with permission from Fassett DR, McCall T, Brockmeyer DL, Schmidt MH. Cervical spine deformity associated with resection of spinal cord tumors. Neurosurg Focus 20 (2):E2, 2006.

Figure 7. Schematic drawings showing lordosis and kyphosis in the cervical spine. Kyphosis tends to be a self-propagating condition because the deformity causes the weight-bearing axis in the cervical spine to move to a more ventral position in front of the vertebral bodies (VBs). In a normal lordotic cervical spine, the weight-bearing axis lies posterior to the VBs, with the anterior spinal column under tension and the posterior elements under compression. With kyphosis, the anterior spinal column is under compression and the posterior elements are under tension. If the integrity of the posterior tension band is violated, as in the case of laminectomy, the structural support of the cervical spine cannot sufficiently resist the biomechanical forces promoting progression of the kyphotic deformity.

With laminoplasty, it is believed that by preserving the lamina and the posterior ligamentous complex, postoperative cervical deformity can be reduced (4, 8, 9). Although laboratory studies have suggested that cervical laminoplasty may produce less instability than laminectomy does (10), the authors of most clinical series to date have reported a high incidence of worsening of cervical alignment (22–53%, mean ~35%) or new kyphotic deformities (2–15%, mean ~10%) after laminoplasty for degenerative disease (8-30). In comparison, the incidence of postoperative kyphosis or worsening of cervical alignment after multilevel laminectomy for spondylitic disease is not significantly different, reported to be approximately 20% and 40%, respectively (31).

Compared with the literature addressing cervical spondylitic disease, the literature regarding kyphotic deformity associated with cervical laminoplasty for tumor resection is very sparse. The two groups of patients differ substantially. Patients with advanced spondylosis are, in general, older and have a more stable spine secondary to partial autofusion of their facet joints compared with the younger tumor patients with flexible and nonarthritic spines. Consequently, the incidence of postoperative kyphosis is projected to be even higher in patients undergoing cervical laminoplasty for resection of spinal tumors. Yeh et al. (32) reported 1 of 3 children who underwent a cervical laminoplasty for tumor resection developed a worsening cervical alignment after surgery. In the same series, only 2 of 9 children developed a worsening alignment postoperatively after cervical laminectomy for tumor resection (32).

In the studies we reviewed, no adult patient developed a kyphotic deformity after laminoplasty requiring fusion unless the facet joints were violated (2, 3). In cadaveric studies, resection of 50% of the facet joint can lead to acute instability (33), and facet capsule resection alone was also shown to result in increased cervical motion (34). As a result, the incidence of postoperative kyphosis after posterior cervical decompression is probably most closely dictated by the extent of facet resection rather than the technique of laminectomy or laminoplasty. This may explain why cervical laminoplasty still has a high incidence of postoperative spinal deformity and why laminoplasty and laminectomy share a similar rate of postoperative cervical kyphosis.

Apart from preservation of the posterior elements, another putative advantage of laminoplasty over laminectomy is that laminoplasty will allow the reattachment of cervical musculature to the lamina, thereby reducing the risk of postoperative spinal deformity (9). Nevertheless, investigators reported significant postlaminoplasty cervical atrophy. In a series of 53 patients, Fujimura et al. (13) found an 80% decrease in the cross-sectional area of the cervical musculature at 5-year follow-up, with 30% loss of the deep cervical musculature 1 year after surgery. Moreover, they found no correlation between the degree of muscle atrophy and cervical curvature postoperatively.

In addition to the extent of facet resection, other factors that have been associated with a higher incidence of postoperative kyphosis after laminoplasty include young age, extent of laminoplasty, preoperative loss of cervical lordosis, tumor resection, and radiation. In pediatric patients, the incompletely ossified VBs and the elastic posterior interspinous ligaments offer poor resistance to compressive forces, which, along with their more horizontally oriented facets and growing spines, predispose children to develop a kyphotic deformity after laminoplasty (2).

Patients who undergo multilevel cervical laminoplasty for intraspinal tumor resection (both intra- and extramedullary) may have a higher incidence of postoperative cervical spine deformity compared with patients who undergo laminoplasty for degenerative disease. With intramedullary lesions, some authors have postulated that it is related to neuromuscular dysfunction and denervation of the paravertebral muscles precipitated by the tumor involvement of the anterior horn cells (32). With extramedullary lesions, the enlargement of the posterior arch and intervertebral foramen, the VB remodeling, and the necessity of extensive facet resections to gain exposure are thought to be contributing factors to the higher rate of postoperative deformity.

With cervical laminectomy, Katsumi et al. (35) found that patients in whom instability did not develop had a mean of 1.2 risk factors, patients in whom instability developed but who did not require stabilization had a mean of 2.5 risk factors, and patients who needed surgical stabilization for instability had at least 3 risk factors. Unfortunately, similar analysis has not been performed with cervical laminoplasty. Nevertheless, we believe that in cervical laminoplasty the cumulative number of risk factors too has an impact on the risk of postoperative deformity. In the case of cervical laminoplasty for tumor resection, one risk factor (tumor resection) is already present, and the surgeon should be aware of the other risk factors present as this may change the choice of initial surgical approach to a laminectomy and fusion in high-risk patients.

As part of risk stratification and preoperative counseling, we recommend that plain radiographs of the cervical spine should be obtained to rule out a preexisting deformity and to serve as a baseline for future comparisons. Patients with preoperative loss of lordosis are counseled that they may have a higher risk of postoperative deformity with either laminoplasty or laminectomy, and that they may need an additional stabilization procedure if deformity occurs. At present, we do not favor laminoplasty over laminectomy at our institution for tumor resection because its clinical efficacy and advantages over laminectomy remain unclear. In the rare case of a patient with preoperative kyphosis, we would consider performing a stabilization procedure at the time of the initial surgery for tumor resection.

Several measures can be taken to reduce the risk of postlaminoplasty deformity. First, efforts should be made to limit the number of levels on which the procedure is performed and to restrict the extent of facet resection to no more than 50% of the medial facet (33, 36-38) without compromising the surgical exposure needed for tumor resection. Whenever possible, one should leave the facets intact and preserve the facet capsules when performing the muscle detachment. We have also occasionally used external cervical orthosis in high-risk patients (e.g., young patients with preoperative loss of cervical lordosis) although we do not have firm evidence to support this practice.

Patients with progressive neurological decline, functional loss, or intractable pain from a postoperative cervical kyphotic deformity are candidates for operative correction. Flexion and extension films are helpful in assessing the flexibility of the deformity, which is important because those patients that reduce on extension may benefit from preoperative traction. Fixed deformities that do not move because of ankylosis as in our case will require an additional surgical release before correction.

Significant correction can be achieved by anterior distraction through either discectomies or corpectomies followed by placement of interbody grafts (39, 40). Herman and Sonntag (40) studied 20 patients with postlaminectomy cervical kyphosis in whom the mean angle was 38 degrees. They found that traction improved the kyphosis by a mean of 8 degrees and open reduction via only an anterior approach resulted in improvement of 28 degrees. Whenever possible, we prefer to preserve the VBs and perform multilevel discectomies and interbody grafting for interspace distraction to achieve optimal correction. In addition, we also prefer to use a plate because it stabilizes the spine and increases fusion rates, especially in multilevel fusions (41). Postoperatively, we generally prescribe a rigid cervical collar for 3 months in cases of deformity correction.

Occasionally, a combined anterior-posterior approach is needed, especially in extensive anterior procedures that involve multilevel discectomies or corpectomies, in patients who require a posterior decompression or release, or in patients with an unstable spine (39, 42). In these cases, the anterior approach allows for deformity correction while the posterior approach supplements the construct stability.

Sagittal cervical spine deformities can be quite common after laminectomy or laminoplasty in children who have undergone tumor resections. On the basis of our review of the literature, there appears to be no benefit to laminoplasty over laminectomy in terms of postoperative spinal alignment and incidence of kyphotic deformity. We recommend that preoperative imaging be performed as part of risk stratification and a stabilization procedure be considered in high-risk patients. Severe postoperative deformities are treated with surgical stabilization, usually through an anterior approach with multilevel discectomies and fusions with plating. Extensive anterior operations may require additional posterior stabilization.

REFERENCES

[1] Cattell HS, Clark GL, Jr. Cervical kyphosis and instability following multiple laminectomies in children. *J Bone Joint Surg Am.* 1967 Jun;49(4):713-20.

[2] Yasuoka S, Peterson HA, Laws ER, Jr., MacCarty CS. Pathogenesis and prophylaxis of postlaminectomy deformity of the spine after multiple level laminectomy: difference between children and adults. *Neurosurgery.* 1981 Aug;9(2):145-52.

[3] Yasuoka S, Peterson HA, MacCarty CS. Incidence of spinal column deformity after multilevel laminectomy in children and adults. *J Neurosurg.* 1982 Oct;57(4):441-5.

[4] Inoue A, Ikata T, Katoh S. Spinal deformity following surgery for spinal cord tumors and tumorous lesions: analysis based on an assessment of the spinal functional curve. *Spinal Cord.* 1996 Sep;34(9):536-42.

[5] Goel VK, Clark CR, Harris KG, Schulte KR. Kinematics of the cervical spine: effects of multiple total laminectomy and facet wiring. *J Orthop Res.* 1988;6(4):611-9.

[6] Panjabi MM, White AA, 3rd, Johnson RM. Cervical spine mechanics as a function of transection of components. *J Biomech.* 1975 Sep;8(5):327-36.

[7] White AA, 3rd, Panjabi MM, Thomas CL. The clinical biomechanics of kyphotic deformities. *Clin Orthop Relat Res.* 1977 Oct(128):8-17.

[8] Hirabayashi K, Satomi K. Operative procedure and results of expansive open-door laminoplasty. *Spine.* 1988 Jul;13(7):870-6.

[9] Hirabayashi K, Toyama Y, Chiba K. Expansive laminoplasty for myelopathy in ossification of the longitudinal ligament. *Clin Orthop Relat Res.* 1999 Feb(359):35-48.

[10] Hidai Y, Ebara S, Kamimura M, Tateiwa Y, Itoh H, Kinoshita T, et al. Treatment of cervical compressive myelopathy with a new dorsolateral decompressive procedure. *J Neurosurg.* 1999 Apr;90(2 Suppl):178-85.

[11] Baba H, Maezawa Y, Furusawa N, Imura S, Tomita K. Flexibility and alignment of the cervical spine after laminoplasty for spondylotic myelopathy. A radiographic study. *Int Orthop.* 1995;19(2):116-21.

[12] Edwards CC, 2nd, Heller JG, Silcox DH, 3rd. T-Saw laminoplasty for the management of cervical spondylotic myelopathy: clinical and radiographic outcome. *Spine.* 2000 Jul 15;25(14):1788-94.

[13] Fujimura Y, Nishi Y. Atrophy of the nuchal muscle and change in cervical curvature after expansive open-door laminoplasty. *Arch Orthop Trauma Surg.* 1996;115(3-4):203-5.

[14] Hukuda S, Ogata M, Mochizuki T, Shichikawa K. Laminectomy versus laminoplasty for cervical myelopathy: brief report. *J Bone Joint Surg Br.* 1988 Mar;70(2):325-6.

[15] Kawai S, Sunago K, Doi K, Saika M, Taguchi T. Cervical laminoplasty (Hattori's method). Procedure and follow-up results. *Spine.* 1988 Nov;13(11):1245-50.

[16] Kimura I, Shingu H, Nasu Y. Long-term follow-up of cervical spondylotic myelopathy treated by canal-expansive laminoplasty. *J Bone Joint Surg Br.* 1995 Nov;77(6):956-61.

[17] Lee TT, Green BA, Gromelski EB. Safety and stability of open-door cervical expansive laminoplasty. *J Spinal Disord.* 1998 Feb;11(1):12-5.

[18] Lee TT, Manzano GR, Green BA. Modified open-door cervical expansive laminoplasty for spondylotic myelopathy: operative technique, outcome, and predictors for gait improvement. *J Neurosurg.* 1997 Jan;86(1):64-8.

[19] Matsunaga S, Sakou T, Nakanisi K. Analysis of the cervical spine alignment following laminoplasty and laminectomy. *Spinal Cord.* 1999 Jan;37(1):20-4.

[20] Miyazaki K, Tada K, Matsuda Y, Okuno M, Yasuda T, Murakami H. Posterior extensive simultaneous multisegment decompression with posterolateral fusion for cervical myelopathy with cervical instability and kyphotic and/or S-shaped deformities. *Spine.* 1989 Nov;14(11):1160-70.

[21] Mochida J, Nomura T, Chiba M, Nishimura K, Toh E. Modified expansive open-door laminoplasty in cervical myelopathy. *J Spinal Disord.* 1999 Oct;12(5):386-91.

[22] Morio Y, Yamamoto K, Teshima R, Nagashima H, Hagino H. Clinicoradiologic study of cervical laminoplasty with posterolateral fusion or bone graft. *Spine.* 2000 Jan 15;25(2):190-6.

[23] Saruhashi Y, Hukuda S, Katsuura A, Miyahara K, Asajima S, Omura K. A long-term follow-up study of cervical spondylotic myelopathy treated by "French window" laminoplasty. *J Spinal Disord.* 1999 Apr;12(2):99-101.

[24] Sasai K, Saito T, Akagi S, Kato I, Ogawa R. Cervical curvature after laminoplasty for spondylotic myelopathy--involvement of yellow ligament, semispinalis cervicis muscle, and nuchal ligament. *J Spinal Disord.* 2000 Feb;13(1):26-30.

[25] Seichi A, Takeshita K, Ohishi I, Kawaguchi H, Akune T, Anamizu Y, et al. Long-term results of double-door laminoplasty for cervical stenotic myelopathy. *Spine.* 2001 Mar 1;26(5):479-87.

[26] Takayasu M, Takagi T, Nishizawa T, Osuka K, Nakajima T, Yoshida J. Bilateral open-door cervical expansive laminoplasty with hydroxyapatite spacers and titanium screws. *J Neurosurg.* 2002 Jan;96(1 Suppl):22-8.

[27] Tomita K, Kawahara N, Toribatake Y, Heller JG. Expansive midline T-saw laminoplasty (modified spinous process-splitting) for the management of cervical myelopathy. *Spine.* 1998 Jan 1;23(1):32-7.

[28] Wada E, Suzuki S, Kanazawa A, Matsuoka T, Miyamoto S, Yonenobu K. Subtotal corpectomy versus laminoplasty for multilevel cervical spondylotic myelopathy: a long-term follow-up study over 10 years. *Spine.* 2001 Jul 1;26(13):1443-7; discussion 8.

[29] Yonenobu K, Hosono N, Iwasaki M, Asano M, Ono K. Laminoplasty versus subtotal corpectomy. A comparative study of results in multisegmental cervical spondylotic myelopathy. *Spine.* 1992 Nov;17(11):1281-4.

[30] Yue WM, Tan CT, Tan SB, Tan SK, Tay BK. Results of cervical laminoplasty and a comparison between single and double trap-door techniques. *J Spinal Disord.* 2000 Aug;13(4):329-35.

[31] Kaptain GJ, Simmons NE, Replogle RE, Pobereskin L. Incidence and outcome of kyphotic deformity following laminectomy for cervical spondylotic myelopathy. *J Neurosurg.* 2000 Oct;93(2 Suppl):199-204.

[32] Yeh JS, Sgouros S, Walsh AR, Hockley AD. Spinal sagittal malalignment following surgery for primary intramedullary tumours in children. *Pediatr Neurosurg.* 2001 Dec;35(6):318-24.

[33] Zdeblick TA, Zou D, Warden KE, McCabe R, Kunz D, Vanderby R. Cervical stability after foraminotomy. A biomechanical in vitro analysis. *J Bone Joint Surg Am.* 1992 Jan;74(1):22-7.

[34] Zdeblick TA, Abitbol JJ, Kunz DN, McCabe RP, Garfin S. Cervical stability after sequential capsule resection. *Spine.* 1993 Oct 15;18(14):2005-8.

[35] Katsumi Y, Honma T, Nakamura T. Analysis of cervical instability resulting from laminectomies for removal of spinal cord tumor. *Spine.* 1989 Nov;14(11):1171-6.

[36] Epstein JA. The surgical management of cervical spinal stenosis, spondylosis, and myeloradiculopathy by means of the posterior approach. *Spine.* 1988 Jul;13(7):864-9.

[37] Raynor RB, Pugh J, Shapiro I. Cervical facetectomy and its effect on spine strength. *J Neurosurg.* 1985 Aug;63(2):278-82.

[38] Sim FH, Svien HJ, Bickel WH, Janes JM. Swan-neck deformity following extensive cervical laminectomy. A review of twenty-one cases. *J Bone Joint Surg Am.* 1974 Apr;56(3):564-80.

[39] Albert TJ, Vacarro A. Postlaminectomy kyphosis. *Spine.* 1998 Dec 15;23(24):2738-45.

[40] Herman JM, Sonntag VK. Cervical corpectomy and plate fixation for postlaminectomy kyphosis. *J Neurosurg.* 1994 Jun;80(6):963-70.

[41] Kaiser MG, Haid RW, Jr., Subach BR, Barnes B, Rodts GE, Jr. Anterior cervical plating enhances arthrodesis after discectomy and fusion with cortical allograft. Neurosurgery. 2002 Feb;50(2):229-36; discussion 36-8.

[42] Sasso RC, Ruggiero RA, Jr., Reilly TM, Hall PV. Early reconstruction failures after multilevel cervical corpectomy. *Spine.* 2003 Jan 15;28(2):140-2.

Chapter 11

RADIONUCLIDE LABELED GLUCURONIDE PRODRUGS FOR IMAGING AND TARGETING THERAPY OF CANCER

Perihan Unak

Ege University; Institute of Nuclear Sciences; Department of Nuclear Applications; 35100 Bornova Izmir Turkey

ABSTRACT

Glucuronide prodrugs may be useful tools to deposit the therapeutic and imaging agents in the target which enhanced enzyme β-glucuronidase. They can be synthesized through enzymatic, metabolic or chemical ways. The enzyme β-glucuronidase, which hydrolyses glucuronide conjugates, reversing one of the main detoxification and excretion pathways, was found to vary in concentration in different cysts and tumor tissues. Thus targeted delivery of cytotoxic agents and their retention in the tumor cells; decreased cytotoxicity and other side effects in normal tissues; decreased interference that caused by multi drug resistance; targeted delivery of therapeutic radionuclides; uptake and retention in the tumor cells with sitotoxic agents which they label; increased efficiency and synergic potentiation of therapeutic effects of sitotoxic agents and radionuclides can be possible.

The aim of this chapter is to provide a brief overview of current status of applications, advantages and up-to-date research and development of radiolabeled glucuronide prodrugs in cancer imaging and targeted therapy.

INTRODUCTION

Scientists has still been maintained a great deal of effort to develop new agents for imaging and therapy to overcome cancer disease. The basic principles of drug design have involved "prodrug" concept, which means a molecule which is not itself active as an anticancer drug, but it can be transformed to an active structure after its administration. Prodrugs can be activated onto the tumor cells by some kind of enzymes. In this perspective, the activation of glucuronide prodrugs by β-glucuronidase has great potential applications in cancer chemotherapy. These drugs enhance tumor selectivity and reduce the systemic toxicity of anti-cancer agents and they may be excellent carriers of therapeutic aglycons for targeting tumor selectively. They may be good carrying agents with radionuclide labeled aglycons both for radionuclide tumor therapy and molecular imaging depend on the radionuclide decay properties. Thus, glucuronide prodrug-mediated radionuclide targeting therapy may have both diagnostic and therapeutic applications for cancer and have beneficial effect such as maximum dose and minimum toxic effect.

The enzyme β-glucuronidase has already been proven to be useful in tumor specific bioactivation of glucuronide prodrugs of anticancer agents.(1, 2) Indeed, several glucuronide prodrugs have already been selectively activated by β-glucuronidase, either present in high concentration in necrotic tumor areas (PMT) (3, 4) or previously targeted to the tumor sites antibody directed enzyme prodrug therapy (ADEPT), gene-directed enzyme prodrug therapy (GDEPT) (5), and consequently demonstrated superior efficacy in vivo compared to standard chemotherapy (6). These results were attributed to the increased drug deposition and retention in the tumor connected with reduced anticancer agent concentration in normal tissues, considerably lowering the destruction of normal cells. Therefore, glucuronide prodrugs are activated by human enzyme β-glucuronidase in antibody-directed enzyme prodrug therapy (ADEPT) and gene directed-enzyme prodrug therapy (GDEPT). These drugs enhance tumor selectivity and reduce the systemic toxicity of anti-cancer agents.

SYNTHESIS METHODS OF GLUCURONIDE PRODRUGS

Both traditional chemical,(7, 8) enzymatic and metabolic methods have been presented for the synthesis of glucuronide conjugates. Each approach has its advantages and disadvantages. In the case of biosynthetic reactions, yields are dependent on the enzyme activity, and it may be difficult to obtain a sufficient amount of product at reasonable cost. While traditional chemical syntheses of glucuronides offer good yields, frequently side products are formed as well. Enzyme-catalyzed reactions are usually more regio- and stereospecific compared to chemical syntheses.

Metabolic Method

Metabolic method is in vivo synthesis mode of the glucuronides in the liver by UDP-glucuronosyltransferases enzyme. The formation of glucuronide conjugates in the living metabolism is known well as a major detoxification pathway for rapidly elimination of toxic chemical agents been administrated. So, the toxic and, in general, water-insoluble materials can easily be transformed to non-toxic and water-soluble forms, and rapidly excreted by the metabolism. The glucuronidation mechanism is firstly started by the hydroxylation of toxic material in the liver by an enzyme specific to its hydroxylation, and then is completed by the transformation of this hydroxylated specie to its glucuronide conjugate by UDP-glucuronyl transferase. Briefly, metabolically synthesized glucuronide extract from urine sample after orally administration of aglycon in an animal model.

Enzymatic Method

UDP-Glucuronosyltransferases:

UDP-glucuronosyltransferases enzymes are present in many tissues, mostly in the liver but also in kidney, small intestines, lungs, skin, adrenals and spleen. The enzyme is mainly located in the membrane of the hepatic endoplasmic reticulum fractions and is therefore ideally positioned to glucuronidate the products of the mixed-function oxidase reactions.

GLUCURONIDATION REACTION

At present, only a small amount of glucuronide metabolites are commercially available. Both traditional chemical and enzymatic methods have been presented for the synthesis of glucuronide conjugates. Each approach has its advantages and disadvantages. In the case of biosynthetic reactions, yields are dependent on the enzyme activity, and it may be difficult to obtain a sufficient amount of product at reasonable cost. While traditional chemical synthesis of glucuronides offer good yields, frequently side products are formed as well. Enzyme-catalyzed reactions are usually more regio- and stereospecific compared to chemical synthesis.

Glucuronidation involves the transfer of glucuronic acid, from the endogenous co-factor UDP-glucuronic acid (UDPGA), to a wide range of endogenous and exogeneous aglycone substrates, possessing functional groups such as –OR, -SR, -NR1R2 or –CR. Many drugs are metabolised through glucuronide conjugation acid (9).

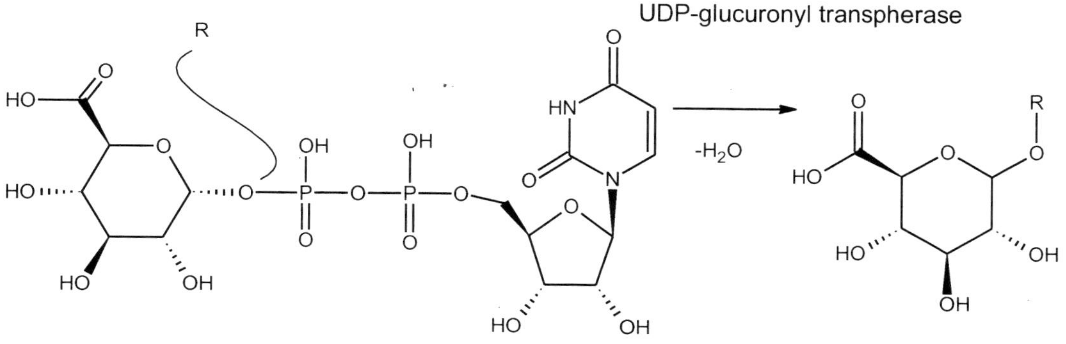

Figure 1. Enzymatic Synthesize Mechanism Of Glucuronides.

Human UDP-glucuronosyltransferases (UGTs) are a family of membrane-bound enzymes of the endoplasmic reticulum. The reaction of UDPGT with a simple phenol, R-OH is represented in the Figure 1. The reaction is reversible, and therefore the possibility of transglucuronylation from one aglycone to another

PROPERTIES OF β-GLUCURONIDASE

All mammalian tissues contain a group specific enzyme that catalyses the hydrolysis of the biosynthetic β-D-glucopyranosiduronic acids of all types to the aglycons and D-glucuronic acid (10, 11). This enzyme is commonly known as β-glucuronidase which hydrolyses conjugated glucuronides, but does not act on α or β-glucosides (12, 13). β-D-glucopyranosiduronic acids will often be referred to as β-glucuronides.

Location of the Enzyme β-Glucuronidase in the Mammalian Cell

The intracellular distribution of β-glucuronidase activity has been studied in homogenates of mouse and rat tissues made in different ways. Subcellular particles were separated by centrifuging at high speeds, or at low speeds after agglutination with slightly acidic buffers, to yield optically clear supernatant liquors. In brief, it was concluded that, whatever the level of β-glucuronidase activity, nearly all the enzyme in the mammalian cell was present in the cytoplasmic granules (mitochondria and microsomes) (14), and was apparently spread over granules of all sizes; little, if any, was in the nuclei or free in the cytoplasm (10, 15).

β-GLUCURONIDASE ACTIVITY IN TUMOURS

Fishman reported first time human cancer tissues are relatively rich in β-glucuronidase (10, 15).

The highest concentration of this enzyme is found in liver, spleen and kidney. It is also present in certain tissues of the endocrine and reproductive systems. Since the early work of Fishman et al (16), it has been known that, as a rule, homogenates of human tumour tissues contain higher β-glucuronidase activity than adjacent uninvolved tissue. β-Glucuronidase activity up to 25 times higher in tumour than in surrounding tissue has been reported (15). This enzyme is also higher in mouse tumours than in the normal tissue of mice (17).

Many tumours show elevated levels of hydrolytic enzymes that may be associated with invasive processes. The RIF-1 murine tumour has levels of β-glucuronidase that are more than four times higher than those in liver (18). Elevated tumour β-glucuronidase levels can be used as a basis for tumor-targeted therapy when systemically administered glucuronides of cytotoxic drugs are deconjugated preferentially at the tumour site. The invasive phenotype of malignant cells also requires the expression of hydrolytic enzymes for digesting the extra cellular matrix of surrounding normal tissues. The enhanced expression of proteolytic and glycosidic enzymes at the cell surface may be part of a combination of properties that marks the malignant phenotype (19) and may be associated with the phenomenon of tumour metastasis (20).

CHEMICAL SYNTHESIS METHODS

Naturally, most of the methods for glucuronide synthesis have their parallel in glucoside synthesis. Glucuronides have their own distinctive chemistry, however, and are usually more difficult to prepare than the corresponding glucopyranosides. A clear majority of all glucuronides have been synthesized *via* acyl-protected intermediates: starting with the commercially available d-glucurono-6,3-lactone ('glucurone') Schmidt and coworkers (21) have in fact drawn up a glycosidation 'league table', in *increasing* ease of glycosyl donation: glycuronates<aldoses< deoxy sugars<ketoses<3-deoxy-2-glyculosonates. That is, of all common sugars, glycuronates require the highest activation for a given aglycone.

Koenigs-Knorr reaction is most used chemical method of glucuronidation for the synthesis of a wide range of alkyl and aryl glucuronides. It based on the or related procedures but often suffer from poor yields and side reactions due to the low reactivity of glucuronic acid derived glycosyl donors and require one or more deprotection steps to liberate free glucuronide. Catalysts used are typically AgI salts, especially Ag_2CO_3, $Hg(CN)_2$ or $CdCO_3$. (22)

Schmidt trichloroacetimidate method is another methode for chemical synthesize of glucuronides. a number of important steroidal secondary alcohols have been synthesized such as androsterone, epiandrosterone, 17-acetoxy-androstane-3a,17b-diol, 11a-hydroxyprogesterone, and 3-benzoylestradiol, 11a-hydroxyprogesterone and 3-benzoylestradiol (23)

Potential Radionuclides for Labeling of Glucuronide Prodrugs for Therapy and Imaging

Table 1. Physical Characteristics of Radionuclides that have potential for Targeted Radionuclide Therapy

Nuclide	Half-Life	Emission	Max Range
^{80m}Br	4.42 h	Auger	<10 nm
^{125}I	60.0 h	Auger	10 nm
^{211}At	7.2 h	Alpha, Auger	65 nm
^{169}Er	9.5 d	Beta	1 mm
^{67}Cu	2.58 d	Beta/gamma	2.2 mm
^{131}I	8.04 d	Beta/gamma	2.4 mm
^{153}Sm	1.95 d	Beta/gamma	3.0 mm
^{198}Au	2.7 d	Beta/gamma	4.4 mm
^{186}Re	3.77 d	Beta/gamma	5.0 mm
^{165}Dy	2.33 d	Beta/gamma	6.4 mm
^{89}Sr	50.5 d	Beta	8.0 mm
^{32}P	14.3 d	Beta	8.7 mm
^{90}Y	2.67 d	Beta	12 mm

Table 1 shows some of the radionuclides, which have different decay characteristics, and emit particles with different LET and different range. Some of these radionuclides emit photons in addition to particle emission which make them suitable for monitoring the therapy with imaging, and for continuous follow-up of the absorbed dose distribution. Also, preadministration of the therapeutic ligands is possible in estimating the absorbed dose per unit administered activity. Where there is no emission of photons, bremstrahlung imaging might be a solution.

Both SPECT or PET radionuclides showed in Table 2 and Table 3 can be used for glucuronides prodrugs for imaging.

Table 2. PET Radionuclides

Radionuclide	Half-life	Positron Energies (keV)	Production
^{11}C	20.5 min	960	Cyclotron
^{13}N	10.0 min	1198	Cyclotron
^{15}O	2.0 min	1732	Cyclotron
^{18}F	110 min	634	Cyclotron
^{82}Rb	1.2 min	3356	^{82}Sr/^{82}Rb

Table 3. SPECT Radionuclides

Radionuclide	Decay Mode	Half Life	Photon Energies(keV)
^{67}Ga	EC	78.3 hrs	93, 185
^{99m}Tc	IT	6.01 hrs	141
^{111}In	EC	67.9 hrs	171, 245
^{123}I	EC	13.2 hrs	159

Table 3 shows some of the radionuclides, which can be used for therapy. Some of the radionuclides such as Sc-47, Rh-105, In-111, I-123, I-131, Nd-147, Pm-151, Sm-153, Ho-166, Gd-159, Tb-161, Er-171, Re-186, Re-188, Tl-201 have potentials in both therapy and diagnosis since they have appropriate decay characteristics for imaging and therapeutic studies. Although they have theoretical therapeutically potentials, In-111, I-123 and Tl-201 are commonly used as diagnostic nuclides. The selection of the optimal radionuclide may depend on the details of the clinical situation, such as the size and type of the tumor, and the particular carrier molecule to be used. Direct comparisons of various radionuclides are required to identify the optimal approach. However, to use of Auger and conversion electron emitters appears to have substantial advantages for single cell killing, in the therapy of micrometastases. Tumor therapy may require a mixture of radionuclides intended to kill both single cells and large tumor masses (24). Auger and conversion electrons can kill cells effectively, with at least 6 logs of cell. Conjugated ligands on the cell surface are only slightly less potent than carrier molecules internalized into the cytoplasm, and this is agree with theoretical considerations. α-particles can kill single cells very effectively, but the short half-lives of the available α-particle emitters are probably a disadvantage. High energy β-particles can also kill single cells if they bind in sufficient amounts, but they have a disadvantage due to their nonspecific toxicity.

Radiolabeled glucuronide derivatives can be used for therapy and tumor imaging depending properties of radioiodine for the beta glucuronidase rich tissues, since glucuronidation leads to rapid and higher incorporation on cancer cell.

RADIONUCLIDE LABELED GLUCURONIDE PRODRUGS

Radioiodinates (I-125 or I-131) and Tc-99m are the most common radionuclides for the labeling of glucuronide prodrugs (25-29); Biber at al., 2006, Ertay et al., 2007, Avcibasi et al., 2008; Enginar et al., 2009). SPECT or PET radionuclides for imaging (table 2 and table 3) or therapy radionuclides (table 4) for targeted radionuclide therapy may also be used for radiolabeling of glucuronides. Toremifene (30), Tamoxifene(31), Codein(29), Morphine(32), Bleomycin A(33), aniline mustard(34) as drug aglycons; aniline and phenol phatelein as aromatic compounds (33); 8-hydroxyquinoline (25, 26) as chelating agent; uracil (35), as nucleotide; exorphine-c as peptide (28, 36); Estradiol (27), diethylstilbestrol (37) as hormons; magnetite (35) as nanoparticles were used to generate radiolabeled glucuronides. General pharmacokinetic profile of radiolabeled glucuronides is fast renal clearance from the body and less liver uptake. Imaging studies with mammary tumor bearing rats showed that ^{99m}Tc-DTPA attached estrogen glucuronide (ESTDTPAG) the breast tumors could be well visualized up to 24 h (Figure 2) (27). Similar results obtained with a peptide glucuronide called exorphin C glucuronide (36). Tumor/muscle ratios were similar for both radiolabeled glucuronides.

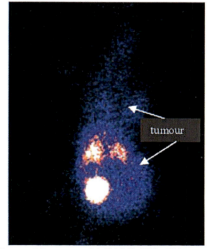

Ref Biber et al, Applied Radiation and Isotopes 64 (2006) 778–788).

Figure 2 The imaging on mammary tumor bearing female Albino Wistar rats after 1 h postinjection of ^{99m}Tc labeled deoxy demethyl homoestradiolyl diethylenetriamine pentaacetic acid (ESTDTPA).

CONCLUSION

Some kinds of cancer cells are reach in enzyme β-glucuronidase respecting to normal cells (38, 39) and glucuronide prodrugs could be converted to antineoplastic agents by these enzymes without seriously damaging surrounding normal tissues.

Radiolabeled glucuronide derivatives can be used for therapy and tumor imaging depending properties of radioiodine for the beta glucuronidase rich tissues, since glucuronidation leads to rapid and higher incorporation on cancer cell.

REFERENCES

[1] Sperker B, Backman JT, Kroemer HK. The role of beta-glucuronidase in drug disposition and drug targeting in humans. *Clin Pharmacokinet*. 1997 Jul;33(1):18-31.

[2] Sperker B, Werner U, Murdter TE, Tekkaya C, Fritz P, Wacke R, et al. Expression and function of beta-glucuronidase in pancreatic cancer: potential role in drug targeting. *Naunyn Schmiedebergs Arch Pharmacol*. 2000 Aug;362(2):110-5.

[3] Angenault S, Thirot S, Schmidt F, Monneret C, Pfeiffer B, Renard P. Cancer chemotherapy: a SN-38 (7-ethyl-10-hydroxycamptothecin) glucuronide prodrug for treatment by a PMT (Prodrug MonoTherapy) strategy. *Bioorg Med Chem Lett*. 2003 Mar 10;13(5):947-50.

[4] de Graaf M, Boven E, Scheeren HW, Haisma HJ, Pinedo HM. Beta-glucuronidase-mediated drug release. *Curr Pharm Des*. 2002;8(15):1391-403.

[5] Chen KC, Cheng TL, Leu YL, Prijovich ZM, Chuang CH, Chen BM, et al. Membrane-localized activation of glucuronide prodrugs by beta-glucuronidase enzymes. *Cancer Gene Ther*. 2007 Feb;14(2):187-200.

[6] Unak T. Potential use of radiolabeled glucuronide prodrugs with auger and/or alpha emitters in combined chemo- and radio-therapy of cancer. *Curr Pharm Des*. 2000 Jul;6(11):1127-42.

[7] Kaspersen FM, Van Boeckel CA. A review of the methods of chemical synthesis of sulphate and glucuronide conjugates. *Xenobiotica*. 1987 Dec;17(12):1451-71.

[8] Stachulski AV, Jenkins GN. The synthesis of O-glucuronides. *Nat Prod Rep*. 1998 Apr;15(2):173-86.

[9] Tephly TR, Burchell B. UDP-glucuronosyltransferases: a family of detoxifying enzymes. *Trends Pharmacol Sci*. 1990 Jul;11(7):276-9.

[10] Fishman WH. The 1993 ISOBM Abbott Award Lecture. Isozymes, tumor markers and oncodevelopmental biology. *Tumour Biol*. 1995;16(6):394-402.

[11] Levvy GA, Marsh CA. Preparation and properties of beta-glucuronidase. *Adv Carbohydr Chem*. 1959;14:381-428.

[12] Anghileri LJ, Miller ES. Beta-glucuronidase activity in tumors. Accumulation of radioiodinated phenolphthalein. *Oncology*. 1971;25(1):19-32.

[13] Ho KJ. A large-scale purification of beta-glucuronidase from human liver by immunoaffinity chromatography. *Biotechnol Appl Biochem*. 1991 Dec;14(3):296-305.

[14] Fishman WH. The influence of steroids on β-Glucuronidase of mouse kidneys, in Dorfman RI (ed): Methods in hormone research. New York, Academic Press. 1965;4:273-326.
[15] Fishman WHaA, A. J. The presence of high β-Glucuronidase activity in cancer tissue. *Journal of Biological Chemistry*. 1947;169:449-50.
[16] Fishman WH. B-Glucuronidase Activity of the Blood and Tissues of Obstetrical and Surgical Patients. *Science*. 1947 Jun 20;105(2738):646-7.
[17] Cohen SL, Bittner JJ. The effect of mammary tumors on the glucuronidase and esterase activities in a number of mouse strains. *Cancer Res*. 1951 Sep;11(9):723-6.
[18] Henle KJ, Monson TP, Nagle WA, Moss AJ. Tumor-targeted cell killing with 8-hydroxyquinolyl-glucuronide. *Radiat Res*. 1988 Aug;115(2):373-86.
[19] Dano K, Andreasen PA, Grondahl-Hansen J, Kristensen P, Nielsen LS, Skriver L. Plasminogen activators, tissue degradation, and cancer. *Adv Cancer Res*. 1985;44:139-266.
[20] Nicolson GL. Cell surface molecules and tumor metastasis. Regulation of metastatic phenotypic diversity. *Exp Cell Res*. 1984 Jan;150(1):3-22.
[21] Thomas Müller RS, Richard R. Schmidt. Utility of glycosyl phosphites as glycosyl donors-fructofuranosyl and 2-deoxyhexopyranosyl phosphites in glycoside bond formation. *Tetrahedron Lett*. 1994;35:4763-6.
[22] Stachulski A.V. and Jenkins G. N., The synthesis of O-glucuronides *Xenobiotica*. 1987;1451(17):173-86.
[23] Harding JR, King CD, Perrie JA, Sinnott D, Stachulski AV. Glucuronidation of steroidal alcohols using iodosugar and imidate donors. *Org Biomol Chem*. 2005 Apr 21;3(8):1501-7.
[24] Mattes MJ. Radionuclide-antibody conjugates for single-cell cytotoxicity. *Cancer*. 2002 Feb 15;94(4 Suppl):1215-23.
[25] Unak T, Unak P. Direct radioiodination of metabolic 8-hydroxy-quinolyl-glucuronide, as a potential anti-cancer drug. *Appl Radiat Isot*. 1996 Jul;47(7):645-7.
[26] Unak T, Unak P, Ongun B, Duman Y. Synthesis and iodine-125 labelling of glucuronide compounds for combined chemo- and radiotherapy of cancer. *Appl Radiat Isot*. 1997 Jun;48(6):777-83.
[27] Biber FZ, Unak P, Ertay T, Medine EI, Zihnioglu F, Tasci C, et al. Synthesis of an estradiol glucuronide derivative and investigation of its radiopharmaceutical potential. *Appl Radiat Isot*. 2006 Jul;64(7):778-88.
[28] Ertay T, Unak P, Biber FZ, Tasci C, Zihnioglu F, Durak H. Scintigraphic imaging with a peptide glucuronide in rabbits: 99mTc- exorphin C glucuronide. *Appl Radiat Isot*. 2007 Feb;65(2):170-5.
[29] Enginar H., Unak P., Lambrecht F. Y., Müftüler F. Z. B., Medine E. I., Yolcular S., Yurt A., Seyitoğlu B., Bulduk I. Radiolabeling of codeine with 131I and its biodistribution in rats. *Journal of Radioanalytical and Nuclear Chemistry*. 2009;280(2):367-74.
[30] Biber Muftuler F. Z., Unak P., H. Enginar, S. Yolcular, A. Yurt, Ç. Acar. Synthesis of Novel Anti Estrogen Glucuronide Radioligand. *The Fifth Conferance Nuclear Science and Its Application*. 2008:149.
[31] Biber Müftüler F. Z., Unak P., Ç. Acar İchedef, İ. Demir, . Synthesis Of Antiestrogen Glucuronide Compound (TAM-G).) *IESS2008, International Enyme and Enzyme Engineering Symposium*. 2008:167.

[32] Enginar H., Unak P., F. Z. Biber Müftüler, F. Y. Lambrecht, B. Seyitoğlu, A. Yurt, S. Yolcular, E. İ. Medine, İ Bulduk. Synthesis, Radiolabelling And In Vivo Tissue Distribution Of Morphine Glucuronide. *The Quarterly Journal of Nuclear Medicine and Molecular Imaging*. 2008;52(1).

[33] Avcibasi U, Avcibasi N, Unak T, Unak P, Muftuler FZ, Yildirim Y, et al. Metabolic comparison of radiolabeled aniline- and phenol-phthaleins with (131)I. *Nucl Med Biol*. 2008 May;35(4):481-92.

[34] Ünak T. Akgün Z., Y. Duman, Y. Yildirim, U. Avcibasi B. Çetinkaya. Radioiodination and preliminary biological tests of aniline-mustard, and its glucuronide conjugate as a potential anticancer prodrug. *Journal of Radioanalytical and Nuclear Chemistry*. 2003;256(3):529-34.

[35] Unak P., Medine E.I., Sakarya S., Yürekli Y., Radyonüklid işaretli manyetik nanopartiküllerin sentezi ve terapötik potansiyellerinin hücre düzeyinde incelenmesi. TÜBİTAK projesi SBAG 3293 (105S486). 2008:135.

[36] Ertay T., Unak P., Özdoğan O., Biber F.Z., Zihnioglu F., Medine E. İ., Durak H. 99mtc-Exorphin-Glucuronide in Tumor Diagnosis: Preparation And Biodistribution Studies in Rats. *Journal Of Radioanalytical And Nuclear Chemistry*. 2006;269(1):21-8.

[37] T. Yılmaz, Unak P., F. Z. Biber Müftüler, Ç. Acar İçhedef, E. İ. Medine, T. Ünak. Dietilstilbstrol'un (DES) Glukuronidasyonu ve 131I ile işaretlenerek radyofarmasötik potansiyelinin incelenmesi. X Ulusal Nükleer Bilimler ve Teknolojileri Kongresi. 2009;1:139-46.

[38] Liotta LA, Rao, C. N. and Barsky, S. H. Tumor invas and the extracellular matrix. *Laboratory Investigation*. 1982;49:636.

[39] Chatterjee SK, Chowdhury, K., Matta, M., Crichard, K., Sharma, M. and Bernacki, J. Role of glycosidases in human ovarian carcinoma cellmediated degradation subendothelial extracellular matrix. *Cancer Research*. 1987;47:4634.

INDEX

A

acid, 30, 33, 53, 68, 127, 148, 151, 157, 200, 241, 242, 243, 245
acidosis, 71, 73, 75
acquired immunodeficiency syndrome, 207
active centers, 53
active transport, 73
acute lymphoblastic leukemia, 82
adaptation, 14, 66, 84, 85, 87
adenine, 201
adenocarcinoma, 7, 14, 33, 34, 35, 37, 38, 41, 43, 46, 48, 50, 51, 53, 54, 56, 57, 62, 96, 153
adenosine, 86, 196
adenovirus, 155, 223, 225
adhesion, 25, 26, 27, 31, 32, 68, 97, 146, 148, 190
adipose, 45, 46
adjustment, 174
adolescents, viii, 58, 99, 100, 103, 105
ADP, 201, 205
adsorption, 53
adulthood, 104
adverse event, 203, 206, 207, 208
aetiology, 210
age, 7, 102, 104, 105, 117, 120, 186, 228, 234
agglutination, 242
aggregation, 223
aggressive behavior, 187, 193
aggressiveness, 78
AIBN, 33
AIDS, 30, 154
alanine, 8
alanine aminotransferase, 8
albumin, 146, 148, 150, 153, 219
alcohols, 243, 247

algorithm, 174
allele, 119
alloys, 63
alpha-fetoprotein, 59
alters, 169
alveoli, 47
amalgam, 4
ammonia, 33, 53
amplitude, 18, 27
amylase, 8
analgesic, 171, 220
anatomy, 57
anemia, 82, 208
angiogenesis, x, 67, 79, 82, 85, 87, 88, 89, 91, 94, 97, 144, 145, 148, 149, 154, 156, 157, 158, 166, 179, 183, 184, 187, 188, 189, 190, 191, 192, 193, 194, 195, 196, 197, 198
angiogenic process, 195
angiotensin converting enzyme, 156
angiotensin II, 153
anhydrase, 68, 71, 73, 76, 80, 83, 87, 88, 90, 91, 93, 94, 95, 96, 97
aniline, 5, 245, 248
ankylosis, 235
anoxia, 198
antagonism, 71
anti-angiogenic agents, 193
antibiotic, 172, 207
antibody, 115, 118, 119, 120, 122, 128, 129, 158, 166, 223, 240, 247
anti-cancer, 114, 240, 247
anticancer activity, 62
anticancer drug, 69, 71, 73, 74, 85, 143, 149, 180, 210, 239
antiemetics, 201, 207
antigen, 20, 29, 61, 63, 88, 110, 111, 114, 115, 119, 120, 122, 124, 126, 131, 214

antioxidant, 10, 12, 14
antitumor, vii, 2, 3, 18, 20, 21, 32, 39, 55, 56, 57, 58, 142, 151, 153, 157, 160, 178, 182, 204, 205, 207, 223
antitumor agent, 151, 153
APC, 112, 113, 115, 122, 126
aplasia, xi, 199, 208
aplastic anemia, 208, 212
apoptosis, 12, 20, 58, 60, 63, 71, 73, 75, 76, 84, 90, 93, 96, 114, 115, 128, 147, 148, 151, 156, 160, 188, 191, 193, 195, 205, 215
aqueous solutions, 169
arginine, 127, 150
aromatic compounds, 245
arrest, 94, 127, 191, 205
arsenic, 7, 8, 16, 56
arteries, xi, 150, 214, 215, 217, 218, 220, 225
arteriovenous shunt, 67, 84
artery, 40, 45, 150, 214, 218, 219, 222, 223, 226
arthrodesis, 238
aryl hydrocarbon receptor, 67
ascites, 69, 79, 95
ascorbic acid, 30
aspartate, 8
assessment, 170, 181, 225, 236
assumptions, 174
astrocytes, 113, 185
astrocytoma, viii, x, 66, 69, 83, 84, 92, 106, 185, 186, 187, 192, 193, 199, 207, 211
ATP, 69, 70, 71, 73, 74, 75, 79, 93, 94, 121
atrophy, 59, 234
authors, xi, 14, 22, 30, 86, 100, 104, 105, 202, 203, 224, 227, 233, 234
autologous bone marrow transplant, 61
automation, 5
availability, vii, 2, 21, 69, 70, 72, 73, 75, 78, 201, 215

B

background, 78, 86, 101, 102
bacteriostatic, 71
barriers, ix, 3, 46, 57, 119, 141, 144, 147, 152, 154, 162, 164, 178
basal ganglia, 186
basal lamina, 187
basement membrane, 145, 147, 148, 158, 189
behavior, 75, 185
Beijing, 225
beneficial effect, 240
benign, xi, 7, 10, 11, 12, 13, 60, 185, 214, 223, 224
benign prostatic hyperplasia, 224
benign tumors, 185

benzodiazepine, 70
beryllium, 16
bicarbonate, viii, 66, 68, 73
bile, 40, 45
bile duct, 40, 45
binding, viii, 66, 67, 82, 85, 88, 89, 91, 93, 98, 129, 148, 156, 172, 178, 189, 190, 191, 192, 195
bioavailability, 215
biodegradation, 5
biological activity, 53
biological behavior, 102
biological processes, 53, 68, 81
biological responses, 189
biological systems, 33
biomechanics, 236
biopolymer, 32, 179
biosynthesis, 74
biotechnology, 180
bladder, 68, 215, 219, 220, 221
blocks, vii, viii, 14, 66, 67, 68, 191
blood, 4, 6, 7, 8, 13, 14, 15, 16, 18, 19, 20, 45, 56, 67, 71, 79, 84, 93, 126, 142, 143, 144, 145, 146, 147, 148, 149, 150, 151, 152, 153, 154, 155, 156, 159, 164, 179, 181, 187, 188, 189, 192, 193, 200, 208, 216, 218
blood flow, 84, 93, 145, 146, 147, 148, 152, 153, 154, 155, 156, 159, 179
blood pressure, 147, 156
blood stream, 146
blood supply, 79, 155, 187, 188, 218
blood vessels, 142, 144, 146, 148, 149, 151, 154, 156, 187, 188, 189, 193
blood-brain barrier, 200
bloodstream, 145, 168
body weight, 34
bone, xi, 3, 22, 23, 29, 32, 58, 60, 61, 79, 119, 145, 156, 199, 202, 208, 231, 237
bone cells, 61
bone form, 32
bone marrow, xi, 3, 58, 60, 79, 119, 145, 156, 199, 202, 208
bone marrow transplant, xi, 119, 199, 208
bones, 61
bowel, 220
brachial plexus, 228, 229
brachytherapy, 204, 215
bradykinin, 158
brain, viii, 6, 66, 68, 69, 70, 71, 73, 74, 75, 82, 84, 86, 88, 91, 93, 95, 99, 100, 105, 111, 112, 113, 114, 117, 124, 128, 131, 154, 184, 186, 187, 188, 192, 193, 194, 196, 198, 203, 209, 210
brain tumor, viii, 66, 73, 74, 75, 82, 86, 91, 105, 117, 131, 154, 186, 194, 196, 198, 203, 209, 210

brainstem, 186
Brazil, 99
breakdown, 115, 127
breast cancer, 18, 60, 79, 87, 88, 92, 123, 159, 177, 187
breast carcinoma, 82, 86, 87
bronchial epithelium, 47
buffer, 19, 30, 33, 34, 35, 36, 46, 47

C

cadmium, 7, 8, 12, 14, 16, 18, 56, 58
calcium, 29, 30, 31, 86
Canada, 154, 203, 211, 213, 216, 223, 224
cancer cells, vii, 14, 69, 70, 71, 72, 78, 79, 84, 86, 93, 96, 112, 116, 118, 123, 142, 143, 146, 147, 150, 154, 205, 246
candidates, 235
capillary, 71, 187
capsule, 51, 169, 219, 221, 234, 237
carbon, 3, 4, 23, 28, 29, 30, 32, 33, 35, 40, 46, 47, 50, 52, 53, 54, 55, 56, 57, 68, 70, 73
carbon dioxide, 68, 73
carcinogenesis, vii, 10, 16, 62, 86, 92, 95
carcinoma, 7, 14, 82, 88, 97, 102, 121, 157, 188, 248
cardiovascular system, 6
carrier, 19, 20, 21, 40, 46, 47, 56, 63, 146, 164, 168, 170, 177, 244
catalyst, 205
catalytic activity, 22, 73, 75, 79
catalytic properties, 97
catheter, 168, 169, 173, 174, 218
cation, 20, 201
CD95, 8, 14, 15, 16, 20, 56
cell culture, 22, 23, 25, 26, 27, 29, 61
cell cycle, 29, 91, 92, 122, 124, 191
cell death, 56, 58, 111, 115, 123, 159, 188, 202, 205
cell killing, 244, 247
cell line, vii, ix, 2, 3, 17, 18, 56, 63, 71, 72, 73, 75, 77, 78, 81, 86, 94, 110, 111, 115, 118, 119, 120, 122, 123, 124, 127, 130, 131, 132, 133
cell lines, vii, ix, 2, 3, 17, 18, 56, 71, 72, 73, 75, 77, 78, 81, 86, 94, 110, 111, 115, 118, 119, 120, 123, 124, 127, 130, 131, 132, 133
cell membranes, 172
cell metabolism, viii, 66, 85
cell surface, 68, 114, 122, 128, 242, 245
cellular regulation, 92
central nervous system, viii, 6, 99, 107, 185, 186, 194, 200, 211
cerebellum, 186
cerebral hemisphere, 102, 186
cervical cancer, 86, 93

cervical laminectomy, xi, 227, 228, 232, 233, 234, 238
cervix, 68, 82, 86, 90
chemical properties, 22, 53, 59
chemical reactions, 53
chemical stability, 78
chemokines, 128, 146
chemotherapeutic agent, ix, 71, 141, 164, 193
chemotherapy, vii, ix, 2, 5, 20, 54, 57, 72, 79, 87, 113, 123, 142, 143, 149, 152, 153, 161, 163, 164, 166, 180, 186, 193, 200, 201, 203, 204, 207, 208, 210, 211, 240, 246
childhood, 99, 101
children, viii, xi, 99, 100, 101, 102, 103, 105, 185, 227, 228, 232, 233, 234, 235, 236, 237
China, 33
chloroform, 88
choroid, 68, 102, 103, 105, 108
chromatography, 3, 33, 246
chromium, 3, 7, 10, 12, 13, 14, 16, 18, 19, 20, 56, 60
chromosomal abnormalities, 106, 191
chromosome, 100, 101, 102, 104, 105, 107, 108, 124, 191, 202
chronic hypoxia, 96
chronic renal failure, 82
circulation, 143, 144, 164, 180, 215
classification, viii, 57, 99, 100, 107, 127, 130, 194
clinical diagnosis, 194
clinical oncology, 58
clinical trials, x, xi, 79, 123, 161, 168, 177, 193, 199, 200, 215, 223
CNS, viii, ix, 99, 102, 110, 111, 118, 119, 120, 124, 130, 131, 132, 133, 134
CO2, 74
coagulation, 175, 179
collagen, 147, 150, 151, 155, 156
collateral, 113, 217
collateral damage, 113
colon, 7, 16, 18, 96, 153, 198
colon cancer, 198
colorectal cancer, 60, 61, 80, 96, 215
combination therapy, 158
complement, 102, 104, 131
complementary DNA, 93
complications, 21, 56, 215, 220, 224
components, 22, 34, 35, 53, 57, 146, 148, 189, 236
composites, vii, 2, 3, 22, 33, 34, 35, 46, 53, 54, 55, 56, 57
composition, 7, 16, 22, 23, 30, 34, 146
compounds, 4, 59, 82, 171, 247
compression, 146, 232, 233
computed tomography, 163, 164, 230

concentration, xi, xii, 3, 4, 5, 7, 8, 12, 13, 14, 16, 18, 19, 20, 22, 23, 24, 25, 26, 27, 28, 30, 32, 35, 54, 56, 71, 73, 76, 81, 163, 169, 170, 171, 172, 173, 174, 175, 176, 178, 201, 214, 215, 216, 217, 219, 220, 239, 240, 242
confidence, 165, 176
confidence interval, 165, 176
congestion, 42, 45, 47, 51
conjugation, 143, 241
connective tissue, 155
constitutive enzyme, 127
consumption, 69, 70
continuity, 20, 33, 45
control, vii, 2, 3, 5, 16, 18, 19, 20, 22, 23, 24, 25, 26, 27, 28, 56, 59, 70, 75, 77, 81, 83, 84, 91, 95, 113, 123, 132, 148, 150, 151, 152, 154, 177, 180, 181, 191, 205, 216, 220
control group, 84
conversion, 244
copper, 3, 7, 8, 10, 14, 16, 56, 58, 59
correlation, vii, x, 7, 14, 16, 56, 65, 66, 75, 83, 84, 87, 93, 97, 147, 155, 166, 167, 170, 171, 183, 184, 191, 193, 196, 210, 234
correlation analysis, 56
correlation coefficient, 16, 167
counseling, 234
CSF, 114, 121, 122
cultivation, 24, 26, 27, 30, 31, 35, 167
culture, 26, 27, 28, 29, 30, 31, 34, 111
cycles, 78, 202, 203, 207, 208, 209, 216, 217, 223
cyclooxygenase, 127, 158
cyclophosphamide, 152, 160
cystoscopy, 221
cytochrome, 10, 70, 124
cytokines, ix, 2, 18, 20, 22, 29, 110, 114, 115, 122, 124, 125, 128, 133, 149, 189
cytometry, 8, 118, 123, 128
cytoplasm, 40, 42, 45, 242, 245
cytotoxic agents, xii, 239
cytotoxicity, xii, 22, 72, 86, 92, 120, 122, 157, 166, 175, 201, 239, 247

D

danger, 12, 185
death, 12, 27, 42, 60, 62, 128, 147, 152, 185, 205
decay, 131, 240, 244
defects, 63, 71, 156
defense, ix, 110, 114, 119, 123, 124, 131, 133, 188
defense mechanisms, 119
defensive strategies, 132
deficiency, 14, 16, 59, 156, 205

degradation, viii, 21, 24, 66, 67, 69, 74, 85, 190, 191, 197, 247, 248
degradation process, 67
dendritic cell, 2, 18, 55, 59, 61, 62, 110, 112, 114, 115, 122
density, 19, 23, 25, 30, 31, 42, 43, 88, 152, 155, 170, 174, 187, 195
deposition, x, 35, 37, 54, 88, 162, 168, 174, 240
deposits, 88
depression, 93
deprivation, vii, 65, 67, 72, 86, 97, 189
deregulation, 191
derivatives, 78, 194, 216, 225, 245, 246
desorption, 33, 53
destruction, 122, 129, 240
detachment, 235
detection, 3, 6, 7, 30, 87, 94, 97, 122, 132, 163, 170, 171
diagnostic markers, 80, 193
dicentric chromosome, 102, 108
differentiation, 7, 29, 30, 82, 84, 87, 92, 94, 96, 148, 193, 216
diffusion, 67, 71, 73, 84, 143, 145, 146, 150, 151, 152, 155, 159, 174, 187
diffusion process, 152
digestion, 10, 151, 155
dimethylsulfoxide, 27
diode laser, 217, 219, 220
diphtheria, 147, 156
disease progression, 69, 71, 205, 215
disorder, 63, 208
disposition, 246
dissociation, 149
distribution, ix, 7, 31, 53, 62, 68, 107, 141, 143, 146, 147, 148, 149, 150, 151, 157, 158, 159, 161, 162, 165, 170, 171, 172, 173, 174, 176, 178, 181, 196, 200, 218, 219, 220, 242, 244
diversity, 117, 247
division, 53, 124, 130
DNA, 12, 22, 59, 93, 103, 122, 166, 172, 190, 191, 198, 200, 201, 202, 205, 209, 210, 211
DNA damage, 191, 198, 205
DNA repair, 59, 166, 202, 205, 209, 210
doctors, 58, 61
dogs, 111, 219, 220
donors, 243, 247
dosing, 152, 160, 177, 209, 215
double helix, 172
drug carriers, x, 157, 161, 167, 178, 181
drug delivery, x, 22, 26, 142, 143, 152, 154, 161, 162, 164, 166, 168, 169, 170, 171, 172, 173, 174, 176, 177, 178, 181, 182, 214, 215, 220, 222, 224
drug design, 239

Index

drug release, 57, 169, 170, 179, 181, 246
drug resistance, xii, 69, 239
drug therapy, 169, 170
drug treatment, 169
drugs, vii, ix, x, xi, 2, 32, 62, 71, 73, 74, 78, 111, 115, 147, 148, 152, 153, 156, 161, 162, 168, 170, 172, 177, 199, 204, 214, 223, 240, 241, 242
DSL, 8
dualism, 53
duplication, 100
duration, 18, 82, 164, 170, 180, 223
dysplasia, 7, 86

E

ECM, 146, 150, 151
edema, 39, 47, 55, 149
elaboration, vii, 2, 3, 6, 57
elastin, 167, 180
electrodes, 4, 5, 95
electromagnetic fields, 20
electron, 33, 195, 204, 244
emboli, 164, 220, 223, 225, 226
embolization, 164, 220, 223, 225, 226
embryonic stem cells, 119
emission, 70, 163, 219, 244
emitters, 244, 246
encapsulation, 57, 168, 169
encoding, 66, 84, 95
endocrine, 156, 242
endothelial cells, 42, 45, 71, 79, 142, 144, 145, 147, 148, 149, 153, 158, 185, 187, 188, 189, 192
endothelium, 147, 148, 156, 196
energy, ix, 14, 19, 22, 68, 69, 70, 71, 74, 75, 88, 89, 92, 161, 172, 216, 245
energy density, 19
energy transfer, 172
enlargement, xi, 151, 152, 214, 234
environment, vii, 8, 32, 65, 67, 73, 75, 76, 78, 80, 115, 168, 169, 173, 189
enzymatic activity, 68, 74
enzyme inhibitors, 69
enzymes, ix, 12, 14, 22, 73, 75, 78, 90, 95, 110, 115, 122, 126, 127, 133, 155, 196, 239, 241, 242, 246
epidemiology, 106
epidermis, 7
epilepsy, 89
epithelia, 68
epithelial cells, 68
epithelium, 7, 10, 35, 37, 51, 54, 102
erythrocyte sedimentation rate, 8
erythrocytes, 8, 14, 15, 16, 19, 40
erythrocytosis, 82

erythropoietin, 83, 86, 87, 88, 90, 92, 93, 97
esophageal cancer, 58
ESR, 15
ethylene, 62
ethylene glycol, 62
etiology, 208
evoked potential, 231
evolution, 94
excision, 201
excitation, 216
excretion, xii, 201, 239
experimental condition, 112
experimental design, 115
exposure, 149, 170, 171, 201, 234, 235
external environment, 169
extracellular matrix, 146, 155, 156, 159, 189, 190, 194, 248
extraction, 70, 88, 219
extravasation, ix, 141, 143, 144, 146, 148, 149, 150, 152, 159, 162, 167, 168, 169, 179

F

family, 10, 20, 55, 68, 79, 84, 93, 94, 114, 124, 185, 241, 246
fatigue, 201, 203, 209
femur, 23, 24
ferrite, 22, 23, 25, 26, 27, 32, 56
fibers, xi, 214, 215, 216, 217, 219
fibrin, 88
fibroblast growth factor, 91, 111
fibroblasts, 18, 30, 55, 146, 197
fibroids, 226
fibrosarcoma, 73, 173, 174, 177
fibrosis, 39, 46, 47, 55
filtration, 154
financial support, 224
fixation, 30, 31, 238
flavonoids, 5
flexibility, 74, 145, 235
floating, 229, 230
fluctuations, 16
fluid, 95, 146, 149, 152, 154, 156, 162, 178, 192
fluorescence, xi, 106, 107, 118, 126, 155, 159, 165, 173, 174, 214, 216, 220
focusing, xi, 144, 199, 200, 228
folic acid, 62
foramen, 234
Fourier analysis, 159
fragments, 53, 152
France, 91, 194
free radicals, 92
frontal lobe, 101, 186

Index

functional changes, 3, 10, 16
fungus, 216
fusion, 231, 234, 235, 237, 238

G

gadolinium, 166, 172, 177
gastrointestinal tract, 6, 12, 16, 18, 19, 57
gelatinase A, 196
gene, viii, xi, 2, 10, 22, 62, 63, 66, 67, 68, 69, 70, 71, 72, 75, 76, 77, 80, 81, 82, 83, 84, 85, 87, 88, 89, 90, 92, 93, 94, 96, 98, 100, 107, 111, 129, 142, 143, 156, 191, 192, 197, 198, 202, 203, 209, 210, 211, 214, 223, 225, 240
gene expression, 22, 72, 77, 80, 81, 85, 88, 89, 90, 94, 191, 197
gene silencing, 211
gene therapy, 2, 62, 223, 225
gene transfer, 198
generation, 26, 74, 149, 157, 193
genes, viii, 2, 60, 66, 67, 68, 69, 71, 72, 76, 80, 82, 83, 84, 85, 94, 95, 100, 103, 115, 124, 190, 191, 193
genetic alteration, 101, 104, 105, 107, 186, 190, 191, 193
genetics, 88, 107, 194
genome, 89, 100, 202
genotype, 96, 119
Germany, 65
gland, 10, 14, 35, 215, 220
glia, 71, 113
glial cells, 185
glioblastoma, viii, x, 66, 69, 70, 71, 76, 80, 83, 84, 85, 94, 95, 101, 105, 106, 107, 110, 184, 186, 187, 189, 191, 193, 194, 195, 196, 197, 198, 199, 204, 210, 211, 212
glioblastoma multiforme, x, 106, 110, 184, 194, 195, 199, 210, 212
glioma, viii, ix, 66, 72, 76, 77, 79, 85, 93, 94, 106, 107, 110, 111, 113, 114, 115, 117, 118, 119, 120, 122, 123, 124, 125, 126, 127, 128, 129, 130, 131, 132, 133, 134, 185, 186, 188, 192, 194, 195, 196, 198, 200, 204, 210, 212
glomerulus, 51
gluconeogenesis, 74
glucose, viii, 6, 8, 66, 67, 68, 69, 70, 71, 72, 73, 74, 75, 76, 86, 92, 93, 94, 95, 96, 190
glucoside, 243
GLUT, 71, 92
glutamate, 6, 94
glutathione, 10, 14, 54
glycerol, 94, 162
glycol, 146, 154, 162, 168

glycolysis, viii, 66, 69, 70, 71, 72, 73, 74, 75, 77, 78, 85, 87, 89, 92, 93
glycosaminoglycans, 146
glycoside, 247
glycosylation, 89
grading, 83, 185
groups, xi, 6, 9, 10, 13, 14, 15, 17, 18, 27, 33, 38, 39, 47, 53, 55, 79, 82, 84, 85, 86, 176, 202, 207, 214, 233, 241
growth factor, x, 18, 69, 79, 81, 82, 89, 92, 94, 96, 97, 111, 146, 153, 156, 157, 158, 183, 184, 189, 190, 191, 192, 196, 197, 198
growth rate, ix, 79, 110, 130, 132
guanine, 201, 202
guidance, 88, 164, 182, 218

H

haemopoiesis, 58
half-life, 144, 164, 165, 168, 201
haploid, 101, 105
head and neck cancer, 91
health, 7, 58, 60
heart disease, 185
heat, 33, 113, 115, 167, 169, 175, 177, 179
heat shock protein, 113, 115
heating, 33, 173, 177
hematuria, 223, 225
hemoglobin, 14, 87, 93, 97
hemorrhage, 51, 167, 223, 225
hemostasis, 218
hepatitis, 30
hepatocellular carcinoma, 95, 223, 225
hepatocytes, 40, 42, 43, 45, 46
hepatoma, 122
herpes, 30, 150, 156, 159
herpes simplex, 150, 156, 159
heterogeneity, ix, 101, 106, 141, 143, 145, 146, 154, 173, 195
histamine, 149, 158
histocompatibility antigens, 118
histone, 110
HIV, 101
HLA, 114
homeostasis, 3, 6, 8, 10, 14, 16, 20
hormone, 8, 82, 247
host, 20, 84, 114, 115, 119, 120, 122, 123, 124, 129, 131, 132, 133, 145, 155, 185, 187, 188, 196
human brain, viii, 66, 68, 69, 77, 80, 81, 83, 86, 95, 107, 117
humidity, 34
humoral immunity, 21
hybrid, 19, 20, 21, 33, 56

hybridization, 100, 106, 107, 108
hydrocarbons, 33
hydrogen, 24, 27
hydrogen peroxide, 27
hydrolysis, 242
hydroxyapatite, 2, 29, 59, 61, 237
hydroxyl, 26
hyperplasia, x, 183, 184, 187, 189, 192, 193, 214, 224
hypertension, 148, 154, 155
hyperthermia, x, 162, 166, 167, 168, 169, 171, 174, 176, 177, 178, 179, 180, 181, 182
hypothesis, 90, 91, 187
hypoxia, viii, x, 66, 67, 68, 69, 70, 71, 72, 73, 75, 76, 77, 78, 79, 80, 81, 82, 83, 84, 85, 86, 87, 88, 89, 90, 91, 92, 93, 94, 95, 96, 97, 98, 115, 152, 167, 183, 184, 185, 187, 188, 189, 190, 191, 192, 193, 194, 195, 196, 197, 198
hypoxia-inducible factor, 67, 69, 79, 83, 86, 87, 89, 91, 92, 93, 95, 96, 97, 185, 196, 197
hypoxic cells, 71, 73, 93, 184, 189, 190
hysterectomy, 226

I

ICAM, 112
ICD, 115
ideal, ix, 161, 168, 170
identification, 79, 122, 164
idiopathic, 18, 208
IFN, 61, 127
IL-17, 114
IL-6, 114
IL-8, x, 183, 190, 192, 198
illumination, 215, 216, 217, 218, 220, 223
image, 103, 153, 172, 173, 229
images, 103, 105, 166, 170, 172, 173, 176, 228, 229, 230
imaging modalities, 164, 170, 171, 174
imbalances, 100, 103, 106, 108
immune function, 126
immune reaction, 20
immune response, 111, 113, 114, 115, 116, 117, 119, 120, 124, 126, 127, 129, 131, 132, 133
immune system, ix, 20, 54, 59, 110, 111, 113, 115, 116, 118, 122, 127, 130
immunity, 20, 21, 61, 114, 115, 116, 119, 120, 122, 128, 131
immunization, 18, 120
immunocompetent cells, 20, 21, 22, 35, 53
immunogenetics, 119
immunogenicity, ix, 110, 116, 117, 118, 120, 129
immunoglobulins, 21

immunohistochemistry, 82
immunomodulatory, 20, 115
immunosuppression, 54, 55
immunotherapy, 2, 20, 57, 113, 115
in situ hybridization, 104, 106, 107
in vitro, viii, 3, 16, 18, 19, 27, 32, 33, 34, 35, 53, 54, 55, 56, 57, 60, 62, 63, 66, 68, 73, 75, 77, 80, 81, 82, 85, 87, 89, 93, 94, 95, 120, 148, 152, 159, 180, 181, 189, 192, 196, 197, 237
in vivo, viii, ix, 3, 20, 29, 32, 33, 34, 35, 37, 54, 55, 56, 66, 69, 73, 75, 80, 83, 84, 89, 94, 95, 110, 119, 120, 122, 126, 131, 132, 148, 154, 155, 159, 172, 177, 178, 179, 196, 197, 223, 240
incidence, x, xi, 104, 107, 116, 183, 186, 211, 227, 228, 233, 234, 235
indices, 3, 5, 7, 8, 9, 10, 13, 14, 15, 16, 19, 20, 21, 24, 25, 27, 28, 31, 38, 39, 43, 46, 55, 56, 58
indolent, 101, 104
inducer, 92
inducible protein, viii, 66, 68, 87
induction, viii, 20, 66, 68, 72, 75, 82, 112, 128, 129, 148, 151, 190, 193, 196, 197, 198, 207, 215
infectious disease, 158
inflammation, 55, 56, 60, 144
infrastructure, 5
inhibition, viii, 16, 34, 38, 56, 59, 66, 69, 70, 71, 72, 73, 74, 85, 88, 92, 149, 150, 157, 158, 159, 166, 192, 197
inhibitor, 71, 72, 76, 77, 80, 86, 92, 93, 96, 97, 110, 123, 148, 149, 150, 156, 158, 159, 197, 198
initiation, viii, 12, 33, 80, 99, 100
injections, 19, 146
innate immunity, 60
insight, 111, 122
instability, 100, 106, 232, 233, 234, 236, 237, 238
instruments, 5
insulin, 96, 198
insulin resistance, 96
integrin, 166, 179, 190, 197
integrity, 167, 191, 202, 233
interaction, xi, 29, 68, 72, 115, 149, 172, 189, 191, 204, 213, 215
interactions, 75, 114, 115, 151, 155, 172, 196
intercellular adhesion molecule, 112
interference, xii, 69, 71, 239
interferon, 114, 204
interferon-γ, 114
interleukin-17, 114
interleukin-8, x, 183, 197
internal environment, 16
interval, 24, 61
intervention, 54, 116
intestinal tract, 7, 10, 11

intestine, 7, 10, 14, 20
intravenously, 148, 163, 201, 215
inversion, 7, 19, 22, 56, 62
involution, 195
iodine, 7, 56, 247
ionizing radiation, 62, 170, 205
ions, 4, 18, 19, 20, 22, 24, 25, 56, 74, 180
ipsilateral, 218
iron, 3, 7, 8, 10, 13, 16, 18, 22, 23, 24, 25, 28, 29, 30, 32, 33, 35, 39, 40, 46, 47, 50, 52, 53, 54, 55, 56, 57, 58, 59, 67
irradiation, vii, x, 2, 54, 199, 204, 212
ischemia, 198
isolation, 60, 88
isomerization, 53
isotonic solution, 24
isotope, 219
isozyme, 94
isozymes, 74
Italy, 199

J

Japan, 141, 152, 232
joints, 233, 234
Jordan, 135

K

Kaposi sarcoma, 177, 188
karyotype, 30, 101, 102, 104, 105
KBr, 33
kidney, 68, 241, 242
kidneys, 51, 56, 217, 247
killer cells, 130, 133
killing, ix, 110, 113, 114, 123, 127, 129, 130, 132
Krebs cycle, 71
kyphosis, 228, 231, 232, 233, 234, 235, 236, 238

L

lactate dehydrogenase, 73, 75, 79
lactic acid, 73, 74, 75, 79, 84, 115
laminectomy, xi, 227, 228, 232, 233, 234, 235, 236, 237
large intestine, 7, 10, 17, 18, 21
lecithin, 32, 33
lesions, 101, 102, 103, 104, 105, 234, 236
leukemia, 82, 87, 96
leukopenia, 201
ligament, 236, 237

ligand, 14, 20, 113, 114, 115, 128, 129, 131, 132, 148, 151, 172, 190, 191
light transmission, xi, 214, 220
likelihood, 87
limitation, 164, 172, 177, 216
line, 14, 22, 23, 34, 73, 105, 118, 130, 133, 173, 175, 176, 209
links, 80, 193, 196
lipid peroxidation, 10, 63
lipids, viii, 62, 66, 70, 162, 169
lipoproteins, 32
liposomes, x, xi, 32, 57, 59, 142, 148, 149, 152, 153, 154, 157, 160, 161, 162, 166, 167, 168, 169, 171, 172, 174, 176, 177, 179, 180, 181, 182, 214, 220, 221, 223
liquid chromatography, 174
liquids, 6, 22, 32
liver, 40, 46, 47, 55, 56, 58, 59, 80, 96, 97, 147, 177, 217, 225, 240, 241, 242, 245, 246
liver cancer, 177
liver cells, 58, 59
liver metastases, 96
local anesthesia, 19
localization, ix, 7, 20, 57, 95, 141, 143, 144, 145, 152, 153, 154, 219
locus, 55, 57, 119
lordosis, 232, 233, 234, 235
lumen, 47, 53, 147, 189
lung cancer, 91, 96, 187, 195
lymph, 87, 180
lymph node, 87, 180
lymphangiogenesis, 158
lymphatic system, 155
lymphocytes, 2, 20, 30, 40, 55, 113, 114, 119, 120, 130, 132, 223
lymphoid, 3, 111, 113, 115
lymphoid tissue, 3
lysine, 67
lysis, 119, 130, 189

M

macromolecules, viii, 66, 70, 148, 149, 153, 154, 155, 158, 178
macrophages, 55, 58, 126, 127
magnesium, 22, 23, 25, 26, 27, 32, 56
magnet, vii, 2, 3, 22, 25, 26, 32
magnetic field, 22, 26, 27, 57, 172
magnetic moment, 172
magnetic resonance, 21, 89, 170, 176, 179, 228, 229
magnetic resonance imaging, 170, 179
magnetization, 33
maintenance, x, 72, 199, 202

major histocompatibility complex, ix, 110, 112
malignancy, xi, 75, 104, 182, 185, 193, 213
malignant growth, 20, 58, 166
malignant melanoma, 180
malignant tumors, 18
mammalian tissues, 242
management, 74, 75, 89, 163, 224, 228, 236, 237, 238
manganese, 162, 171, 172, 176
manipulation, viii, 66, 72, 168
marker genes, viii, 66
marrow, 22, 23, 24, 26, 27, 28, 29, 32, 56, 59, 61
matrix, 88, 151, 154, 155, 189, 196, 242
matrix metalloproteinase, 154, 196
maturation, 29, 55
measurement, 7, 30, 159, 163, 165, 178
media, 123, 159
median, 186, 207, 216
melanoma, 18, 121, 147, 155, 156, 157, 187, 188, 195
melting, 162
membranes, 14, 34, 53, 149, 169, 181
memory, 58, 122
men, xi, 8, 10, 11, 15, 106, 213, 214, 215
mercury, 4, 5, 7, 56
mesenchymal stem cells, 60
meta-analysis, 18, 114
metabolic pathways, 70, 75, 78
metabolism, 8, 12, 20, 56, 62, 67, 69, 70, 71, 73, 74, 75, 78, 88, 89, 92, 93, 94, 96, 97, 178, 190, 240
metabolites, 72, 94, 127, 241
metal nanoparticles, 22, 32
metals, 5, 12, 14, 62, 63
metamorphosis, 180
metaphase, 101, 103
metastasis, 67, 79, 82, 85, 88, 89, 94, 185, 189, 242
methanol, 23, 123, 125, 126
methylation, x, 199, 201, 202, 203, 209, 210, 211
MHC, ix, 110, 112, 113, 114, 118, 119, 124, 130, 132
mice, 14, 22, 23, 26, 27, 28, 34, 40, 41, 43, 44, 46, 47, 48, 49, 50, 51, 52, 56, 61, 63, 82, 92, 97, 116, 119, 122, 132, 147, 153, 156, 157, 181, 197, 242
microdialysis, 94
micronutrients, 16, 62
microscope, 33, 154
microscopy, 30, 31, 155, 219
microsomes, 242
microspheres, 150, 151, 177, 223
microstructure, 159
migration, 55, 148, 153, 189, 192, 193, 198
Ministry of Education, 152
minority, 209

misunderstanding, 208
mitochondria, 70, 71, 92, 124, 242
mitogen, viii, 66, 69, 79, 149, 190
mitosis, 205
MMP, 189
MMP-2, 189
MMPs, 189
model, 24, 33, 53, 63, 80, 85, 120, 122, 123, 129, 133, 148, 160, 164, 168, 173, 174, 178, 179, 181, 192, 193, 195, 196, 205, 217, 222, 225, 240
modeling, 29, 32
models, xi, 73, 74, 80, 111, 117, 119, 124, 130, 133, 134, 159, 167, 169, 177, 181, 188, 213, 215, 216
modules, 159
mole, 3, 4, 5, 6, 33, 74, 75
molecular biology, 101
molecular targeting, x, 161
molecular weight, 151, 165
molecules, vii, ix, 2, 3, 12, 18, 20, 22, 32, 33, 53, 54, 56, 62, 69, 79, 110, 112, 113, 114, 115, 119, 123, 124, 127, 130, 132, 133, 146, 153, 164, 170, 172, 174, 178, 245, 247
monoclonal antibody, 88, 118, 126, 128, 185
monolayer, 51
morbidity, 6, 8, 61, 214
morphogenesis, 88
morphology, 29, 54, 61, 145, 193
morphometric, 34, 149
mortality, 16, 79, 204, 214
mortality rate, 204
motion, 234
motor skills, 113
movement, 150
MRI, 103, 105, 166, 170, 171, 172, 173, 174, 178, 180, 181
mRNA, viii, 66, 69, 71, 72, 76, 77, 78, 80, 81, 82, 83, 84, 92, 97, 100, 108, 127, 192
mucous membrane, 3, 10, 11, 15, 16
multiple myeloma, 177
muscle atrophy, 234
muscles, 234
mutant, 10, 197
mutation, 100, 120, 191
mycelium, 32
myelodysplasia, 208
myocardium, 58

N

NaCl, 22, 23, 24, 26, 28
nanocomposites, 34
nanomaterials, 33
nanomedicine, vii, 2, 5

nanometers, 30
nanoparticles, vii, x, 2, 3, 5, 22, 24, 25, 26, 27, 28, 29, 30, 31, 32, 33, 35, 39, 40, 46, 47, 50, 52, 53, 54, 55, 56, 57, 59, 60, 63, 142, 143, 146, 150, 151, 152, 153, 161, 165, 245
nanotechnology, 60, 182
natural killer cell, 40
NCS, 148
Nd, 244
neck cancer, 87, 97, 179
necrosis, x, xi, 27, 39, 42, 46, 55, 56, 88, 114, 122, 149, 157, 183, 184, 187, 188, 189, 193, 194, 195, 196, 205, 213, 215
negative consequences, 13
neoangiogenesis, 157
neoplasm, 105, 185
neoplastic tissue, 153
neovascularization, 79, 191, 195
nerve, 6
nervous system, vii, 193, 194
Netherlands, 57
network, 150, 151, 154
neuroblastoma, 196
neurofibroma, 228
neurons, 71, 113
neurotransmitter, 6
neutropenia, 201, 202, 203, 207, 208
neutrophils, 129
nitric oxide, 14, 90, 92, 93, 114, 127, 158, 159
nitric oxide synthase, 93, 127, 159
NK cells, 114, 127, 129, 130
nodes, 21, 38
noise, 170, 174
nuclei, 242
nucleic acid, 172
nucleotides, viii, 66, 70
nucleus, viii, 32, 40, 42, 53, 66, 67, 156, 185, 190
nuclides, 244
nutrients, vii, 65, 67, 84, 145, 187, 192

O

observations, xi, 79, 101, 149, 213, 214, 215, 223
older people, 117
oligodendroglioma, 186, 207
oncogenes, 191
optical density, 15, 26, 27, 30, 31
optical fiber, xi, 213, 215, 216
optimization, 152, 168
order, 19, 69, 74, 110, 146, 164, 167, 169, 170, 171, 174, 177, 187, 204, 208, 215
organ, 32, 42, 55, 119
organelles, 158

organic compounds, 4
organism, vii, 2, 3, 16, 18, 20, 21, 22, 32, 39, 55, 56, 62
ossification, 232, 236
ovarian cancer, 177, 188, 196
ovarian tumor, 87
overlay, 173
oxidation, 4, 7, 30, 33, 53
oxidative stress, 62, 72, 86, 115
oxides, 18, 22, 25, 32, 46, 56, 57
oxygen, vii, xi, 14, 33, 54, 65, 67, 68, 69, 70, 72, 73, 74, 75, 78, 84, 85, 87, 90, 92, 93, 95, 97, 145, 166, 184, 185, 187, 189, 190, 192, 213, 215, 216, 225
oxygen consumption, 72

P

p53, 84, 96, 107, 111, 121, 191, 197, 198, 205, 223, 225
paclitaxel, 62, 151, 152, 160
pain, 228, 231, 235
palliative, 163, 223
pancreas, 20
pancreatic cancer, 87, 92, 159, 246
parameter, 29, 86
parameters, xi, 30, 58, 163, 214
parenchyma, 40, 42, 45, 46, 51, 113
parenchymal cell, 80, 113
particles, x, 18, 22, 23, 25, 30, 32, 33, 54, 56, 57, 58, 59, 61, 150, 151, 161, 164, 171, 242, 244, 245
passive, 32, 73, 114, 146, 150, 187, 205
pathogenesis, 100, 102, 104
pathology, 5, 10, 13, 14, 16, 19, 20, 61, 107, 111, 193, 196
pathways, viii, xii, 67, 72, 73, 75, 79, 88, 91, 92, 94, 99, 100, 103, 106, 114, 115, 122, 123, 127, 131, 132, 149, 153, 177, 190, 191, 194, 205, 239
PCR, 72, 81, 119, 203
penicillin, 5
peptides, 14, 112, 114, 119, 166
perfusion, 147, 152, 162, 164, 166, 167, 168, 178, 216
peripheral blood, 16, 20, 59
permeability, ix, 60, 79, 89, 95, 141, 142, 143, 144, 145, 146, 149, 150, 152, 153, 154, 155, 157, 158, 159, 162, 164, 165, 166, 167, 169, 178, 181
permeation, 167
peroxide, 14, 23
PET, 163, 170, 171, 244, 245
PGE, 127
pH, 22, 24, 68, 73, 74, 75, 78, 96, 155, 162, 169, 180, 181, 200

phagocyte, 21
pharmaceuticals, 2, 164, 170
pharmacokinetics, ix, 111, 141, 154, 165, 177, 178
pharmacology, 61, 201
phenol, 5, 88, 241, 245, 248
phenolphthalein, 246
phenotype, viii, x, 66, 69, 75, 80, 96, 107, 111, 132, 183, 187, 189, 193, 195, 242
phosphates, 29
phosphatidylcholine, 33, 35, 53
phospholipids, 32, 33, 53, 56, 180
phosphorylation, 67, 72, 93
photobleaching, 159
photons, 244
physicochemical properties, 60, 181
physiological factors, 162
physiology, 162, 164, 166, 169, 193, 194
plasma, 3, 6, 58, 61, 91, 94, 144, 164, 165, 168, 172, 201
plasma proteins, 144, 172
plasminogen, 189
platinum, 71, 218
plexus, 68, 102, 103, 105, 108
pneumoconiosis, 61
pneumonia, 209
pneumonitis, 208
polymer, 32, 148
polymerase, 106, 201, 205
polymerase chain reaction, 106
polymers, x, 161, 177
polymorphisms, 210
polypeptide, 67, 121
polyploidy, 102, 108
polyps, 7
pons, 113
poor, vii, 2, 3, 67, 69, 70, 73, 85, 87, 96, 144, 151, 164, 170, 171, 184, 187, 193, 204, 234, 243
population, 6, 8, 9, 30, 58, 61, 62, 102, 130, 194, 210
porosity, 152
precursor cells, 186
pressure, 145, 146, 148, 149, 152, 154, 156, 158, 159, 162, 178
prevention, 14, 16, 59
priapism, 223, 225
primary brain tumor, x, 70, 183, 186, 192
primate, 225
priming, 152, 159
probe, 33, 60, 175
prodrugs, xii, 239, 240, 244, 245, 246
production, ix, 22, 59, 61, 69, 71, 73, 74, 75, 78, 84, 110, 114, 117, 132, 159, 170, 191

prognosis, vii, x, 12, 14, 54, 65, 66, 69, 70, 79, 84, 85, 87, 88, 90, 91, 96, 106, 184, 186, 187, 192, 199
proliferating fraction, 130
proliferation, vii, 29, 65, 67, 69, 70, 74, 75, 79, 82, 92, 95, 97, 117, 122, 130, 184, 185, 189, 191, 192, 194, 195
promoter, viii, x, 66, 67, 85, 93, 98, 100, 185, 192, 199, 202, 203, 209, 211
propagation, 78
prophylaxis, 6, 63, 202, 207, 209, 236
proportionality, 172
prostaglandins, 113, 127
prostate, xi, 16, 87, 97, 154, 187, 197, 213, 214, 215, 216, 217, 218, 219, 220, 221, 222, 223, 224, 225
prostate cancer, xi, 87, 154, 187, 197, 213, 214, 215, 220, 224
prostate carcinoma, 97, 225
prostate gland, xi, 214, 221
prostatectomy, 215
protective mechanisms, 18
protein synthesis, 72, 93
proteins, viii, 66, 67, 68, 70, 72, 76, 84, 85, 92, 112, 119, 120, 123, 124, 131, 132, 150, 151, 153, 156
proteoglycans, 146
protocol, 19, 162, 211
protons, 24, 73
proto-oncogene, 90, 103
pruning, 149, 150
pyrolysis, 33

Q

quality of life, 163
quantum dot, 32

R

radial distance, 175
radiation, ix, 68, 69, 71, 72, 80, 90, 93, 94, 110, 113, 115, 123, 154, 161, 163, 170, 177, 180, 202, 203, 204, 205, 208, 209, 210, 211, 212, 215, 223, 234
Radiation, vi, ix, 65, 86, 92, 109, 159, 161, 168, 199, 204, 211, 245
radiation therapy, 68, 71, 93, 94, 163, 177, 180, 204, 209, 210, 215
radical mechanism, 33, 53
radio, 20, 69, 73, 80, 123, 163, 193, 219, 245, 246
radioactive isotopes, 163
radioisotope, 170
radiosensitization, 92, 179

radiotherapy, x, 69, 73, 79, 86, 87, 89, 91, 92, 113, 142, 168, 179, 180, 186, 193, 199, 200, 202, 203, 204, 207, 208, 209, 211, 215, 224, 247
radius, 176
range, 3, 4, 5, 19, 20, 24, 27, 77, 105, 114, 164, 173, 177, 186, 204, 208, 216, 241, 243, 244
reactant, 54
reactive oxygen, 216
reactivity, 22, 33, 53, 243
reagents, 5, 124
real time, x, 161
recall, 202
receptors, 70, 115, 148, 149, 157, 166, 185, 189, 190, 192, 196, 197
recognition, 85, 113, 131, 162, 172
reconstruction, 238
recovery, 159
rectum, 7, 16, 17, 18, 215, 219, 220
recurrence, 204, 209, 224
redistribution, 12, 14
regeneration, 5, 42, 56
region, viii, 8, 9, 34, 58, 61, 66, 67, 68, 85, 100, 104, 105, 106, 175
regression, 25, 30, 158, 173, 188, 193, 195, 196
regression analysis, 30
regression equation, 25
regulation, 12, 59, 68, 69, 71, 72, 76, 78, 79, 81, 84, 85, 86, 89, 91, 94, 95, 96, 97, 122, 158, 190, 192, 195, 196, 197, 198
regulators, 10, 59, 72, 91
rehabilitation, 61, 63
rejection, 119
relationship, 88, 93, 114, 119, 128, 142, 154, 164, 172, 174
relativity, 8
relaxation rate, 181
relevance, vii, 2, 210
remission, 82
renal cell carcinoma, 225
repair, 91, 201, 202, 205, 210
reparation, 12, 22
replication, 133, 155, 201
reproductive organs, 97
resection, x, xi, 163, 199, 200, 208, 227, 228, 231, 232, 233, 234, 235, 237
resistance, ix, 3, 16, 20, 32, 56, 68, 69, 71, 73, 76, 78, 79, 90, 95, 110, 133, 146, 202, 210, 232, 234
resolution, 103, 154, 164, 170, 171, 172
respiration, 71, 75
respiratory, 74
retention, xii, 142, 144, 153, 168, 169, 174, 220, 239, 240
reticulum, 112, 241

reverse transcriptase, 119
rhythm, 5
ribose, 201, 205
risk, xi, 10, 58, 62, 87, 114, 154, 213, 214, 215, 223, 224, 228, 234, 235
risk factors, 10, 224, 228, 234
RNA, 88
roentgen, 30
room temperature, 7, 53
Russia, 1, 6, 8, 9, 57

S

safety, 32, 60, 154
sampling, 7, 100, 174
scatter, 198
scattering, 159
scavengers, 150
sclerosis, 39, 55
search, vii, 2, 3, 14, 18, 54, 106, 222
secrete, 55, 95, 190
secretion, 35, 55, 192
sediment, 19
sedimentation, 16
selectivity, xi, 35, 54, 57, 69, 74, 180, 213, 215, 220, 240
selenium, 3, 5, 7, 8, 10, 14, 16, 56, 59, 62
self-assembly, 53
senescence, 117, 205
sensitivity, 3, 4, 5, 33, 56, 69, 156, 170, 171, 181
sensors, 90
separation, 4, 124
sepsis, 207, 220
septum, 47
serine, 148, 190
serotonin, 6, 158
serum, 6, 8, 14, 16, 22, 30, 34, 114, 120, 150, 163, 192, 198, 220, 223
shape, 30, 35, 37, 40, 54, 91, 144, 145, 159
shock, 20, 123, 197
Siberia, 9
side effects, ix, x, xi, xii, 74, 141, 142, 161, 163, 168, 177, 207, 213, 239
signal transduction, 72, 156, 191
signaling pathway, 191
signalling, 79, 86, 89, 97, 156
signals, x, 5, 8, 13, 90, 144, 148, 183, 184
signs, 14, 42, 43, 46, 47, 220, 228
siRNA, 70, 86
skin, 10, 12, 13, 215, 217, 218, 220, 223, 241
small intestine, 68, 241
smooth muscle, 90, 147, 195
smooth muscle cells, 90, 147, 148, 195

Index

sodium, 22, 24, 25, 26, 34, 159
soft tissue sarcomas, 179
software, 219
solid phase, 24, 58
solid tumors, viii, ix, 20, 21, 73, 79, 84, 95, 99, 141, 142, 143, 144, 145, 146, 149, 154, 155, 156, 157, 160, 179, 181, 182, 193
solubility, 22, 78
solvents, 22
SPA, 22
space, 144, 146, 148, 150, 151, 152, 162, 165, 167
spasticity, 228
species, 119, 155, 216
spectrophotometry, 3
spectrum, 31, 33, 34, 53
speculation, 119
speed, 33, 35, 53, 216
sphincter, 220
spinal cord, 186, 227, 228, 231, 232, 233, 236, 238
spinal cord tumor, 227, 228, 232, 233, 236, 238
spinal stenosis, 238
spinal tumor, 233
spine, viii, 99, 100, 228, 229, 232, 233, 234, 235, 236, 237, 238
spleen, 217, 241, 242
sprouting, 195
squamous cell, 86, 87, 88, 89
squamous cell carcinoma, 86, 87, 88, 89
stability, 67, 68, 78, 92, 97, 168, 181, 200, 235, 236, 237
stabilization, 18, 21, 71, 190, 234, 235
starvation, 115
stasis, 80, 167
statistics, 8, 24, 30, 34, 185, 224
stem cells, 29, 32, 56, 60, 62, 119
stenosis, 229, 232
steroids, 247
stimulus, x, 127, 183, 193
stomach, 6, 7, 10, 14, 21, 56, 59, 60, 63, 68, 93, 200
stomach ulcer, 7
strain, 12, 119
strategies, ix, 33, 60, 70, 80, 85, 87, 110, 141, 152, 185, 203, 204, 209, 215, 216
stratification, 234, 235
strength, 22, 26, 27, 228, 238
stress, vii, 8, 10, 20, 60, 65, 66, 68, 72, 84, 85, 92, 123
stress granules, 92
stressors, 191
stroma, 37, 96, 157
stromal cells, 29, 30, 31, 156
structural changes, 47
structuring, 53

styrene, 148
substrates, 4, 5, 7, 16, 29, 32, 241
suicide, 60, 61
sulfonamide, 74
sulfonamides, 71, 74, 95
Sun, 91, 135, 197
supervision, 16, 21, 39, 55
supply, vii, 65, 67, 74, 84, 184
suppression, 61
surface area, 153
surgical intervention, 111
surgical resection, 104, 177, 185, 186, 193
surveillance, 214, 224
survival, vii, viii, x, xi, 6, 65, 66, 67, 69, 76, 78, 79, 82, 87, 88, 89, 90, 92, 95, 107, 110, 114, 117, 124, 128, 132, 149, 168, 184, 185, 186, 190, 191, 192, 194, 199, 202, 203, 204, 208, 210, 211, 212, 213, 214, 216
survival rate, x, 6, 107, 184, 186, 199, 203, 204
survivors, 110, 210
susceptibility, 129
sustainable development, 58
Sweden, 8
swelling, 185, 220
switching, 217
Switzerland, 65
symptoms, 209, 214
syndrome, 82, 87, 96, 121
synergistic effect, 74
synthesis, viii, 30, 32, 33, 58, 59, 66, 70, 197, 240, 241, 243, 246, 247
synthetic polymers, 144
syphilis, 30
systolic blood pressure, 148

T

T cell, 61, 111, 113, 114, 115, 117, 118, 119, 120, 121, 122, 124, 126, 127, 128, 129, 132
T lymphocytes, 122
target organs, 56
targets, 2, 18, 58, 67, 80, 85, 166, 191, 194
teaching, 21
technetium, 171, 179
technical assistance, 86
temperature, 19, 22, 33, 53, 162, 167, 169, 172, 173, 174, 175, 176, 177, 178, 179, 181, 182
temporal lobe, 101, 186
tension, 70, 97, 190, 225, 232, 233
TGF, 113, 114, 124, 125, 126, 131, 132, 133, 148, 149, 156, 157, 191
therapeutic agents, 124
therapeutic approaches, viii, 66, 69, 71, 73, 85, 107

therapeutic interventions, 124, 132
therapeutic practice, 3
therapeutic targets, viii, 66
therapeutics, ix, 60, 110, 111, 153, 156, 197, 210
therapy methods, vii, 2
thermal analysis, 33
threonine, 148, 190
thresholds, 179
thrombocytopenia, 201, 202, 203, 207, 208, 209
thrombosis, 187, 188, 193
thymus, 21, 117
thyroid, 163
tissue perfusion, 216
titanium, 16, 19, 30, 58, 61, 237
TNF, 14, 55, 112, 114, 149, 190
TNF-α, 14, 149, 190
total energy, 19
toxic effect, 3, 43, 46, 51, 54, 56, 57, 200, 201, 202, 203, 240
toxic metals, 8, 12
toxic side effect, 168, 177
toxic substances, 5
toxicity, xi, 3, 22, 23, 27, 28, 32, 33, 57, 59, 62, 63, 78, 177, 199, 202, 204, 207, 208, 209, 215, 216, 218, 240, 245
toxin, 147, 156
trace elements, vii, 2, 3, 5, 16, 22, 56, 57, 58
transcription, viii, 66, 67, 68, 69, 70, 73, 76, 84, 85, 91, 92, 98, 184, 190, 191, 192, 193, 197, 198
transcription factors, 84, 184
transcripts, 82
transduction, 129
transection, 236
transformation, 8, 12, 70, 71, 73, 75, 79, 82, 87, 92, 184, 186, 240
transforming growth factor, 113, 114, 124, 156, 192
transgene, 155, 223
transition, 75, 162, 169, 172, 181
transition metal, 172
transition temperature, 162, 169
translation, 61, 72, 92, 190
translocation, viii, 66, 67
transmission, 101
transplantation, 20, 34, 57, 58, 62, 119
transport, 62, 93, 143, 146, 147, 149, 150, 152, 153, 155, 156, 174, 178
trauma, 166
treatment methods, 54
trial, 91, 180, 181, 201, 203, 207, 209, 210, 211, 212, 225, 226
tricarboxylic acid, 74
triggers, 71, 73, 75, 84, 149
tryptophan, 127

tumor depth, 150
tumor growth, vii, 12, 34, 38, 56, 67, 71, 72, 73, 79, 82, 95, 130, 142, 159, 169, 174, 188, 192, 198
tumor metastasis, 87, 247
tumor necrosis factor, 14, 20, 55, 61, 112, 114, 129, 151, 157
tumor progression, viii, 12, 21, 61, 66, 69, 78, 84, 86, 87, 187, 193, 194, 207
tumor resistance, 89
tumorigenesis, ix, 74, 76, 99, 100
tumours, 67, 71, 80, 85, 97, 106, 107, 178, 180, 194, 237, 242
Turkey, 239
turnover, 155
type 1 collagen, 146
tyrosine, 80, 190, 191, 192, 193
Tyrosine, 121

U

UK, 201
ulcer, 63
ultrasound, 164, 170, 171, 181, 182
ultrastructure, 93, 154
underlying mechanisms, 211
uniform, 40, 42, 53, 174, 176
United States, 186, 194
urea, 8, 127
urethra, 219, 221
uric acid, 5
urinary retention, 214, 220, 221
urinary tract, 214
urine, 4, 6, 7, 220, 240
urokinase, 189
uterine cancer, 97
uterine fibroids, 223

V

vaccine, 2, 18, 171
vacuole, 45
vanadium, 16
vapor, 30
variables, 174
vascular bundle, 187
vascular endothelial growth factor (VEGF), x, 79, 83, 92, 124, 158, 183, 184
vascular system, 196
vascular wall, 143, 164
vasculature, ix, 67, 80, 84, 141, 142, 143, 144, 145, 146, 147, 148, 149, 150, 151, 152, 153, 158, 163, 164, 166, 167, 178, 179, 188, 193, 195, 196

vaso-occlusion, 187
vasopressor, 90
vector, 143, 147, 155, 156
VEGF expression, 79, 82, 97, 190
VEGF protein, 196
vehicles, 168, 170, 177
vein, 40, 42, 45
ventricle, 102, 107
versatility, 110, 156
vessels, viii, 47, 66, 69, 79, 90, 142, 144, 145, 146, 147, 148, 149, 150, 153, 154, 158, 163, 164, 187, 188, 189, 194, 196, 218
vestibular schwannoma, 82, 88
viral vectors, 151
viruses, 2, 147, 155
vision, 31
visualization, 164, 170
vitamin C, 5
vitamin D, 94
vitamins, 5
vomiting, 207, 209

W

wells, 30, 34
women, 8, 9, 10, 11, 15
workers, 105, 149
wound healing, 90

X

xenografts, 97, 147, 155, 158, 159

Y

Y-axis, 118

Z

zinc, 3, 7, 8, 10, 12, 14, 16, 20, 22, 56, 58, 59, 60, 62, 225